Dental Indices

Ready Reckoner

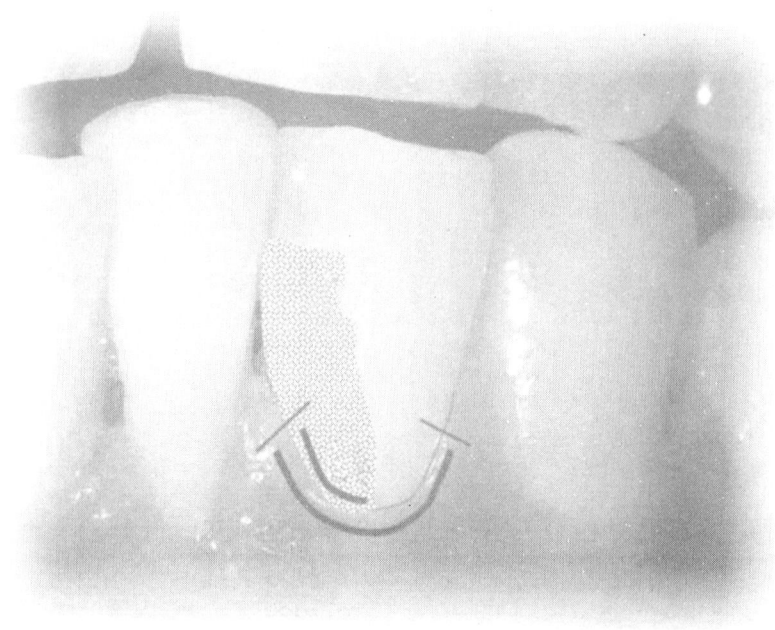

Dental Indices
Ready Reckoner

P Kalyana Chakravarthy MDS

Assistant Professor
Department of Public Health Dentistry
Manipal College of Dental Sciences
Manipal University, Manipal
Karnataka, India

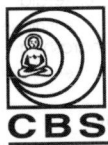

CBS Publishers & Distributors Pvt Ltd

New Delhi • Bengaluru • Chennai • Kochi • Mumbai • Pune
Hyderabad • Kolkata • Nagpur • Patna • Vijayawada

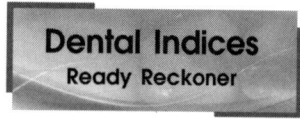

Dental Indices
Ready Reckoner

ISBN: 978-81-239-2398-7

Copyright © Author and Publishers

First Edition: 2014

Published by Satish Kumar Jain for

CBS Publishers & Distributors Pvt Ltd
4819/XI Prahlad Street, 24 Ansari Road, Daryaganj, New Delhi 110 002, India.
Ph: 23289259, 23266861/67   Fax: 011-23243014   Website: www.cbspd.com
                                                              e-mail: delhi@cbspd.com; cbspubs@airtelmail.in
Corporate Office: 204 FIE, Industrial Area, Patparganj, Delhi 110 092
Ph: 4934 4934   Fax: 4934 4935   e-mail: publishing@cbspd.com; publicity@cbspd.com

Branches

- **Bengaluru:** Seema House 2975, 17th Cross, K.R. Road,
  Banasankari 2nd Stage, Bengaluru 560 070, Karnataka
  Ph: +91-80-26771678/79   Fax: +91-80-26771680   e-mail: bangalore@cbspd.com
- **Chennai:** 20, West Park Road, Shenoy Nagar, Chennai 600 030, Tamil Nadu
  Ph: +91-44-26260666, 26208620   Fax: +91-44-42032115   e-mail: chennai@cbspd.com
- **Kochi:** 36/14 Kalluvilakam, Lissie Hospital Road, Kochi 682 018, Kerala
  Ph: +91-484-4059061/65   Fax: +91-484-4059065   e-mail: kochi@cbspd.com
- **Mumbai:** 83-C, Dr E Moses Road, Worli, Mumbai-400018, Maharashtra
  Ph: +91-22-24902340/41   Fax: +91-22-24902342   e-mail: mumbai@cbspd.com
- **Pune:** Bhuruk Prestige, Sr. No. 52/12/2+1+3/2 Narhe, Haveli
  (Near Katraj-Dehu Road Bypass), Pune 411 041, Maharashtra
  Ph: +91-20-64704058/59, 32392277   Fax: +91-20-24300160   e-mail: pune@cbspd.com

Representatives

- **Hyderabad** 0-9885175004   • **Kolkata** 0-9831437309, 0-9051152362
- **Nagpur** 0-9021734563   • **Patna** 0-9334159340   • **Vijayawada** 0-9000660880

Printed at: India Binding House, Nodia, UP

Foreword

It gives me immense pleasure to write the Foreword to the book titled *Dental Indices—Ready Reckoner* by Dr P Kalyana Chakravarthy, Assistant Professor, Department of Public Health Dentistry, MCODS, Manipal.

Dental diseases are the most prevalent and most neglected of all the chronic diseases affecting the mankind. Prevention of any disease rests on the knowledge of the disease manifestation, distribution, etiology and other related factors. Epidemiological study of any disease requires the condition to be measured and quantified accurately, based on scientific principles to understand the disease. The quantitative measurement of disease most commonly relies upon index. Hence, dental index is the main tool of epidemiological oral health survey, to measure the prevalence, incidence and severity of a particular condition. In this direction, *Dental Indices—Ready Reckoner* is an excellent piece of work by Dr Kalyana. The book explicitly deals with a complete coverage of various indices related to dental ailments to determine the baseline data to assess the needs of population to evaluate the effects and results of community program.

A good number of books on public health dentistry are currently available in libraries and market, but till date no book is written on dental indices alone for dental students. The data in this book is indeed comprehensive, with well-compiled chapters, scientifically accurate with thorough review of recent literature; positively providing a stimulus for new investigators, wishing to advance in the science of public health dentistry.

Further, the chapters on indices for assessing root caries, bone loss criteria, plaque and gingivitis for geriatric individuals and notes on pediatric indices published in this book will definitely serve as a valuable resource not only for undergraduate and postgraduate students, but also to every dental professionals alike. I have no hesitation in recommending this book to dental fraternity at large.

I compliment the author Dr P Kalyana Chakravarthy and his team of contributors for their commendable work in bringing out this edition in a presentable way and wish success in their endeavors.

Dr Nirmala N Rao MDS
Dean
Professor of Oral Pathology
Manipal College of Dental Sciences
Manipal University
Manipal, Karnataka, India

Contributors

Gowtham Suresh MDS

Assistant Professor—Periodontist and Implantologist
Department of Dental Surgery
PSG Institute of Medical Sciences and Research
Coimbatore, Tamil Nadu

Chapter 3: Indices to Assess Periodontitis

Sweta Singh MDS

Assistant Professor
Department of Public Health Dentistry
Babu Banarasi Das College of Dental Sciences
Lucknow, Uttar Pradesh

Chapter 10: Indices to Assess Dental Fluorosis and Enamel Defects

Thippeswamy HM MDS

Reader
Department of Public Health Dentistry
JSS Dental College
Mysore, Karnataka

Chapter 14: Indices to Assess Tooth Wear

Saurabh Singh MDS

Assistant Professor
Department of Pedodontics and Preventive Dentistry
Manipal College of Dental Sciences
Manipal, Karnataka

Chapter 17: Indices for Children and Adolescents

Preface

Research… The one sole factor through which one would expect to take dentistry to the next level, is seeing an upward trend with its inclusion and extensive promotion in the undergraduate curriculum. This book aims at bringing light to the available material and give the user an access to the most primary and important indices since their conception. The book is a treasure for postgraduates and research-oriented dental fraternity.

The recent stringent guidelines related to publications and research requirements for dental faculty by the regulating bodies, has led to exponential rise in the research projects and publications from the new generation dentists. Hence, we came up with the idea of compiling a book which includes as many indices as possible to cover almost all the areas of dental disorders. Lot of effort was made to review the literature and procure them. Literature related to a few indices was omitted due to they being in foreign languages or due to inability to procure or retrieve the original manuscripts of the proposed authors.

Almost all the information on various indices discussed in this book has been obtained from original literature as proposed by the respective authors. This ensures that there is proper description of required instruments, criteria and procedures to calculate the score without any misinterpretation, also, citation for each index has been placed for the readers and researchers to refer to the literature and also to understand the circumstances under which these indices were developed and proposed.

Some obsolete indices have also been included which are primarily relevant to the academicians. This would also help researchers to develop newer indices keeping in mind the limitations of those indices. Few indices for which literature was not available are discussed from review articles for which appropriate citation is provided.

I hope this endeavor would help all the researchers in oral health to achieve their goals and increase their knowledge on dental indices. I wish to welcome constructive suggestions along with any information related to any indices. I assure they will be acknowledged in future editions.

P Kalyana Chakravarthy

Acknowledgements

It is hard to beat a person who never gives up
—Thomas Jefferson

A lot of hard work and commitment has gone into this book which would not have been possible without the guidance of the able few and the blessings of my parents.

My wife, Dr Deepika and her family, for constant encouragement and dedication to see me through this project.

The entire idea was put into action because of the support offered by the Dean, Dr Nirmala Rao, and my mentors, Dr Shashidar Acharya, Dr Megashyam Bhat and Dr Sree Vidya, who helped me focus my views for the project.

I sincerely thank Dr Gowtham Suresh for his encouragement, contributions, critical appraisal of the contents, illustrations and proofreading.

I appreciate all the efforts from Dr Thippeswamy HM, Dr Sweta Singh and Dr Saurabh Singh for their valuable contributions and views in their respective chapters.

I am deeply indebted to my friends Dr Varun Reddy and Dr M Arun Shyam for their support in finding critical literature.

Mr YN Arjuna, Senior Director — Publishing, Editorial and Publicity, and Mr Mandal of CBS P&D for their constant support.

In all my work, there is a part of it where things would have gone other ways if not for the divine presence.

P Kalyana Chakravarthy

Contents

Introduction and Classification

Epidemiology is the study of health and disease in populations, and of how these states are influenced by heredity, biology, physical environment, social environment and human behavior. It focuses on groups of people, often whole populations, rather than on individuals or patients. The goal of epidemiological study is to identify the risk of disease that follows certain exposures, so that appropriate preventive interventions may be carried out at the public health and individual levels. To achieve this goal, epidemiological study uses a number of different research designs. All of them, however, include people with and without the disease in question.

The measurement of the degree of disease in a population, therefore requires that are much more standardized and objective. The researcher judges the condition of the oral tissues as they are at a particular time, not on how they might be in the future. This application of standard criteria, which can require suppression of intuitive clinical judgment, is the fundamental requisite in performing quality research.

The tissues involved in oral epidemiology are readily accessible to direct examination by a variety of methods: by inspection, probing, palpation or radiographic methods. The ready access of the oral cavity to examination gives the oral epidemiologist an advantage not enjoyed by most researchers in other fields.

As a result, oral diseases can be quantified more precisely than can most other chronic conditions. The quantitative measure of these oral diseases most commonly rely on indices or indexes.

The measurement of oral diseases usually requires that they are measured by the degree of intensity and not just simply by the prevalence of the condition. While the disease can be present in many individuals, the intensity can vary greatly between them. Such difference in intensity can only be determined by index.

An index as defined by Russell AL is a numerical value describing the relative status of a population on a graduated scale with definite upper and lower limits, which is designed to permit and facilitate comparison with other populations classified by the same criteria and methods. Based on this definition both proportions and rates can be classified as indices. Indeed the word index is often used to apply to the simplest form of quantification of disease.

Ideally, an index should possess the following:

Validity: The index must measure what it is intended to measure, so it should correspond with clinical stages of the disease under study at each point.

Reliability: The index should be able to measure consistently at different times and under a variety of conditions. The term reliability is virtually synonymous with reproducibility, repeatability and consistency, meaning the ability of the same or different examiners to interpret and use the index in the same way.

Clarity, simplicity and objectivity: The criteria should be clear and unambiguous, with mutually exclusive categories. Ideally, it should be readily memorized by an examiner after some practice.

Quantifiability: The index must be amenable to statistical analysis, so that the status of a group can be expressed by a distribution, mean, median or other statistical measures.

Sensitivity: The index should be able to detect reasonably small shifts, in either direction, in the condition.

Acceptability: The use of the index should not be painful or demeaning to the subject

Probably no index used in oral epidemiology satisfies all the above conditions.

Classification of Indices

In general there are two types of dental indices.

1. The first type of index measures the number or proportion or people in a population with or without a specific condition at a specific point in time or internal of time.
2. The second type of dental index measures the number of people affected and the severity of the specific condition at a specific time or interval of time.

- **Irreversible index:** It is the one that measures cumulative conditions that cannot be reversed, e.g. an index that measures dental caries.
- **Reversible index:** Index that measures conditions that can be changed. Reversible index scores can increase or decrease on subsequent examinations, e.g. indices that measure periodontal conditions.

Depending upon the extent to which areas of oral cavity are measured:

a. **Full mouth indices:** These indices measure the patient's entire periodontium or dentition, e.g. Russell's periodontal index.
b. **Simplified indices/partial recording indices:** These indices measure only a representative set of teeth, e.g. Greene and Vermillion's oral hygiene index-simplified (OHI-S).

A variant of this type is that the examination/measurement is done on full mouth basis but only the highest scores are recorded in that sextant/quadrant/mouth.

For example, Dean's index and Greene and Vermillion's oral hygiene index (OHI)

Indices may be categorized according to the entity which they measure like:

1. **Disease index:** The 'D' (decay) portion of the DMF index best exemplifies a disease index.
2. **Symptom index:** The indices measuring gingival/sulcular bleeding essentially symptom indices.
3. **Treatment index:** 'F' (filled) portion of the DMF index best exemplifies a treatment index.
4. **Treatment need index:** TN in CPITN index best exemplifies the treatment need index.

Dental indices can also be classified under special categories as:

a. **Simple index:** Index that measures the presence or absence of a condition, e.g. plaque index.
b. **Cumulative index:** Index that measures all the evidence of a condition (past and present), e.g. DMF index for dental caries.

Types of dental indices according to use:

a. **Individual assessment**
- Evaluation and monitoring the progress and maintenance of oral health.
- Measures effects of personalized disease control programs over time.
- Monitors progress of disease healing, patient education, motivation, e.g. Patient hygiene performance index.

b. Clinical trial

- Determines the effect of an agent or procedure on the prevention, progression, or control of a disease
- Comparison of an experimental group with a control group, e.g. Gingival index, Plaque index

c. Epidemiologic survey

- Survey for the study of disease characteristics of populations.
- Not designed for evaluation of an individual patient, e.g. CPITN

Useful and effective index will:

a. Be simple to use and calculate.
b. Require minimal equipment and expense.
c. Require a minimal amount of time to complete.
d. Not to cause discomfort to the patient.
e. Have a clear cut criteria.
f. Be as free as possible from subjective interpretation.
g. Be reproducible by the same examiner or different examiner.

h. Be amenable to statistical analysis and have validity and reliability.

In order to provide specific preventive regimes and improved treatment for the challenges presented by the various oral diseases, it is essential that data be collected first. The first step in this direction is by a pragmatic reporting method. The following sections deal with indices for various oral diseases, the use of which will help the researcher achieve the goal.

Bibliography

1. Barnes GP, Parker WA, Lyon TC, Fultz RP. Indices Used to Evaluate Signs, Symptoms and Etiologic Factors Associated with Diseases of the Periodontium. J Periodontol 1986:643–51.
2. Davies, GN The different requirements of periodontal indices for prevalence studies and clinical trials. International Dental Journal 1968;18, 560–69.
3. Striffler DF, Young WO, Burt BA. Dentistry, Dental Practice and the Community. In methods for assessing the distribution of oral diseases 1974, 3rd edn, pp 75–114.

Indices to Assess Dental Caries

Dental caries is a chronic disease process that usually progresses slowly and infrequently is self-limiting. It can affect enamel, dentin, and cementum which manifests clinically along a continuum from initial loss of mineral to complete tooth destruction. Carious lesions can occur in either the coronal or root surfaces of teeth and in smooth (proximal surfaces) surfaces or pit and fissure areas (occlusal pits and fissures). This portrait of dental caries describes the basic attributes of the disease. But, more importantly, it is the formulation of a functional definition of dental caries, i.e. one by which epidemiologists can assess population characteristics and disease patterns, etiology, and test preventive and restorative therapies.

Various indices/indexes for measuring caries were suggested during the 1920s to the early 1930s. It was only with Dean's studies of naturally occurring fluoridated water in the 1930s that a practical method was developed and used. Dean et al., 1942 counted the numbers of teeth in the mouth with obvious caries. Filled teeth and teeth missing due to caries were added in, so that the index score included all teeth that had been attacked by caries during the past. In the following section, various indices to assess dental caries will be discussed.

2.1A Decayed Missing Filled Teeth (DMFT) Index

The first description of what is now known as the DMF index came from extensive studies of dental caries among children in Hagerstown, Maryland, USA, in the 1930s. After that, the DMF index became the most used of all dental indexes. It was given by Klein H, Palmer CE and Knutson JW in 1938.

Instruments used were mouth mirror and fine pointed pig tail explorer under favorable lightning conditions. Observations were made on all teeth and in addition unerupted and extracted permanent teeth were noted. Pits and fissures in which the explorer caught and which after thorough inspection were not considered definitely carious were noted as separately and were not considered as caries. Teeth designated as carious were those, which showed actual, although frequently small cavities. Remaining roots were considered as equal to carious teeth.

Rules for Recording

- A tooth is considered to be erupted when the occlusal surface or incisal edge is exposed.
- Decayed missing and filled should be recorded separately.
- No tooth should be counted more than once.
- Tooth lost or filled due to causes other than caries are not included.

- Deciduous teeth are not taken into account.
- Tooth is considered present even the crown is destroyed and only the roots are left.

WHO Criteria for Computing DMF Index (1987)

Caries is recorded as present when a lesion in a pit or fissure, or on a smooth tooth surface, has a detectably softened floor, undermined enamel, or softened wall

- All third molars are included
- Temporary restorations are considered as 'D'
- Only carious lesions are considered as 'D'

When any doubt exists, caries should not be recorded as present.

- Individuals 30 years and older, M component should include teeth missing due to caries and any other reason.
- <30 years M component includes missing due to caries only.

WHO Criteria for Computing DMF Index (1997)

Caries is recorded as present when a lesion in a pit or f issure, or on a smooth tooth surface, has an unmistakable cavity, undermined enamel, or a detectably softened floor or wall. A tooth with a temporary filling, or one which is sealed but also decayed, should also be included in this category. In cases where the crown has been destroyed by caries and only the tooth is left, the caries is judged to have originated on the crown and therefore is scored as crown caries only. The CPI probe should be used to confirm visual evidence of caries on the occlusal, buccal, and lingual surfaces. Where any doubt exists, caries should not be recorded as present.

Advantages

Simple, rapid, versatile, universally accepted, statistically manageable and reliable index.

- Gives total lifetime caries experience of an individual and group of individuals.
- D component gives treatment needs in terms of teeth to be filled, extracted or endodontically treated.
- M component gives tooth mortality.
- F component gives the account of fillings done among the population.

Limitations

- The DMF index today is really outdated as a measure of caries incidence and severity, and may actually be more valid as a measure of treatment received.
- It is philosophically questionable to use an index for a disease that is so dependent upon the treatment judgments of many practitioners, and the combination of previous treatment (i.e. the M and F components) with current treatment need (the D component) is not used elsewhere in public health surveillance.
- DMF values are not related to the number of teeth at risk.
- The DMF index gives equal weight to missing, untreated decayed or well-restored teeth.
- The DMF index is invalid when teeth have been lost for reasons other than caries. Teeth can be lost for periodontal reasons in older adults, and for orthodontic reasons in teenagers. Decision rules, which go along with criteria, are required to determine how to deal with these instances.
- The DMF index can overestimate caries experience in teeth with 'preventive restorations'. In an epidemiological survey, such teeth must be included in the F component of DMF, although had they not been filled in the first place they might have been diagnosed as sound teeth. DMF scores will thus be inflated (Bader et al., 1993).
- Composite and resin restorations not only may have been placed on non-carious teeth,

but are often hard for an examiner to detect, thus leading to underestimation.

- DMF scores cannot be compared from one group to another without considering the criteria by which caries was considered present or absent.
- DMF data are of little use for estimating treatment needs.
- DMF cannot account for sealed teeth. Sealants did not exist in 1938, so are obviously not included in the description of the index. Sealants and other composite restorations for cosmetic purposes have to be dealt with separately.
- DMF values are not related to the number of teeth at risk. So it does not directly give an indication of the intensity of attack of caries.
- Reaches saturation level at particular point of time when all the teeth are involved and prevents further registration of caries attack even when caries activity is continuing.
- Cannot be used for root caries.
- Rate of caries progression cannot be assessed.

2.1B DMFS Index

Klein H, Palmer CE and Knutson JW in 1938 proposed the DMFS index. This index follows the same criteria's and method as DMFT but instead of individual teeth, surfaces are recorded. For posterior teeth (molars and premolars) 5 surfaces and for anterior teeth (Incisors and canines) 4 surfaces will be recorded. Remaining roots were considered as equal to five carious surfaces. Records for filled teeth were made in a similar manner, i.e. filled surfaces were considered as past carious surfaces. Full crowns were considered equal to five filled surfaces. If 28 teeth are examined maximum score is 128 and if 32 teeth are examined maximum score is 148.

Advantages

- More sensitive, index of choice in clinical trials for caries preventive agents
- More precise.
- Gives true status of the caries attack.

Problems with MS component: In the format originally proposed for the DMFS index in 1931, it was suggested that 'lost teeth are debited as deeply carious ones by adding three points to the total count of cavities', rather than the full value possible for the tooth; it was further suggested that crowns be assigned three surfaces 'as such teeth are commonly decayed on three surfaces', while those which serve as abutments for bridges may be rated lower. Bodecker proposed the current format of the DMF index in 1939, it was pointed out that assigning five surfaces to crowned and extracted teeth would overestimate the true caries experience of such teeth, and it was recommended that a total of three surfaces should be assigned to crowned or extracted teeth, provided that the tooth had been extracted before 35 years of age.

Various methods of accounting for the 'M' component of the DMFS index have been proposed since 1939. For cross-sectional studies, one of the more common methods is to ignore such surfaces, as though the affected teeth were not present at baseline (designated as DM_1FS, equivalent to the DFS index). Alternatives for cross-sectional studies are to assign three surfaces for any extracted tooth ($DM_{3a}FS$, or to take the more common approach of assigning the maximum of four surfaces for an extracted anterior tooth or five for an extracted posterior tooth (DM_5FS). An examiner may also assign an arbitrary number of surfaces based upon the general status of an individual's dentition; however, this carries with it the risk of examiner bias.

Other modifications of DMF index reported in the literature:

The simplified indices selected were the ones proposed by Guimarães in 1971. These are known as "DMF in 6 teeth" (DMF6T) and "DMF in 2 quadrants" (DMF2Q).

- The DMF6T index corresponds to the mean number of permanent teeth attacked by caries in six selected teeth (16, 11, 24, 37, 32 and 45).

- The DMF2Q index corresponds to the mean number of permanent teeth attacked by caries in the upper left and lower right quadrants. It is calculated by multiplying the DMFT value obtained from the two quadrants by two.

These indices can be utilized especially when a rapid diagnosis of the situation of dental caries is desired, provided that such diagnoses are coherent with the objectives of the study. These are reliable alternatives that can be applied in epidemiological surveys of oral health.

Veigas AR 1969 — Proposed three simplified methods as per the prevalence of caries in 7–12-year-old children when only a part of each child's mouth is examined.

1. Requires only the examination of right lower first molar (RLM): Low prevalence areas.
2. Requires the examination of upper right and left central incisors along with RLM (2UCIS).
3. Method 1 for 7-year-old and method 2 for 11-year-old.

Bibliography

1. Broadbent JM, Thomson WM. For debate: problems with the DMF index pertinent to dental caries data analysis. Community Dent Oral Epidemiol 2005; 33: 400–9.
2. Cypriano S, Rosario de Souza ML, Wada RS. Evaluation of simplified DMFT indices in epidemiological surveys of dental caries. Rev Saude Publica 2005;39(2).

3. Klein H, Palmer CE, Knutson JW. Pub Health Reports 1938;53:751–65.
4. Klein H, Palmer CE. Pub Health Reports 1940: No. 28 (July 12):55.
5. Striffler DF, Young WO, Burt BA. Dentistry, Dental Practice and the Community. In methods for assessing the distribution of oral diseases. 3rd edn;75–114.
6. Veigas AR. Simplified indices for estimating the prevalence of dental caries experience in children of 7–12 years of age. J Public Health Dent 1969;19:76–91.

2.2 Simplified Caries Index

A simplified caries index was designed by RM Grainger 1967 to provide an epidemiologic tool that would assess the dental caries experience of a population with a minimum of decisions required of the examiner. Specifically, this caries index categorizes the dentition into five zones that represent increasing severity of caries experience, and it records the existence of dental caries or fillings in the highest rated zone. The criteria are illustrated in Table 2.1.

Bibliography

1. Ralph V. Katz, Wayne R. Radi, George P. Barnes. Evaluation of a Simplified Caries Index for Use by the US Army Dental Corps. J Dent Res 1976; 55:935.
2. WHO: International Dental Epidemiological Methods Series, Manual No. 3 (first draft) Geneva, Switzerland: World Health Organization 1967, pp.1,26.

Table 2.1: Criteria for classification of individuals according to severity zone of dental caries

Severity zone	Severity zone definition (surfaces involved)
5	Proximal surfaces of mandibular anterior teeth (excluding distal surfaces of cuspids)
4	Labial surfaces of maxillary and mandibular incisors and cuspids (excluding those of maxillary cuspids)
3	Proximal surfaces of maxillary anterior teeth (excluding distal surfaces of cuspids)
2	Proximal surfaces of molars and premolars (including distal surfaces of cuspids)
1	Pit and fissure surfaces of posterior teeth and labial surfaces of maxillary cuspids
0	None dental caries or fillings observed

2.3 Dental Caries Severity Classification Scale (D1–D3)

This index was first published by the World Health Organization (WHO) in 1979 (WHO, 1979), and will be referred to as the D1–D3 scale. (There is a D4 for pulpal involvement, but that recording is seldom contentious). It permits identification of lesion initiation, progression and regression. Teeth to be dried prior to the examination. The scoring criteria are given in Table 2.2.

Limitations

• Requires meticulous examiner training
• Very lengthy and detailed examination.

Bibliography

1. World Health Organization, A guide to oral health epidemiological investigation. Geneva. WHO, 1979.

2.4 Modified DMFT Index

According to the WHO criteria, if both caries and a filling are present on the same tooth, only the caries will be scored, since each tooth is counted only once. In other words, caries took priority over fillings. Thus, it was realized that recording the F component of the DMFT index, especially in a population group that has been provided with restorative care of poor quality, does not reflect the true scope of restorative services rendered. Furthermore, many of the teeth examined demonstrated a significant and extensive destruction of the crown, and were thus indicated for extraction or root canal treatment. Yet, according to the DMFT index, these had to be coded under the same "Decayed" (D) category as those with simple carious lesions. Since such information is essential for planning dental health care programs of restorative care for population groups, modified DMFT was developed. It was given by Joseph Z Anaise in 1984.

The examinations were carried out in the schools and performed by the examiner using a standard plane mirror and a sharp thin probe (Martin No. 4) in front of a standard artificial light only. Dental caries were recorded and diagnosed using only visual and tactile methods of detection. M and F components are recorded as usual as per WHO criteria. There are 4 divisions for D component. The criteria were presented in Table 2.3.

Table 2.2: Dental caries severity classification scale [D1–D3]		
Score	Stage	Criteria
0	Sound	No evidence of treated or untreated clinical caries (slight staining allowed in otherwise sound teeth)
D1	Initial caries	No clinically detectable loss of substance. For pits and fissures, there may be significant staining, discoloration or rough spots in the enamel that do not catch the explorer, but loss of substance cannot be positively diagnosed. For smooth surfaces, these may be white, opaque areas with loss of luster
D2	Enamel caries	Demonstrable loss of tooth substance in pits or fissures, or on smooth surfaces, but no softened floor or wall or undermined enamel. The texture of the material within the cavity may be chalky or crumbly, but there is no evidence that cavitation has penetrated the dentin
D3	Caries of dentin	Detectably softened floor, undermined enamel or a softened wall, or the tooth has a temporary filling. On approximal surfaces, the explorer point must enter a lesion with certainty
D4	Pulpal involvement	Deep cavity with probable pulpal involvement. Pulp should not be probed. (Usually included with D3 in data analysis)

Table 2.3: Modified DMFT index

Code	Criteria
C	Unfilled teeth that are carious
CF	Restored teeth that are either secondarily carious around the margins of the restorations or primarily on a tooth surface other than the restored one
IX	Carious teeth either filled or unfilled that in the examiner's opinion are indicated for extraction, i.e. caries has so destroyed the crown that it cannot be restored; only the roots remain
IRC	Carious teeth either filled or unfilled that in the examiner's opinion are indicated for pulp treatment or root canal treatment, i.e. caries has progressed to an extent that there is an obvious exposure of the pulp and the teeth can be endodontically treated; caries has progressed to an extent that during carious material removal the pulp would be affected and the teeth should be treated endodontically
M	Teeth which were missing (as a result of caries) at the time of examination
F	Filled teeth which showed no sign of secondary caries

The DMF index has been modified by subdivision of decayed teeth (D) into Decayed and unfilled, secondarily decayed filled teeth (DF) and decayed but indicated for extraction (I). In addition to these four categories of decayed teeth, the remaining two categories of the DMFT index ("F"-filled teeth, with no decay and "M"-missing teeth) are recorded as usual, according to the criteria recommended by WHO. The DMFT score is then the summation of all six categories and the calculation of the individual components as well as the sum remain essentially the same as the original DMFT index.

Advantages

- Provides description of previous dental care.
- Shows the extent of dental services needed by the population.
- More detailed account of the population dental needs can be recorded at no additional cost and without an obligation to use an additional index.

Bibliography

1. Anaise JZ. Decayed Missing Filled teeth among Jewish and Arab school children in Israel. Community Dent Oral Epidemiol 1980;8:61–5.
2. Anaise JZ. Measurement of dental caries experience—modification of the DMFT index. Community Dent Oral Epidemiol 1984;12:43–6.

2.5 Moller's Index

It was given by Moller JJ in 1966 and later tested by Moller JJ and Poulsen S in 1973. The basis for development of the system was to make available a system which could be used in many different situations. The advantage of the system seems to be its flexibility in meeting the varying needs of different types of clinical studies on dental caries.

Standardized system of diagnosing, recording and analyzing dental caries data includes:
- Standardization of diagnostic criteria.
- Standardization of the equipment used for examination (including the circumstances under which the examination is carried out).
- Standardization of the recording procedures and the field records.

Equipment used were unscratched plane mouth mirrors and standardized dental probes (Holst probe, CG Brincker, Copenhagen). Each probe is used only once, after which it is sent to the manufacturer for restandardization. It is recommended that the use of the probe during the clinical examination be limited to only those areas where carious lesions are suspected but not verified by clinical inspection. The reason for this is that the actual probe pressure applied by different examiners varies considerably and seems beyond standardization. The scoring criteria were described in Table 2.4.

- Examination under high quality day operating lamp, with isolation.
- Pre-cleaning of the teeth, isolation with cotton rolls and saliva ejector, and drying with compressed air is highly recommended, since it has been shown that this adds substantially to the number of carious lesions detected.
- Radiographic examination for proximal surfaces are carried out wherever possible. The exposure, development and diagnosis of the radiographs should be carried out under standard conditions.
- For posteriors, 5 surfaces are examined and while for anteriors, 4 surfaces are examined.
- For the primary dentition the examination is performed accordingly. Examination of the teeth is performed in routine order, from maxillary right to maxillary left, and from mandibular right to mandibular left. For each tooth the examination is performed by examining each surface in the following sequence: (1) occlusal surface, (2) mesial surface, (3) vestibular surface, (4) distal surface and (5) lingual or vestibular surface. The diagnosis is given by the examiner using the respective coding for each tooth or tooth surface and is recorded.

- All the teeth are included except the third molars

The dental designation used on the record forms is in accordance with the Haderup nomenclature. According to the Haderup system of dental designation, '+' signifies the maxilla, '−' the mandible. If the symbol is placed to the right of the figure, the right side is indicated, and vice versa. 'O' before the figure indicates a primary tooth. However, the two-digit system proposed by FDI can be adapted without any changes in the present system. If the tooth is used as the observation unit, only the first box in each row should be filled in, according to the respective coding, and the rest should be filled in with O. If the tooth surface is used as the observation unit, all 5 or 4 boxes (representing one tooth) should be filled in according to the coding for the respective tooth surfaces.

The coding used is as follows:
- 0 – sound
- 1 – caries 1
- 2 – caries 2
- 3 – caries 3
- 4 – caries 4
- 5 – filled
- 6 – missing due to caries

Table 2.4: Diagnostic criteria and respective coding for Moller's index

Pits and fissures smooth surfaces	Vestibular or lingual	Proximal surfaces (radiographs)	Score
Sound (normal)	Sound (normal)	Enamel surface contour distinct and unbroken	0
Discoloration; no definite sticking	White opaque area with loss of luster, no loss of substance	Enamel surface is broken; shadow between the enamel surface and a border not more than one fourth through the enamel	1
Sticking with/ without discoloration; no dentin involvement	Discontinuity in the enamel; loss of substance, no dentin involvement	Shadow has reached dentinoenamel junction	2
Definite cavity with dentin involvement	Dentin involvement	A shadow between the dentinoenamel junction and a border not more than half way through dentin	3
Probable pulp complication	Probable pulp complication	Shadow more than half way through the dentin	4

- 7 – tooth or tooth surface not erupted
- 8 –missing for reason other than caries
- 9 – congenitally missing
- '–' not recordable
- There was no specific coding used for recording secondary caries. It should be stated in the criteria for assessment whether secondary caries has been recorded as a filling or as a carious lesion.
- Arrested caries should be recorded as caries because one cannot distinguish with certainty between acute and arrested caries, at least not on radiographs nor clinically in pits and fissures. A tooth is usually recorded as present when any part of it projects through the gingiva. By using the tooth surface as the observation unit, partial eruption can be recorded.

Bibliography

1. Moller JJ and Poulsen S. A standardized system for diagnosing, recording and analyzing dental caries data. Scand J Dent Res 1973;81:1–11.

2.6 DMFT Treatment Time index

The following problems with use of the DMF Index in predicting treatment needs (time) have been encountered: (1) DMF is an accretion index measuring this history of caries experienced and may not accurately represent present treatment needs. (2) Elimination of the filled component from the index still leaves the problem of treatment needed to replace missing teeth. (3) The M component is not a useful predictor since it does not differentiate between missing teeth that need replacement and those which do not. (4) There is a wide variety of treatment representing a range of treatment times that is commonly applied to a tooth that is designated "D". Hence to overcome the above problems Beck JD and Field HM (1980) evaluated the ability of certain modifications of the DMFT components to predict the amount of treatment time needed. From the patient records they collected information like normal, missing, needing replacement, replaced, carious, etc. for each

tooth and tooth surface prior to beginning treatment. The restorative, rehabilitative, and surgical treatment(s) performed on each tooth were recorded. These were then converted into Relative Productivity Units (RPU). One RPU represents 10 min treatment time. This is based on the time it would take a dentist with one chair side assistant to perform the treatment in question. The RPU times were derived from the procedure times collected at the Dental Manpower Development Center in Louisville, Kentucky, and from the Professional Budget Plan of Madison, Wisconsin.

Bibliography

1. Beck JD and Field HM. Pilot results of DMF Treatment Time Index. Community Dent Oral Epidemiol 1980;8:52–5.

2.7 White Spot Lesion Index

The labial surfaces of all bonded teeth were visually examined and registered as:
1. No white spot formation,
2. Slight white spot formation (thin rim),
3. Excessive white spot formation (thicker bands), and
4. White spot formation with cavitation.

Bibliography

1. Cited in Gorelick L, Geiger AM, Gwinnett AJ. Incidence of white spot formation after bonding and banding. American Journal of Orthodontics 1982;81:93–8.

2.8 Caries along Wire Index (CarWI)

Artun proposed a system for assessment of enamel caries along the retainer wire and around the composite at each end in subjects wearing bonded lingual retainer following orthodontic treatment. The scoring criteria were described in Table 2.5.

Table 2.5: CarWI	
Score	Criteria
0	Surface appears intact
1	Whitish demineralization without cavitation
2	Cavitation

CarWI was scored both incisally and gingivally along the retainer wire in areas corresponding to all interproximal surfaces from the mesial aspect of one canine to the mesial aspect of the other canine and in areas corresponding to all lingual surfaces from canine to canine. CarWI was scored after thorough scaling along the wire.

Bibliography

1. Artun J. Caries and periodontal reactions associated with long-term use of different types of bonded lingual retainers. Am J Orthod 1984;86(2):112–8.

2.9 Functional Measure Index (FMI)

FMI was given by Sheiham A, Maizels J and Maizels A in 1987 as modification of DMFT

- First composite index to measure dental health rather than disease.
- Filled and sound teeth are weighted equally while Decayed and missing teeth are given zero weights.

$$FMI = \frac{Filled + Sound}{28}$$

Score range 0–1.

Advantages

- More reliable indicator of dental health status than conventional DMFT.
- More efficient in revealing the antecedent and behavioral factors that are associated with dental health status.

Bibliography

1. Sheiham A, Maizels J, Maizels A. New composite indicators of dental health. Community Dent Health 1987;4:407–14.

2.10 T-Health index/ Tissue Health Index (THI)

The T-Health index represents the total amount of a subject's healthy dental tissue at a particular point in time. By giving more weight to healthy teeth, the T-Health index attempts to measure the influence of primary prevention.

- It is a composite indicator of dental health given by Sheiham A, Maizels J and Maizels A in 1987.
- THI is number of sound equivalent teeth at a given point of time.
- An arbitrary set of weights was originally proposed to calculate the T-Health index: 1 for sound teeth, 0.5 for filled teeth, 0.25 for decayed teeth, and 0 for missing teeth.

$$THI = \frac{(0.25 \times DT) + (0 \times MT) + (0.5 \times FT) + (1 \times ST)}{28}$$

- Score ranges from 0 – 1.

Use — to assess dental health rather than disease

Advantages

- More reliable indicator of dental health status than the conventional DMFT.
- Marcenes and Sheiham found that a modified set of weights, which assigned a score of 0.25 for filled and decayed teeth, performed similarly to the original set of weights.

Bernabe E et al., in their study with the 36 sets of weights used to calculate the T-Health index, assigning twice the weight of a decayed tooth to a filled tooth whilst keeping the weight for a filled tooth d≤ 0.20 provided the strongest association with levels of perceived oral health and did not vary according to the extent of restorative treatment.

Bibliography

1. Bernabe E, Suominen-Taipale AL, Vehkalahti MM, Nordblad A, Sheiham A. The T-Health index: a composite indicator of dental health. Eur J Oral Sci 2009; 117:385–9.

2. Marcenes WS, Sheiham A. Composite indicators of dental health: functioning teeth and the number of sound equivalent teeth (T-Health). Community Dent Oral Epidemiol 1993;21:374–8.

3. Sheiham A, Maizels J, Maizels A. New composite indicators of dental health. Community Dent Health 1987;4:407.

2.11 Dental Health Index (DHI)

DHI was given by Carpay JJ, Neiman FH, König KG, Felling AJ and Lammers JG in 1988.
- Any number of teeth may be examined and the denominator is adjusted accordingly.
- It is developed to minimize the difference between the Sound(+1) and Affected or extracted teeth (−1)

$$DHI = \frac{ST \quad (DT + FT + MT)}{ST + DT + FT + MT}$$

Score ranges from −1 to +1

Advantage: Fewer teeth can be used to arrive at a value

Disadvantage: Although time is saved by scoring a subset of teeth, partial recording methods are usually less accurate.

Bibliography

1. Carpay JJ, Nieman FH, König KG, Felling AJ, Lammers JG. The dental condition of Dutch schoolchildren assessed by a new dental health index. Community Dent Health 1988;5(3):231–41.

2.12 International Caries Detection and Assessment System (ICDAS)

Coronal Primary Caries Detection Criteria

- Codes for coronal caries range from 0 to 6 depending on the severity of the lesion.
- Minor variations between the visual signs associated with each code depending on a number of factors
  - Including the surface characteristics (pits and fissures vs smooth surfaces)
  - Whether there are adjacent teeth present (mesial and distal surfaces)
  - Whether or not the caries is associated with a restoration or sealant.

The basis of the codes is essentially the same throughout and described in Table 2.6.

Depending on the surface [pits and fissures, smooth surface (mesial or distal), free smooth surfaces and caries associated with restorations and sealants (CARS)] the above codes are mentioned in detail (Tables 2.7 and 2.8).

Table 2.6: Description for ICDAS criteria

Code 0	Sound
1	First visual change in enamel (seen only after prolonged air drying or restricted to within the confines of a pit or fissure)
2	Distinct visual change in enamel
3	Localized enamel breakdown (without clinical visual signs of dentinal involvement)
4	Underlying dark shadow from dentin
5	Distinct cavity with visible dentin
6	Extensive distinct cavity with visible dentin

Table 2.7: Pit and fissure caries (ICDAS)

Code	Condition	Criteria
0	Sound tooth surface	No evidence of caries, developmental defects (enamel hypoplasia's, fluorosis, tooth wear (attrition, abrasion and erosion), extrinsic/intrinsic stains, will be recorded as sound
1	First visual change in enamel	Wet: no evidence of any change in color attributable to carious activity but prolonged air drying a carious opacity or discoloration
2	Distinct visual change in enamel	When wet there is a (a) carious opacity (white spot lesion) and/or (b) brown carious discoloration
3	Localized enamel breakdown due to caries with	Carious opacity (white spot lesion) and/or brown carious discoloration which is wider than the natural fissure/fossa that is not consistent with

contd...

Table 2.7: Pit and fissure caries (ICDAS) (Contd.)

Code	Condition	Criteria
	no visible dentin or underlying shadow	the clinical appearance of sound enamel. Dentin is NOT visible in the walls or base. If in doubt, the WHO/CPI/PSR probe can be used gently.
4	Underlying dark shadow from dentin with or without localized enamel breakdown	Shadow of discolored dentin visible through an apparently intact enamel surface, seen more easily when the tooth is wet, shadow must clearly represent the caries on the surface being examined.

Code 3 and 4, histologically may vary in depth with one being deeper than the other and vice versa.

Code	Condition	Criteria
5	Distinct cavity with visible dentin	Cavitation in opaque or discolored enamel exposing the dentin beneath, wet tooth may have darkening of the dentin visible through the enamel, frank cavitation
6	Extensive distinct cavity with visible dentin	Obvious loss of tooth structure, the cavity is both deep and wide and dentin is clearly visible on the walls and at the base. An extensive cavity involves at least half of a tooth surface or possibly reaching the pulp.

Table 2.8: Smooth surface (mesial and distal): Visual inspection from the occlusal, buccal and lingual directions

Code	Condition	Criteria
0	Sound tooth surface	There should be no evidence of caries (either no or questionable change in enamel translucency after prolonged air drying (suggested drying time 5 seconds)). Surfaces with developmental defects such as enamel hypoplasia; fluorosis; tooth wear (attrition, abrasion and erosion), and extrinsic or intrinsic stains will be recorded as sound.
1	First visual change in enamel	When seen wet there is no evidence of any change in color attributable to carious activity, but after prolonged air drying a carious opacity (white or brown lesion) is visible that is not consistent with the clinical appearance of sound enamel. This will be seen from the buccal or lingual surface.
2	Distinct visual change in enamel	In addition to the previous criteria, when viewed from the occlusal direction, this opacity or discoloration may be seen as a shadow confined to enamel, seen through the marginal ridge.
3	Initial breakdown in enamel due to caries with no visible dentin	Once dried for approximately 5 secs, distinct loss of enamel integrity, viewed from buccal/lingual direction. If in doubt, or to confirm the visual assessment, the CPI probe can be used gently across the surface to confirm the loss of surface integrity.
4	Underlying dark shadow from dentin with or without localized enamel breakdown	This lesion appears as a shadow of discolored dentin visible through an apparently intact marginal ridge, buccal or lingual walls of enamel. This appearance is often seen more easily when the tooth is wet. The darkened area is an intrinsic shadow which may appear as grey, blue or brown in color.
5	Distinct cavity with visible dentin	Cavitation in opaque or discolored enamel (white or brown) with exposed dentin in the examiner's judgment.
6	Extensive distinct cavity with visible dentin	Obvious loss of tooth structure, the extensive cavity may be deep or wide and dentin is clearly visible on both the walls and at the base. The marginal ridge may or may not be present. An extensive cavity involves at least half of a tooth surface or possibly reaching the pulp.

Table 2.9: Free smooth surface (buccal and lingual) and direct examination of mesial and distal surfaces (with no adjacent teeth)

Code	Condition	Criteria
0	Sound tooth surface	There should be no evidence of caries [either no or questionable change in enamel translucency after prolonged air drying (approximately 5 seconds)]. Surfaces with developmental defects such as enamel hypoplasia; fluorosis; tooth wear (attrition, abrasion and erosion), and extrinsic or intrinsic stains will be recorded as sound.
1	First visual change in enamel	When seen wet there is no evidence of any change in color attributable to carious activity, but after prolonged air drying a carious opacity is visible that is not consistent with the clinical appearance of sound enamel
2	Distinct visual change in enamel	There is a carious opacity or discoloration that is not consistent with the clinical appearance of sound enamel (Note: the lesion is still visible when dry). The lesion is located in close proximity (in touch or within 1 mm) of the gingival margin
3	Initial breakdown in enamel due to caries with no visible dentin	Once dried for 5 seconds there is carious loss of surface integrity without visible dentin.
4	Underlying dark shadow from dentin with or without localized enamel breakdown:	This lesion appears as a shadow of discolored dentin visible through the enamel surface beyond the white or brown spot lesion, which may or may not show signs of localized breakdown. This appearance is often seen more easily when the tooth is wet and is a darkening and intrinsic shadow which may be grey, blue or brown in color.
5	Distinct cavity with visible dentin	Cavitation in opaque or discolored enamel exposing the dentin beneath.
6	Extensive distinct cavity with visible dentin	Obvious loss of tooth structure, the cavity is both deep and wide and dentin is clearly visible on the walls and at the base. An extensive cavity involves at least half of a tooth surface or possibly reaching the pulp.

Caries-associated with restorations and sealants (CARS) detection criteria (Table 2.9):

- Sound tooth surface with restoration or sealant: Code 0, A sound tooth surface adjacent to a restoration/sealant margin.
- First visual change in enamel: Code 1
- Distinct visual change in enamel/dentin adjacent to a restoration/sealant margin: Code 2, If the restoration margin is placed on enamel the tooth must be viewed wet. If the restoration margin is placed on dentin: Code 2 applies to discoloration that is not consistent with the clinical appearance of sound dentin or cementum.
- Carious defects of <0.5 mm with the signs of code 2: Code 3, cavitation at the margin of the restoration/sealant <0.5 mm.

- Marginal caries in enamel/dentin/cementum adjacent to restoration/sealant with underlying dark shadow from dentin: Code 4, view tooth wet and then dry, This lesion should be distinguished from amalgam shadows.
- Distinct cavity adjacent to restoration/sealant: Code 5, in addition to code 4, a gap > 0.5 mm in width.
- Extensive distinct cavity with visible dentin: Code 6, extensive cavity may be deep or wide and dentin is clearly visible on both the walls and at the base.

ICDAS two-digit coding method restorations/sealants with the first digit, followed by the appropriate caries code

0 = Sound
1 = Sealant, partial

2 = Sealant, full
3 = Tooth colored restoration
4 = Amalgam restoration
5 = Stainless steel crown
6 = Porcelain/gold/PFM crown or veneer
7 = Lost or broken restoration
8 = Temporary restoration
9 = Used for the following conditions
96 = Tooth surface cannot be examined: Surface excluded
97 = Tooth missing because of caries (tooth surfaces will be coded 97)
98 = Tooth missing for reasons other than caries (all tooth surfaces will be coded 98)
99 = Unerupted (tooth surfaces coded 99)

Special Considerations

- In case of doubt the examiner should score low.
- Distinguish among unerupted teeth, teeth extracted because of caries and those extracted or missing for other reasons.
- Non-vital teeth should be scored in the same manner as vital teeth.
- Banded or bracketed teeth. All visible surfaces should be examined, when completely covered by a band or bracket and there is no evidence of caries the tooth status code is "0".
- In the case of supernumerary teeth, the examiner should decide which tooth is the legitimate occupant of the space. Only that tooth should be scored.
- When both a primary and permanent tooth occupy the same space, only the permanent tooth is coded.
- All surfaces restored with full coverage should be coded as crowned. Less than full coverage, the surfaces involved in the restoration will be scored separately.
- If part of a restoration is lost on a surface, the surface should be coded as "7" (first number), even when not all the restoration is missing.

- It is important that there is a code to record the instances where there are non-carious cavities.
- Where more than one carious lesion exists on a surface, the worst lesion should be scored, though scoring pits and fissures separately to free smooth surfaces is an option.
- A root surface adjacent to a crown margin that is free of decay should be scored sound.
- If more than one lesion is present on the same root surface, the most severe lesion is scored.
- All tooth surfaces of retained roots should be scored as (06).

Root Caries Criteria

- *Code E:* Root surface cannot be visualized directly as a result of gingival recession or by gentle air-drying, then it is excluded. Surfaces covered entirely by calculus can be excluded or, calculus can be removed prior to determining the status of the surface.
- Code 0: No unusual discoloration nor does it exhibit a surface defect either at the cementoenamel junction or wholly on the root surface. The root surface has a natural anatomical contour, OR exhibit a definite loss of surface continuity or anatomical contour that is not consistent with caries process, e.g. attrition abrasion or erosion.
- Code 1: A clearly demarcated area on the root surface or at CEJ that is discolored, but there is no cavitation (< 0.5 mm).
- Code 2: There is a clearly demarcated area on the root surface or at CEJ that is discolored, there is cavitation (loss of anatomical contour ≤ 0.5 mm) present.

Figures 2.1 to 2.3 show the steps in assessment of primary caries on the root surface, caries associated with root restorations and root caries activity.

Special Considerations

- When both a coronal and root surface are affected by a single carious lesion that

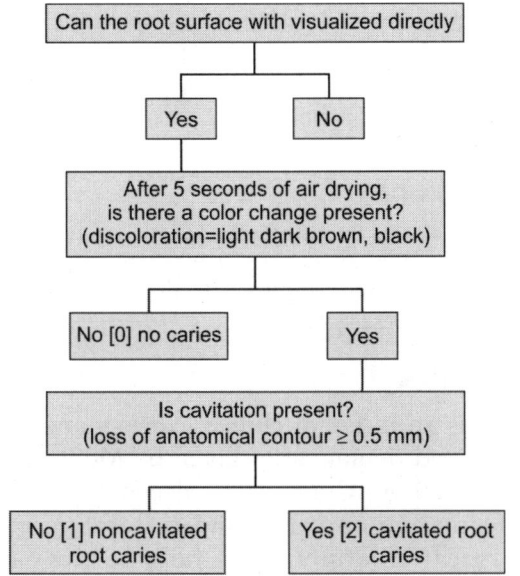

Fig. 2.1: Decision tree for primary caries on the root surface

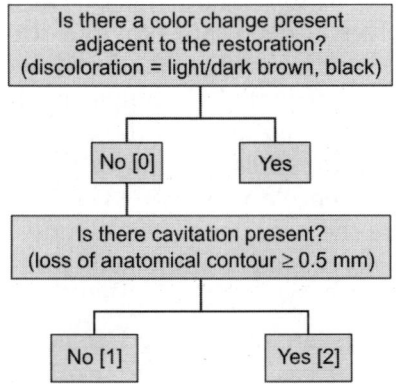

Fig. 2.2: Decision tree for caries associated with root restorations

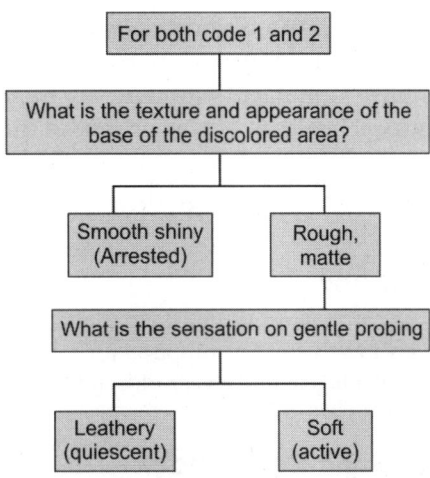

Fig. 2.3: Decision tree for root caries activity

involve at least 1/3 of the distance across the adjacent surface, that adjacent surface also should also be scored as caries.

- If more than one lesion is present on the same root surface, the most severe lesion is scored.
- Non-vital teeth are scored the same as vital teeth.

Bibliography

1. International Caries Detection and Assessment System Coordinating Committee. Criteria Manual. Workshop held in Baltimore, Maryland, March 12th–14th 2005.
2. Ismail AI, Sohn W, Tellez M, Amaya A, Sen A, Hasson H, Pitts NB. The International Caries Detection and Assessment System (ICDAS): an integrated system for measuring dental caries. Community Dent Oral Epidemiol 2007; 35: 170–8.

2.13 Significant Caries Index (SiC)

- It was introduced by Douglas Bratthall in 2000 and recommended by WHO in 2005.
- The SiC is not a new index, but rather is a form of data presentation to help give a better picture of caries distribution in the population in order to bring attention to those individuals with the highest caries scores in each population.
- It is the mean DMF score for the third of the population that is most affected by caries,

extends at least 1 mm past the CEJ in both the incisal and apical directions, both surfaces should be scored as caries.

- For lesion affecting both crown and root surfaces that does not meet the 1 mm or greater extent of involvement, only the coronal or root surface that involves the greater portion (more than 50%) of the lesion should be scored as caries.
- When a carious lesion on a root surface extends beyond the line angle of the root to

intended to be used alongside the mean DMF of the whole population to give a more complete summary of its caries distribution.

• New oral health goal was proposed that, by the year 2015, the SiC Index should be less than 3 DMFT among the 12-year-old, globally.

Bibliography

1. Bratthall D. Introducing the Significant Caries Index together with a proposal for a new global oral health goal for 12-year-olds. Int Dent J. 2000 Dec;50(6):378–84.

2.14 Specific Caries Index

This index was proposed by Shashidhar Acharya in 2006. This criteria's for this index is based on GV Black, classification of cavity preparation (Table 2.10).

Advantages

• Provides information on caries prevalence, location and type of caries lesion in an individual based on clinical examination.
• Criteria are simple and easy to use.
• Reproducibility is fair to good.
• Ensures optimal utilization of scarce dental manpower as well as materials.

Limitations

• Cases of large lesions which cover more than one surface, only assumption can be made regarding the originating lesion.

• Lack of provision for assessing root caries
• Inability of this index if used alone to capture information useful for treatment planning.

Bibliography

1. Acharya S. Specific Caries Index: A new system for describing untreated dental caries experience in developing countries. J Public Health Dent 2006;66(4):285–7.

2.15 PUFA

This is an index of clinical consequences of untreated dental caries given by Monse B et al in 2010. Classical indices provides information on caries and restorative and surgical treatment but fails to provide information on the clinical consequences of untreated dental caries, such as pulpal involvement and dental abscess, which may be more serious than the caries lesions themselves. A deep caries cavity with pulpal involvement is usually considered under the code 'caries of dentin' and pulpal involvement is not mentioned at all in the caries scoring system in the latest edition of Oral Health Surveys. Hence a new index was developed to assess the prevalence and severity of oral conditions related to untreated caries called PUFA.

PUFA is an index used to assess the presence of oral conditions resulting from

Table 2.10: Criteria for specific caries index

Score	
0	No carious lesion detected
1	Carious lesion occurring on the occlusal, buccal pits and fissures of molars and premolars and the lingual pits of the anterior teeth
2	Proximal caries affecting the molars and premolars
3	Carious lesion situated on the proximal surface of the anteriors and not involving the incisal angles
4	Carious lesion situated on the proximal surface of the anteriors and involving the incisal angles
5	Carious lesion situated on the cervical region of the tooth
6	Carious lesions situated on the occlusal cusp tips of molars and on the incisal edges of the incisors
6A	Grossly decayed tooth/root stumps indicated for extraction

6 and 6A remain the same i.e., 6

untreated caries. The index is recorded separately from the DMFT/dmft and scores the presence of either a visible pulp, ulceration of the oral mucosa due to root fragments, a fistula or an abscess. Lesions in the surrounding tissues that are not related to a tooth with visible pulpal involvement as a result of caries are not recorded. The assessment is made visually without the use of an instrument. Only one score is assigned per tooth. In case of doubt concerning the extent of odontogenic infection, the basic score (P/p for pulp involvement) is given. If the primary tooth and its permanent successor tooth are present and both present stages of odontogenic infection, both teeth will be scored. Uppercase letters are used for the permanent dentition and lowercase letters used for the primary dentition. The codes and criteria for PUFA index are described in Table 2.11.

The PUFA/pufa score per person is calculated in the same cumulative way as for the DMFT/dmft and represents the number of teeth that meet the PUFA/pufa diagnostic criteria. The PUFA for permanent teeth and pufa for primary teeth are reported separately. Thus, for an individual person the score can range from 0 to 20 pufa for the primary dentition and from 0 to 32 pufa for the permanent dentition. The prevalence of PUFA/pufa is calculated as percentage of the population with a PUFA. (PUFA/pufa score of one or more). The PUFA/pufa experience for a population is computed as a mean figure and can therefore have decimal values.

The Untreated Caries, PUFA Ratio is calculated as $[PUFA+pufa/D+d] \times 100$

Bibliography

1. Monse B, Heinrich-Weltzien R, Benzian H, Holmgren C, van Palenstein Helderman W. PUFA – An index of clinical consequences of untreated dental caries. Community Dent Oral Epidemiol 2009.

2.16 Caries Assessment Spectrum and Treatment (CAST)

This index was developed because of the need to find a reliable, pragmatic, cohesive and easy-to-read reporting system for presenting results obtained from using both ICDAS II and PUFA indices.

The newly proposed index is more than a combination of the two previously mentioned indices, as it also aggregates the "M" and "F" component of the DMF index. As mentioned previously, PUFA complements ICDAS II, as there is no overlap between them. The fusion of the three indices resulted in the development of the new Caries Assessment Spectrum and Treatment (CAST) index. It covers the total dental caries spectrum, from no carious lesion, through caries protection (sealant) and caries cure (restoration) to carious lesions in enamel and dentine, and the advanced stages of carious lesion progression in pulpal and tooth-surrounding tissue. It comprises assessing stages of primary and, so called, secondary carious lesion progression in Enamel, Dentine and the Pulp, as well as Lost

	Table 2.11: Criteria for PUFA
P/p	Pulpal involvement is recorded when the opening of the pulp chamber is visible or when the coronal tooth structures have been destroyed by the carious process and only roots or root fragments are left. No probing is performed to diagnose pulpal involvement.
U/u	Ulceration due to trauma from sharp pieces of tooth is recorded when sharp edges of a dislocated tooth with pulpal involvement or root fragments have caused traumatic ulceration of the surrounding soft tissues, e.g. tongue or buccal mucosa.
F/f	Fistula is scored when a pus releasing sinus tract related to a tooth with pulpal involvement is present.
A/a	Abscess is scored when a pus containing swelling related to a tooth with pulpal involvement is present.

Table 2.12: CAST index

Characteristic	Code	Description
	0	Sound. No visible evidence of a distinct carious lesion is present
Sealed	1	Sealed. Pits and fissures have been at least partially sealed with a sealant material
Restored	2	A cavity has been restored with an (in)direct restorative material currently without a dentine carious lesion and no Fistula/Abscess present
Enamel	3	Distinct visual change in enamel. A clear caries related discolouration (white or brown in colour) is visible, including localized enamel breakdown without clinical visual signs of dentine involvement
Dentine	4	Internal caries-related discolouration in dentine. The lesion appears as shadows of discoloured dentine visible through enamel which may or may not exhibit a visible localized breakdown
	5	Distinct cavitation into dentine. No (expected) pulpal involvement is present
Pulp	6	Involvement of pulp chamber. Distinct cavitation reaching the pulp chamber or only root fragments are present
	7	Fistula/Abscess. A pus containing swelling or a pus releasing sinus tract related to a tooth with pulpal involvement due to dental caries is present
Lost	8	The tooth has been removed because of dental caries
Other	9	Does not match with any of the other categories

and Restored teeth resulting from dental caries (Table 2.12).

Furthermore, CAST has been developed such that the severity of the consequences of the dental caries process increases with increase in codes. Different to common caries indices, a restored tooth is considered a sound, well functioning tooth, and is therefore positioned at the beginning of the list of codes. Clearly, only the primary carious lesion assessment criteria from the two-digit ICDAS II index are needed and their Caries-Associated with Restorations and Sealants (CARS) criteria are not scored separately but are included in the primary carious lesion assessment criteria. This is because the so-called secondary carious lesions do not differ in their onset from primary carious lesions, so separate scoring would be superfluous.

Bibliography

1. Frencken JE, de Amorim RG, Faber J, Leal SC. The Caries Assessment Spectrum and Treatment (CAST) index: rational and development. Int Dent J 2011;61(3):117–23.

2.17 Relative Increment of Decay (RID)

This index was given by Donald R Porter and John A Dudman in 1960 in order to make comparisons of increments of dental caries activity between individuals or groups of individuals. The following information must be known for such comparisons:
- The period of observation or time
- The number of units or surfaces showing change
- The number of units or surfaces which were available or at risk during the interval.

The general principle underlying the construction of any index of the time rate of change of decay must be based solely on observations made at some time A and at some later time B and upon the time interval from A to B. The surface is taken as the basic unit of observation. A grosser unit would be the tooth itself, a finer unit the anatomic area or lesion. At a given time, a surface is classified as being in one and only one of four possible states:
1. Present and decay-free
2. Present and decayed
3. Present and filled
4. Missing

The index rate of decay is based on observations of individual surfaces at time A and time B, and the increase in decay is based on a count of the surfaces which have changed from one state to another. The sixteen categories of possibilities for any surface experience in a given time interval is given in Table 2.13

Status at	Status at time b			
time A	Decay free	Decayed	Filled	Missing
Decay free	N_{1-1}	N_{1-2}	N_{1-3}	N_{1-4}
Decayed	N_{2-1}	N_{2-2}	N_{2-3}	N_{2-4}
Filled	N_{3-1}	N_{3-2}	N_{3-3}	N_{3-4}
Missing	N_{4-1}	N_{4-2}	N_{4-3}	N_{4-4}

Table 2.13: RID

The individual boxes in above table contain the number (N) of units representing status at the two times. The N's are labelled so as to facilitate the location by row and column. The index is built from these counts: first, a measure of the absolute increment of decay (surfaces becoming carious), then a measure of the number of surfaces available for decay during the interval. Their ratio is the relative increment of decay during the interval A–B. Dividing by the length of the interval A–B will yield the relative increment of decay per unit time, which is used as the index of rate of decay.

Absolute increment of decay: Only five of the counts of surfaces in this table give information as to the increment of decay: N_{1-2}, N_{4-2}, N_{1-4}, N_{4-3} and N_{1-3}. These are the counts of the surfaces which went from decay-free or missing to decayed during the interval, the counts of the surfaces which went from decay-free to filled or missing, and the counts of those which went from missing to decayed. Of these, only the first two (N_{1-2} and N_{4-2}) give positive information of new decay. The other counts might indicate new decay, but surfaces could fall into these categories for reasons other than decay; for example, a surface could be filled because of decay in adjacent surfaces, or a surface could go from decay-free to missing because of exfoliation or extraction with no decay.

Advantages

1. The RID index was designed to permit the comparison of dental caries increments of children of any age or type of dentition.

2. By using this tool, the rates of dental caries activity of children in mixed dentition can be compared with those of children in primary or permanent dentitions.

3. The RID index can be used in longitudinal studies because it is an expression of the total dental caries activity in given time intervals.

Disadvantages

1. The expression is a pure number and not a descriptive number, as is the DMF index.

2. The expression is a figure with a decimal which may not seem meaningful.

3. The RID index presupposes, as do most other indexes, that each surface has an equal likelihood of becoming carious. Many surfaces are unlikely ever to become carious in some individuals and are prone to caries in others.

4. The RID index does not take into consideration filled surfaces which became carious at subsequent examinations. Because of the complications arising in this assessment when the surface is the unit of measure, these changes were not included.

5. The index does provide a weighting factor for surfaces changing to filled without certainity of decay.

The need of an expression of dental caries activity in an absolute figure which allows comparison of dental carious increments of the certain age group children with the other age groups is met by the RID index. This unique feature alone justifies its use for studies when such values are desired.

Bibliography

1. Porter D and Dudman JA. Assessment of Dental Caries Increments I. Construction of the RID. Index. J Dent Res 1960;39:1056–61.

2.18 Extrapolated Carious Surface Increment Index

Extrapolated Carious Surface Increment (ECSI) Index was proposed by Wagg BJ in 1974 in order to provide information on the ability of a particular treatment to arrest existing lesions or, more specifically, to provide a means of measuring caries progression as well as caries incidence. It is intended to supplement rather than to replace existing indices. As this index measures the rate it is not appropriate for prevalence studies.

Principle: A caries index should concern itself exclusively with dental caries. Fillings and extractions are not dental caries but rather the results of dental caries. Hence they are not included in the index as such, but a judgment is made as to the most likely state of caries which led to the filling or extraction and it is this extrapolated value which features in the index.

Recognizably distinct degrees of caries are defined in Table 2.14.

This scale is similar to that used by Marthaler and by Moller, Holst and Sorensen but is reduced by one point since it is considered that it is not possible to define with certainty the extent of the early enamel lesion. These principles are applicable both to clinical and to radiographic diagnosis, although the opinion has been expressed that a lesion is not demonstrable radiographically until it has at least reached the amelodentinal junction; if this opinion is accepted the minimum score to be attributed to a radiographically visible lesion should be 2.

Calculation: The use of the ECSI Index presupposes that the original observations have either been made according to the four-point scale above or are convertible into it. Because it is a measurement of rate there can, strictly speaking, be no baseline ECSI Index, but the baseline data are converted into ECSI terms as follows:

- Sound surfaces are scored zero
- Carious surfaces are scored according to the above scale,
- Unerupted teeth are treated as though they had erupted with all surfaces sound.
- Teeth extracted prior to the baseline examination are scored 3 and teeth which are shown radiographically to be congenitally absent or are known to have been extracted for orthodontic reasons are eliminated from the study.

Where a surface is restored by means of a filling, this is assumed to be equivalent to a lesion of Grade 2, This is taken to be an absorbing state, i.e. a filling cannot decay further and become equivalent to a lesion of Grade 3. There is, however, an exception to this rule which is detailed below. When a tooth is present in an early examination but missing in a subsequent one, efforts should be made via clinical judgment, the subject's clinical records or by direct interrogation to discover the reason. If the reason is orthodontic extraction or accidental loss, the tooth concerned remains in the analysis permanently in the state in which it was last recorded. In the case of a tooth extracted because of caries, however, the most likely explanation of its loss is that of pulpal involvement, i.e. a lesion of Grade 3, Reference is then made to the last examination at which it was present and the most seriously affected surface at that time recorded as 3 for the

Table 2.14: Criteria for extrapolated carious surface increment index	
Score	
0	Surface on which no carious attack can be demonstrated,
1	Surface on which carious attack is judged to be confined to the enamel,
2	Surface on which the carious attack is judged to involve both enamel and dentin but not yet to involve the pulp.
3	Surface on which the carious attack is of such severity that it has involved the pulp.

purpose of the current examination, all other surfaces being presumed to have remained in their previous state. Extraction like restoration, is an absorbing state; an extracted tooth cannot decay further. If the most seriously affected surface was filled (therefore by definition a lesion of Grade 2) then it is assumed that the restoration was ineffective and caries beneath it involved the pulp. In this case alone, the filling is not an absorbing state but it is considered to have progressed to a lesion of Grade 3.

Crowns and endodontically treated teeth are regarded as carious extractions unless it is known that purely cosmetic considerations were involved, in which case they are counted as 'accidental loss'. Reversals, or apparent improvements in caries state, are of two types. The first category is of those reverse transitions which are clearly impossible and must be the result of diagnostic or clerical error. These are an extracted tooth becoming present, an erupted tooth becoming unerupted and a filled surface becoming sound. The second category is of those reverse transitions which, although probably due to diagnostic error, are not impossible. A particular example of this is of a carious surface becoming sound. To this type of transition the term 'recovery' is given, the older term 'reversal' being confined to the category of impossibilities. Recoveries are treated as negative increments because it must be assumed that the majority result from diagnostic error and for every negative error which is detectable there is likely to be a positive one which is not. Reversals are corrected where possible as described later; if correction is not possible, reversals are ignored and the tooth concerned is assumed to remain in its previous state as with orthodontic extractions.

Calculation

Three types of transition are considered:

1. Tooth present or unerupted at examination A and present at examination B: The ECSI increment for each surface is obtained by subtracting the surface score at examination A from that at examination B, teeth unerupted at examination A are treated as though they were present with all surfaces sound. Fillings are treated as Grade 2 lesions.

2. Tooth present or unerupted at examination A and extracted because of untreated caries prior to examination B: If examination A and B arc consecutive, then the ECSI increment for the tooth is equal to 3-x, where 3 is the assumed state of the most seriously decayed surface immediately prior to extraction and x is the highest surface score at examination A. If the surface most seriously affected at examination A was filled, it is assumed that the filling was ineffective and the surface had attained a score of 3 immediately prior to extraction. If examinations A and B are not consecutive, the ECSI increment is equal to $(3 - x) + y$, where x is now the highest surface score at the last examination at which the tooth was present or unerupted (examination Q) and y is the ECSI increment for that tooth calculated between examination A and examination Q. Thus a tooth which was sound at examination A, had an occlusal lesion of Grade 2 and a proximal lesion of Grade 1 at examination Q and had been extracted prior to examination B would give an ECSI increment of $(3 - 2) + 3 = 4$.

3. Other transitions: Impossible transitions such as extracted teeth becoming sound are defined as reversals and make no contributions to the ECSI, nor do such transitions as sound to orthodontic extraction or sound to accidental loss. Restoration of proximal lesions represents a special case, since it will usually be necessary to involve the occlusal surface in the restoration, irrespective of its caries state.

For purposes of calculating the ECSI, the following rules have been adopted.

- A sound occlusal surface at examination 7A becoming involved in a proximal-occlusal filling at examination B. In this case the proximal surface is taken as being equivalent to a lesion of Grade 2 and the occlusal surface as being sound. Since the clinical records will show the occlusal surface as filled, however, an absorbing state exists and the occlusal surface cannot subsequently be recorded as carious.

- A carious occlusal surface at examination A becoming involved in a proximal-occlusal filling at examination B. There is currently no provision for recording two lesions on the same surface, so the assumption is made that the situation defined above is equivalent to a lesion of Grade 2 on each surface and that this is an absorbing state for both of these surfaces unless the tooth is subsequently extracted.

4. Correction of recording errors: In the majority of cases, the appearance of a reversal in a later examination will identify the recording error made previously. For example, a tooth which was originally recorded as extracted and subsequently found to be present must have been unerupted in the first examination and it is quite legitimate to correct the data accordingly. Another source of error is the wrong identification of a tooth adjacent to a missing tooth. This is particularly true of the premolars; where clinicians are denied access to data from previous examinations it may frequently occur that a single premolar is identified as a first premolar on one occasion and a second premolar on another. If bitewing radiographs are available it is usually a simple matter to correct the data retrospectively. In their absence, or where doubt still remains, it does not matter for the purpose of the ECSI whether or not an error of identification has been made so long as there is consistency from one examination to the next.

Bibliography

1. Wagg BJ. ECSI – A new index for evaluating caries progression. Community Dent Oral Epidemiol 1974;2:219–24.

2.19 def Index

The index was given by Allen O Gruebbel in 1944. It is an index of caries status because extracted and exfoliated teeth are ignored. "def" are used to indicate decayed deciduous teeth indicated for filling (d), decayed deciduous teeth indicated for extraction (e), and filled deciduous teeth (f).

It was proposed that the term observable dental caries prevalence be used in connection with the symbol "def" to indicate dental caries experience which can be observed in deciduous teeth present in the mouth at the time of the examination. The observable dental caries prevalence in deciduous teeth is computed by adding the number of decayed deciduous teeth indicated for filling (d), the number of decayed deciduous teeth indicated for extraction (e) and the number of filled deciduous teeth (f) for each child examined.

Jackson (1950) recommended that dmf index be used for a full mouth dentition from 3 to 5 years inclusive and for primary molars from 3 to 8 years inclusive. Another solution to the problems caused by natural shedding of primary teeth is the use of the df index a solution which is basically the same as that of the def index. The only difference being that the d component of the df index is subdivided so that d = d + e, where def = df. In addition to giving an indication of the type of treatment required, the *def* index also reflects the extent and severity of disease.

Modifications

1. dmf index — for children before the age of exfoliation, for children over 7 years primary molars and canines only are used for dmft or dmfs.

2. def index applied only to primary molars after 9 years.

Bibliography

1. Haugejorden O. Dental caries indices for primary teeth: the need to comply with international recommendations. Community Dent Oral Epidemiol, 1978;6:126–8.
2. Gruebbel AO. A Measurement of Dental Caries Prevalence and Treatment Service for Deciduous Teeth. J Dent Res 1944;23:163.
3. Jackson D. The Measurement of caries suscepti-bility. Br Dent J. 1950; 89:157–168.

2.20 Stone's Index

This index was given by Stone HH, Lawton FE, Bransby ER and Hartley HO in 1949 to evaluate the incidence of caries in national children's home aged 3–16 years (Table 2.15).

Bibliography

1. Stones HH, Lawton FE, Bransby ER and Hartley HO. British Dental J 1949;86:263.
2. Stones HH, Lawton FE, Bransby ER and Hartley HO. British Dental J 1950;9:199

2.21 Caries Severity Index (CSI)

This index is given by Aubrey Chosack in 1986. The index was developed with aim that it could be used in surveys of dental caries and give information in addition to def figures.

Criteria for different surfaces are described in Tables 2.16 to 2.19).

In cases of proximal caries "3", this will not count also as occlusal caries unless the caries

Table 2.15: Criteria for stone's index

Score	
0	Teeth free from caries
1	One point to one or more cavities in the same tooth detectable by sharp probe or bite-wing radiograph, where the lesion had not penetrated through the enamel to involve the dentine.
2	One or more cavities in the same tooth where the dentine was involved, but where a total of less than a quarter of the crown is estimated to have been destroyed
3	One or more cavities in the same tooth resulting in a total destruction of more than quarter of the crown

Table 2.16: Criteria for occlusal surfaces and pit and fissure caries on buccal and palatal surfaces of molars

Score	
1	Early pit and fissure caries where the explorer catches or resists removal with moderate to firm pressure and may be with softened base or an opacity as an evidence of demineralization. Softened enamel adjacent to the pit or fissure which may be scraped away.
2	Cavitation of at least 1mm across the smallest diameter at the tooth surface
3	Cavitation with breakdown or undermining of at least half a cusp

Table 2.17: Criteria for buccal — lingual and palatal smooth surfaces caries

Score	
1	A white lesion not extending to the embrasure areas, found to be soft and sticky by penetration with explorer
2	Cavitation of at least 1mm but less than 2 mm across the smallest diameter, or a soft sticky white lesion extending into one embrasure

Table 2.18: Criteria for proximal surfaces of molars

Score	
1	Discontinuity in enamel in which an explorer will catch and there is a softness
2	Cavitation with early breakdown of the marginal ridge or obvious discoloration indicating undermining of the ridge
3	Breakdown of the marginal ridge with cavitation extending to the mesial or distal extensions of the occlusal fissures

Table 2.19: Criteria for proximal surfaces on incisors and canines

Score	
1	Discontinuity in enamel in which an explorer will catch and there is a softness
2	Cavitation with breakdown or obvious discoloration, indicating undermining for at least 1 mm on the buccal or lingual surfaces
3	Cavitation with breakdown of the incisal edge or undermining of the edge as indicated by obvious discoloration

extends past the distal or mesial extensions of the fissures; in which case occlusal caries will be scored as in section A.

Only the largest caries involvement is scored for any one surface and scores of two or more lesions on one surface is not combined.

Calculation: Caries seen on the buccal, lingual and palatal surfaces in all teeth continuous with occlusal or proximal caries is only scored for these surfaces when normal pits or fissures of these surfaces are affected or included, or when the caries extends along at least half the gingival third of these surfaces. Only the largest caries involvement is scored for any one surface. Scores of two or more lesions on one surface are not combined.

A filled surface is given a score of 1. Secondary caries at the margin of a restoration is given a score of 2. The score for each tooth is the total of the scores of all its surfaces. Although a theoretical score of 15 is possible for molars and 12 for canines and incisors, part of the tooth material loss may have occurred because of fracture of an unsupported surface, rather than caries of that surface. Thus a maximum of 12 is scored for molars and a maximum of 9 for canines and incisors. If caries has resulted in complete breakdown of the crown, leaving only roots, the maximum score is recorded for this tooth. A full crown restoration gives a total score of 5 for that tooth. A total tooth score of 6 is given to a tooth extracted because of caries. These scores are based on clinical experience of the earlier levels of caries severity resulting in these types of treatment. The caries severity index (CSI) for the population is the mean of the scores for the caries teeth. Teeth free of caries are not included in this calculation.

Bibliography

1. Chosack A. A dental caries severity index for primary teeth. Community Dent Oral Epidemiol 1986;14:86–9.

2.22 Caries Analysis System (CAS)

The dmfs/t index may not be the most useful and appropriate index for caries studies because of high population variance and non-normal caries distribution. Furthermore, the index does not differentiate between caries patterns that could suggest different etiologies and consequently different preventive measures. To overcome these drawbacks Caries Analysis System was given by Douglass JM, Wei Y, Zhang BX, Tinanoff N in 1994.

It focuses on only those subjects with caries, thus emphasizing the extent of the disease in affected children. It differentiates between various caries patterns and examines the percentage of affected children, the degree to which these children are affected, and the proportion of total caries each disease pattern represents. These parameters—Prevalence, Severity and Distribution, respectively — uniquely describe caries experience and patterns.

Method: Dental examinations were done using mirror and number 23 explorer. Caries diagnosis was based on the modified method of Radike and the results for each child were recorded such that each tooth surface could be indicated as sound, carious, filled, or missing. No radiographs were taken for caries diagnosis.

Table 2.20: Caries analysis system (CAS)

Fissure pattern	Includes occlusal fissures, buccal pits of mandibular second molars and lingual grooves of maxillary second molars, represented surfaces susceptible to caries due to their anatomy.
Maxillary anterior	The caries pattern that often develops when an infant sleeps with the feeding bottle.
Posterior proximal	Comprises of all contacting posterior smooth surfaces, including the distal surfaces of the canines that are protected from routine mechanical disturbances.
Posterior buccal/ lingual smooth	Includes all buccal/ lingual surfaces of the molars without pits and fissures, representing surfaces that generally are affected only in extreme disease.

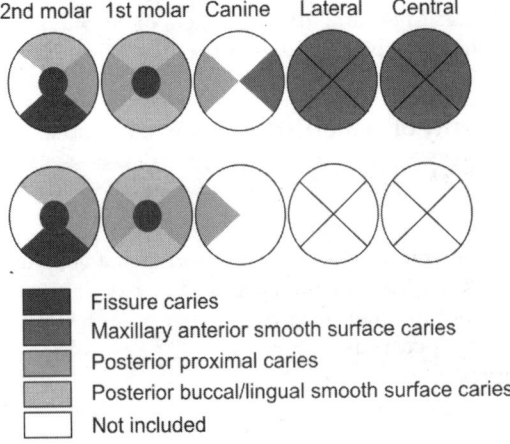

Fissure caries
Maxillary anterior smooth surface caries
Posterior proximal caries
Posterior buccal/lingual smooth surface caries
Not included

Fig. 2.4: Caries scoring criteria for caries analysis system

The caries data was categorized into four patterns (Table 2.20 and Fig. 2.4). These patterns were chosen to represent caries potentially caused by different factors.

Errors in identifying the potential etiologies of carious lesions (e.g., fissure pattern versus posterior proximal pattern) might occur in teeth that had large lesions involving more than one surface. All carious, restored and missing surfaces were included as they represented both current and past disease. Several surfaces were excluded from the analyses. The buccal surfaces of canines were excluded because of the high prevalence of developmental defects. The lingual surfaces of the maxillary canines, the lingual and mesial surfaces of the mandibular canines, as well as the mandibular incisors were excluded because they become affected only in cases of rampant caries. The distal surfaces of the second molars were excluded as these surfaces change character from free smooth surfaces to contacting posterior proximal surfaces. In total, 5.7% of the carious surfaces were excluded, of which 25% were canine buccal surfaces.

The data were calculated to determine prevalence, severity and distribution with help of equations are shown in Table 2.21. It should be noted that children could be included in more than one category.

Bibliography

1. Douglass JM, Wei Y, Zhang BX, Tinanoff N. Dental caries in preschool Beijing and Connecticut children as described by a new caries analysis system. Community Dent Oral Epidemiol 1994;22;94–9.

Table 2.21: Calculation to determine prevalence, severity and distribution for CAS

Parameter	Definition	Example equation
Prevalence	Percentage of subjects affected by a caries pattern	$\dfrac{\text{Number of subjects with fissure pattern}}{\text{Total number of subjects}}$
Severity	Percentage of surfaces by affected in a specific caries pattern	$\dfrac{\text{Total number of carious fissures pattern surfaces}}{\text{Number of fissure pattern surfaces in subjects with fissure caries}}$
Distribution	Percentage of total caries comprised by a caries pattern	$\dfrac{\text{Total number of carious fissure pattern surfaces}}{\text{Total number of carious surfaces}}$

2.23 Criteria for Classification of Individuals According to Severity Zone of Dental Caries (Poulsen and Horowitz)

Poulsen and Horowitz criteria are shown in Table 2.22

Table 2.22: Poulsen and Horowitz criteria

Severity zone	Definition (surfaces involved)
5	Proximal surfaces of mandibular anterior teeth (excluding distal surfaces of cuspids)
4	Labial surfaces of maxillary and mandibular incisors and cuspids (excluding those of maxillary cuspids)
3	Proximal surfaces of maxillary anterior teeth (excluding distal surfaces of cuspids)
2	Proximal surfaces of molars and premolars (including distal surfaces of cuspids)
1	Pit and fissure surfaces of posterior teeth and labial surfaces of maxillary cuspids
0	None of the above

Revised criteria for classification of individuals to severity of dental caries is shown in Table 2.23.

Table 2.23: Revised Poulsen and Horowitz criteria

Severity zone	Definition (surfaces involved)
3 (formerly 5 and 4)	Proximal surfaces of mandibular anterior teeth (excluding distal surfaces of cuspids) or labial surfaces of maxillary or mandibular incisors and cuspids
2 (formerly 3 and 2)	Proximal surfaces of all maxillary teeth or proximal surfaces of mandibular teeth posterior to and including distal surfaces of cuspids
1	Pit and teeth fissure surfaces of posterior
0	None of the above

Bibliography

1. Poulsen S, Horowitz HS. An evaluation of a hierarchical method of describing the pattern of dental caries attack. Community Dental Oral Epidemiol 1974;2:7–11.

2A Root Caries Indices

The need for developing a universally adopted method in the reporting of root caries was suggested by the increasing interest in root caries as a disease process and particularly by the age shifts within the population.

Essentially three methods of reporting the findings on root caries were in the literature. They are:

- Percent of study population exhibiting root caries lesions (one or more lesions)
- Number of root caries lesions/person
- Number of root caries lesions teeth present

2A.1 Root Caries Index

The root caries index (RCI) is a method for reporting root caries that measures the severity of the disease, and delineates the true intraoral population at risk (i.e. the denominator). It is given by Ralph V Katz in 1979.

- Root caries is defined as soft progressive, destructive lesions, either totally confined to the root surface or involving undermining of enamel at the CEJ but clinically indicating the lesion initiated on the root surface.
- Only teeth with gingival recession are examined.
- Method — mesial, distal, buccal, lingual are examined.
- For multiple types of root surface are exposed the most severely affected root surface is recorded.
  - Missing (M) — when whole tooth is missing and not the surface
  - No association of recession (NoR) — when CEJ cannot be observed.
  - Recession present, surface Decayed (R-D)
  - Recession present, surface Filled (R-F)
  - Recession present, surface Normal or sound (R-N)

Table 2.24: Diagnostic conventions proposed for RCI 1986

Convention no 1	If diagnosis of caries or filling is uncertain then score it as sound
Convention no 2	All caries detected at CEJ shall be scored as D regardless of the condition of adjacent enamel
Convention no 3	Coronal filling must extend more than 3 mm beyond CEJ to score as filled (except cast crowns)
Convention no 4	To score filling involving multiple surfaces, it should extend across at least 1/3rd of each additional surface
Convention no 5a	Recurrent decay should be regarded as independent disease category called "Recurrent Tooth Decay"
Convention no 5b	Recurrent decay associated with coronal filling extending less than 3 mm onto the root/crown should be recorded as independent disease category called "Root Decay Contiguous with Coronal Filling"
Convention no 6	For any root surface that is decayed, the events of an additional but separate root lesion is recorded as an independent disease category called "Additional Root Caries Lesion"
Convention no 7	Any root surface which appears sound but has more than 20% of its area inaccessible to clinical examination due to calculus and heavy plaque deposits shall be scored as unreadable

If calculus is present in the absence of any other findings on a recessed root surface, it is scored as sound with the assumption that decay not found under band of calculus (Table 2.24).

$$\text{RCI Score} = \frac{(RD) + (RF)}{RD + RF + RN} \quad 100$$

Advantages: The RCI represents a measurement that can be

- Readily understood (e.g. the percent of teeth at risk attacked by disease).
- Reported by tooth (like the DMF index) or by tooth surface (like the DMFS index).

- Analyzed by standard epidemiologic techniques (e.g. use of relative risk and attributable risk analysis
- Reported either by person at risk or by tooth-type (e.g. attack rate for molars, premolars, or simply for specific tooth).

Bibliography

1. Ralph V Katz. Assessing Root Caries in Populations: The Evolution of the Root Caries Index. J Public Health Dent. 1980;40:7–16.

2A.2 Root Surface Caries Severity Index

This was given by Billings RJ in 1986. The criteria are described in Table 2.25.

Table 2.25: Root surface caries severity index

Grade	Surface defect	Surface texture	Pigmentation
I (incipient)	None	Soft, can be penetrated by dental explorer	Light tan to brown
II (shallow)	Less than 0.50 mm in depth	Soft or irregular, rough, can be penetrated by a dental explorer	Tan to dark brown
III (cavitation)	Cavitation greater than 0.50 mm in depth, no pulpal involvement	Soft, can be penetrated by a dental explorer	Light brown to dark brown
IV (pulpal)	Deeply penetrating with pulpal or root involvement		Brown to dark brown

2A.3 Root Surface Caries Index

De Paola et al., 1989 described this index for quantification of different kinds of dental root surface caries (Table 2.26).

Types of designations:

(1) Caries description
(2) Restoration description
(3) Non-caries description

Bibliography

1. DePaola PF, Hyg MS, et al. Methodological issues relative to the quantification of root surface caries. Gerodontology. 1989; 8: 3-8

2A.4 Root Caries Criteria as Given by Banting DE, Ellen RP and Fillery ED in 1980

Following a thorough scaling and polishing, a visual examination by mouth mirror and explorer was conducted. Radiographs were taken only when there were proximal surfaces "at risk" with visible gingival recession, thus assuming that surfaces with loss of attachment but no visible recession (i.e. with periodontal pockets) were not at risk.

Root caries was recorded if

- There was a discrete, well-defined, and discolored soft area,
- The explorer entered easily and displayed some resistance to withdrawal, and
- The lesion was located either at the cementoenamel junction or wholly on the root surface.

Restored lesions were counted as root caries only if it was obvious that the lesion originated at the cementoenamel junction or was completely confined to the root surface; otherwise, these lesions were scored as cervical enamel lesions.

Bibliography

1. Banting DE, Ellen RP, Fillery ED. Prevalence of root caries among institutionalized older persons. Community Dent Oral Epidemiol 1980;8:84–88.r

2A.5 Root Caries as Assessed by NIDCR (refer page 33) and ICDAS (refer page 16) criteria's: The criteria's for root caries are described in the relevant sections

Table 2.26: Root surface caries index		
Caries description	*Designation*	*Code*
Well-defined, yellowish or light brown softened surface without cavitation before probing	Incipient caries	C1
Well-defined yellowish or light brown softened surface broken or with discontinuity	Frank cavitation	C2
Darkly stained and almost black leathery or hardened consistency penetration difficult no resistance on withdrawal with or without cavitation	Arrested caries	AC
Soft, yellowish or light brown caries at the interface between the restoration and the root surface	Secondary caries	CF
Restoration description	*Designation*	*Code*
Restoration involving the root surface only	Root restoration	F
Restoration primarily in enamel but extends onto the root	Overlapping restoration	R1
Restoration primarily on the root but extends onto the enamel	Overlapping restoration	R2
Non-caries description	*Designation*	*Code*
Wedge-shaped defect with highly polished exposed dentin, softly angled early but sharply angled later	Root abrasion	A
Shallow, broad, smooth, disc-like depression, secondary to chemical action	Root erosion	E

2B Important Criteria's used in the Literature for Caries Assessments (Ismail AI, 2004):

2B.1 Backer-Dirks et al. in 1961

For approximal caries, the clinical examination by mirror and explorer was completely abandoned, because of poor accuracy which makes it almost impossible to standardize diagnosis. Pits and fissures were cleaned with a new sharp explorer and dried with compressed air. The diagnosis was made with a small hand light of high intensity. Incident and transmitted light was used. Caries was estimated in 4 different grades. Caries I signifies a minute black line at the bottom of the fissure. In caries II, there is also a white zone along the margins of the fissure. Caries III denotes the smallest perceptible break in the continuity of the enamel (cavity) with or without undermined margins. Caries IV is a large cavity more than 3 mm wide.

2B.2 Marthaler, 1966

The basic rule in this criteria is "First look! Probe only when doubtful".

Grade 1: Slightly brown narrow line or (on smooth surfaces Class V) white spot with hard surface, smallest extent not exceeding 2 mm

Grade 2: Clearly brown or black line or (on Class V lesions) white spot, smallest extent exceeding 2 mm.

For Class III lesions (proximal of anterior teeth), the lesion has a dark brown discolored surface.

Grade 3: Cavity, discontinuity of the enamel surface.

Grade 4: Cavity with the narrowest extent of the entrance broader than 2 mm.

2B.3 Radike in 1968

(I) **Frank lesions**—The detection of these lesions on the basis of gross cavitation usually does not present a problem in diagnosis. When cavitation is present, the diagnosis is positive.

(A) Cavitation in this context can be defined as a discontinuity of the enamel surface caused by loss of tooth surfaces.

(B) Cavitation which is the result of the caries process must be distinguished from fractures and smooth lesions or erosion and abrasion.

(II) **Lesions not showing cavitation**—The most difficult part of the examiner's task is the detection of lesions without frank cavitation. These are lesions close to the decision point between carious and sound. The criteria for detection of these lesions are summarized in three categories, each presenting its special problems.

(A) Detection of pit and fissure lesions of the occlusal, facial, and lingual surfaces.

(1) Area is carious when the explorer "catches" or resists removal after insertion into a pit or fissure with moderate to firm pressure and when accompanied by one or more of the following signs of caries:

  (a) A softness at the base of the area.

  (b) Opacity adjacent to the pit or fissure as evidence of undermining or demineralization

  (c) Softened enamel adjacent to the pit or fissure which may be scraped away with the explorer.

(2) Area is carious if there is loss of the normal translucency of the enamel, adjacent to a pit, which is in contrast to the surrounding tooth structure. This condition is considered to be reliable evidence of undermining. In some of these cases, the explorer may not catch or penetrate the pit.

(B) Detection of lesions on smooth area[s] of facial and lingual surfaces

(1) Area is carious if surface is etched or if there is a white spot as evidence of subsurface demineralization, and if the area is found to be soft by:

  (a) Penetration with explorer

  (b) Enamel can be scraped away with explorer

(2) Area is sound when there is apparent evidence of demineralization (etching or white spots) but no evidence of softness.

(C) Detection of lesions on proximal surfaces: It was not possible to attain agreement on a single set of criteria, since procedures used for diagnosis of proximal surfaces varied considerably. Some examiners depended largely upon visual-tactile methods, some depended largely upon radiographs and transillumination, while others used a combination of these procedures. The following is intended to be a composite of the best elements from all procedures:

(1) For area exposed to direct visual and tactile examination, these are diagnosed as under "B" above for smooth areas.

(2) For hidden areas not exposed to direct visual-tactile examinations:

(a) **Visual examination:** If the marginal ridge shows an opacity as evidence of undermined enamel, the proximal surface is carious.

(b) **Tactile examination:** Any discontinuity of the enamel in which an explorer will enter is carious if it also shows other evidence of decay, such as softness, shadow by transillumination, or loss of translucency.

(c) **Radiography:** Any definite radiolucency indicating a break in the continuity of the enamel surface is carious.

(d) **Transillumination:** Use mostly for anterior teeth: A loss of translucency producing a characteristic shadow in a calculus-free and stain-free proximal surface is adequate evidence of caries.

2B.4 Clinical and Radiographic Criteria for Dental Caries were Reported by Murray JJ and Shaw L in 1975

Clinical and Radiographic criteria for dental caries are discussed in Table 2.27.

Bibliography

1. Murray JJ and Shaw L. Errors in diagnosis of approximal caries on bite wing radiographs. Community Dent Oral Epidemiol 1975;2:276–82.

2B.5 NIDCR 1987

Coronal Caries

Frank lesions are detected as gross cavitation. Incipient lesions may be subdivided into three categories according to location, each with special diagnostic considerations. These categories are:

(A) Pits and fissures on occlusal, buccal, and lingual surfaces. These areas are diagnosed as carious when the explorer catches after insertion with moderate to firm pressure and when the catch is accompanied by one or more of the following signs of decay:

(1) Softness at the base of the area

(2) Opacity adjacent to the area, providing evidence of undermining or demineralization

(3) Softened enamel adjacent to the area which may be scraped away with the explorer (Care should be taken to avoid removal of enamel that could be remineralized)

(B) Smooth areas on buccal (labial) or lingual surfaces. These areas are carious if they are decalcified or if there is a white spot as evidence of subsurface demineralization and if the area is found to be soft by:

(1) Penetration with the explorer, or

(2) Scraping away the enamel with the explorer. These areas should be diagnosed as sound when there is only visual evidence of demineralization, but no evidence of softness.

(C) Proximal surfaces: For areas exposed to direct visual and tactile examination, as when there is no adjacent tooth, the criteria are the same as those for smooth areas on facial or lingual surfaces. For areas not available to direct visual-tactile examination, the following criterion applies: A discontinuity of the enamel in which the explorer will catch is carious if there is softness. Visual evidence of undermining under a marginal ridge is not acceptable evidence of a proximal

	Table 2.27: Murray JJ and Shaw L		
Score	Clinical criteria	Score	Radiographic criteria
C1	A pit, fissure or smooth surface in which there is discoloration in both incident and transmitted light, with minute discontinuity in the enamel surface which does not allow definite 'sticking' of the probe on gentle pressure	R1	A radiolucent area reaching the inner half of the enamel, but not extending beyond the amelodentinal junction
C2	A cavity in a pit, fissure or a smooth surface in which a probe sticks with gentle pressure and requires a definite pull for its removal	R2	A radiolucent area in enamel and dentin but not involving the pulp
C3	A large open cavity, probably with pulpal involvement. (If there was any doubt as to whether a lesion should be scored Cl, C2 or C3, in all cases the lower score was assigned)	R3	A gross carious lesion with definite pulpal involvement. (If there was any doubt as to whether a lesion should be scored R1, R2 or R3, in all cases the lower score was assigned)
		5	Filled
		6	Missing, unerupted, extracted, or congenitally absent
		7*	Overlap, unreadable
		8	Presumed present but not on radiograph, unreadable
		9*	Not completely readable, but presumed sound. Less than half the width of the enamel overlapped

* The differentiation of overlapped surfaces into those with under half the width of enamel overlapped (Category 9) and those over half this area (Category 7) was to achieve compatibility with the radiographic caries score of RI. Any surface with under half the enamel overlapped could be presumed sound and this enabled many more surfaces to be included in the final analysis.

lesion unless a surface break can be entered with the explorer.

Root caries: Active caries lesions in root surfaces are yellow/orange, tan, or light brown. Lesions in remission tend to be darker, sometimes almost black. When root caries is covered by small amounts of plaque, the discoloration of the lesions usually shows through. The tactile criterion of softness to an explorer tip must be met for a definite diagnosis of root caries.

2B.6 Ekstrand et al. 1998

0 = no or slight change in enamel translucency after prolonged air drying

1 = opacity (white) hardly visible on the wet surface, but distinctly visible after air drying

1a = opacity (brown) hardly visible on the wet surface, but distinctly visible after air drying

2 = opacity (white) distinctly visible without air drying

2a = opacity (brown) distinctly visible without air drying

3 = localized enamel breakdown in opaque or discolored enamel and/or grayish discoloration from the underlying dentin

4 = cavitation in opaque or discolored enamel, exposing the dentin beneath

2B.7 Nyvad et al. in 1998

(1) **Active caries (intact surface):** Surface of enamel is whitish/yellowish opaque with loss of luster; feels rough when the tip of the probe is moved gently across the surface; generally covered with plaque. No clinically detectable loss of substance.
Smooth surface: Caries lesion is typically located close to gingival margin.
Fissure/pit: Intact fissure morphology; lesion extending along the walls of the fissure.

(2) **Active caries (surface discontinuity):** Same criteria as score 1. Localized surface defect (microcavity) in enamel only. No undermined enamel or softened floor detectable with the explorer.

(3) **Active caries (cavity):** Enamel/dentin cavity easily visible with the naked eye; surface of cavity feels soft or leathery on gentle probing. There may or may not be pulpal involvement.

(4) **Inactive caries (intact surface):** Surface of enamel is whitish, brownish, or black. Enamel may be shiny and feels hard and smooth when the tip of the probe is moved gently across the surface. No clinically detectable loss of substance.
Smooth surface: Caries lesion typically located at some distance from gingival margin.
Fissure/pit: Intact fissure morphology; lesion extending along the walls of the fissure.

(5) **Inactive caries (surface discontinuity):** Same criteria as score 4. Localized surface defect (microcavity) in enamel only. No undermined enamel or softened floor detectable with explorer.

(6) **Inactive caries (cavity):** Enamel/dentin cavity easily visible with the naked eye; surface of cavity may be shiny and feels hard when probed with gentle pressure. No pulpal involvement.

2B.8 Fyffe et al. in 2000

White-spot lesion—Visual assessment of dried tooth indicates intact surface, no clinically detectable loss of substance, with a white or cream-colored area of increased opacity presumed carious by the trained examiner. Brown-spot lesion—Visual assessment of dried tooth indicates intact surface, no clinically detectable loss of substance, with a brown/black discoloration, presumed carious by the trained examiner.

Enamel cavity—In the opinion of the trained examiner, there is a lesion with demonstrable loss of surface but no visual, clinical evidence of the lesion penetrating dentin.

Dentin lesion (uncavitated)— Surfaces are regarded as falling into this category if, in the opinion of the trained examiner, there is a caries lesion into dentin but no visible evidence of cavitation.

Dentin cavity—Surfaces are regarded as falling into this category if, in the opinion of the trained examiner, there is a carious cavity into dentin.

Pulp involved—Surfaces are regarding as falling into this category if, in the opinion of the trained examiner, there is a carious cavity that involves the pulp, necessitating an extraction or pulp treatment.

Arrested dentinal decay— Surfaces are regarding as falling into this category if, in the opinion of the trained examiner, there is arrested caries in dentin.

Bibliography

Ismail AI. Visual and Visuo-tactile detection of dental caries. J Dent Res.2004; 83(Spec Iss C):C56-C66.

3

Indices to Assess Periodontitis

Periodontitis is a chronic inflammatory disease caused by infection of the supporting tissues around the teeth. Generally, the clinical diagnosis of periodontitis is based on measures of the presence and extent of periodontal pockets, loss of clinical attachment, the pattern and extent of alveolar bone loss, or a combination of these measures. The broader term "periodontal diseases" includes other conditions, such as gingivitis, a reversible condition that is diagnosed by the presence and extent of gingival inflammation, frequently measured as bleeding on probing (BOP). However, the following discussion will focus mainly on the indices accounting for periodontal pockets, loss of clinical attachment, the pattern and extent of alveolar bone loss, recession or a combination of these measures.

3A Indices for Measuring Pocket Depth and Loss of Attachment

3A.1 Periodontal Index (PI)

This was developed by Russell AL over a period of ten years in 1956. It is essentially an epidemiological tool. Hence this method is inappropriate in diagnosis for the individual dental patient, but is useful and valid in the field.

The rationale for this method was based on the data published by Sandler and Stahl (1954) who compared the gingival recession scores with the individual scores for bone loss, using X-rays. They concluded that for the individual patients, estimates of recession were unreliable in diagnosis of bone loss. However, it was seen that the average degree of bone loss for a given degree of recession is quite constant.

PI estimates periodontal disease by presence/absence of gingival inflammation, pocket formation and masticatory function. PI is probably the most widely used index. It is a composite index, as it records both reversible and irreversible changes.

Method

All the teeth present are examined. All gingival tissue circumscribing each tooth is examined. Russell's scoring is in order related to stages of the disease: inflammation, pocket formation and loss of function (Table 3.1). Required field equipment has been reduced to a minimum. Mouth mirror and explorer are supplemented occasionally by a straight Jacquette scaler or the chip blower for demonstration of a periodontal pocket. Adequate light is essential, preferably from a source corrected to the approximate color of sunlight.

Table 3.1: Scoring criteria for PI		
Criteria for field studies	*Additional X-ray criteria*	*Score*
Negative (neither overt inflammation in the investing tissues nor loss of function due to destruction of supporting tissues)	Radiographic appearance normal	0
Mild gingivitis (overt area of inflammation in the free gingivae but this area does not circumscribe the tooth)		1
Gingivitis (inflammation completely circumscribes the tooth but there is no apparent break in the epithelial attachment)		2
(not used in field study)	Early notch like resorption of the alveolar crest	4
Gingivitis with pocket formation (the epithelial attachment is broken and there is a pocket. There is no interference with normal masticatory function the tooth is firm in its socket and has not drifted.	Horizontal bone loss involving the entire alveolar crest up to half of the length of the tooth root (distance from apex to cemento-enamel junction)	6
Advanced destruction with loss of masticatory function (tooth may be loose; tooth may have drifted; tooth may sound dull on percussion with a metallic instrument; the tooth may be depressible in its socket)	Advanced bone loss involving more than half of the length of the tooth root or a definite intrabony pocket with definite widening of the periodontal membranes. There may be root resorption or rarefaction at the apex	8

Calculation

The PI score per individual is obtained by adding all the individual scores and dividing by the number of teeth present or examined.

PI score = Sum of individual scores/No. of teeth present

These numbers would be meaningless unless they had some systematic relationship to clinical conditions or prognosis on treatment. Given below is relationship between clinical diagnoses made for treatment planning in clinical center, dental clinic National Institute of Health.

Clinically normal supportive tissue	0–0.2
Simple gingivitis	0.3–0.9
Beginning of destructive PD	0.7–1.9
Established destructive PD	1.6–5.0
Terminal disease	3.8–8.0

This has been modified to prevent overlapping

Advantages

1. Simple to use
2. Precise and method has proved to provide adequate data of periodontal disease.

Disadvantages

1. It tends to under estimate the true level of disease.
2. Number of periodontal pockets without supragingival calculus is under estimated.
3. Variations due to subjective method
4. Scoring criteria are not continuous
5. Overlapping of scores.
6. Radiographs are necessary to estimate bone loss
7. No treatment need assessment

The PI was used extensively in epidemiologic surveys of numerous populations, including the first two national surveys in the United States. The PI was flawed, conceptually and methodologically, in that gingivitis is no longer considered to be the equivalent of early periodontitis, and the index did not measure features specific for periodontitis (in contrast to gingivitis), such as PD, CAL, and radiographic bone loss. Consequently, the index is no longer considered valid.

Bibliography

1. Russell AL. A System of Classification and Scoring for Prevalence Surveys of Periodontal disease. J Dent Res. 1956;35:350.

3A.2 Periodontal Disease Index (PDI)

The PDI is a clinical modification of Russell's PI index for epidemiological surveys of periodontal disease. The PDI is concerned with an accurate assessment of the periodontal status of the individual person. Emphasis is placed on recording of the attachment level of periodontal tissue relative to CEJ.

The components of periodontal index:
1. Gingival and periodontal component
2. Plaque component
3. Calculus component

Gingival and periodontal component: The scoring criteria were defined in Table 3.2. Maximum accuracy depends on standardized optimal and standardized thickness of measuring probe. Only six selected teeth are scored for assessment of the periodontal status of the mouth: however, for short term clinical trials and where a limited number of patients are available, all the teeth in the mouth can be included.

Index teeth: 16, 21, 24, 36, 41 and 44

It has been shown by Jamison and others that these 6 teeth provide basis for a surprisingly accurate assessment of the total periodontal status of the individual as expressed in scoring of all the teeth. The gingiva is scored as follows. It is basically a combination of PMA and PI.

Since all these criteria are subjective, proper examination is essential. The gingiva around the teeth is first dried superficially by gently touching with absorbing cotton to assess changes in color, form, consistency or density. The score of 3 is based on evidence of ulceration of the gingiva with bleeding, if the gingiva is touched gently with the side of a periodontal probe, or if there is severe redness and marked change in contour. The score of 3 is given even if these changes do not extend all around the tooth. The next step in scoring is recording of crevicular depth related to CEJ. The University of Michigan # 0 probe (Premises Mfg. Co., Philadelphia) is used.

The probe should be held with a light grasp similar to the manner of holding a pencil and balanced well in the hand so it can be moved and directed by very small forces. The end of the probe should be placed against the enamel surface coronally to the margin of the gingiva so that the angle formed by the working end of the probe and the long axis of the crown of the tooth is approximately 45°. A minimal force should be used to pass the probe in apical direction maintaining contact with the tooth. The angle between the probe and the tooth

Table 3.2: PDI		
Score		*Criteria*
Gingival status	0	Absence of signs of inflammation
	1	Mild to moderate inflammatory gingival changes, not extending around the tooth.
	2	Mild to moderately severe gingivitis extending all around the tooth.
	3	Severe gingivitis characterized by marked redness, swelling tendency to bleed and ulceration.
Periodontal status	4	Gingival crevice extending apical to CEJ not more than 3 mm.
	5	Gingival crevice apical to CEJ 3–6 mm.
	6	Gingival crevice more than 6 mm from CEJ.

may have to be decreased slightly when the probe touches the gingiva to avoid pressure on the gingiva when the probe is inserted in the gingival crevice. Since the surfaces of the enamel and the cementum have different inclines, the change in direction of the movement of the point of the probe is detectable when it moves from the enamel to the cementum. The texture or surface characteristics are also different since the cementum is distinctly rougher than enamel. A very important point is to use a light grip on the probe otherwise the keen sense of touch in the fingertips becomes impaired. The probe should always be pointed towards the apex of the tooth or the central axis of multi-rooted teeth. After the distance from the free gingival margin to the cementum enamel junction has been measured, an attempt should be made to move the probe along the cemental surface. This of course can be achieved only if there has been loss of periodontal attachment. If calculus covers the cementum enamel junction it has to be removed before the CE junction can be localized. Occasionally it is also necessary to remove heavy deposits of supragingival calculus to gain access to the gingival crevice. The University of Michigan #0 probe is graduated at 3, 6 and 8 mm from the end, making it necessary to estimate intervening measurements. This is because reproducibility is better and eye strain is less than having marks every mm. All measurements are rounded to nearest mm except that anything close to ½ a mm is always rounded to the lower whole number.

Crevicular Measurements

The distance from the free gingival margin to the cementum enamel junction and the distance from the free gingival margin to the bottom of the gingival crevice or pocket is measured for the buccal and mesial aspect of each tooth examined. The buccal measurements should be made at the middle of the buccal surfaces. The mesial measuring should be made at the buccal aspect of the interproximal contact area with the probe touching both teeth if there is a neighbor tooth present and the probe pointing in the direction of the long axis of the tooth to be scored.

Modification for the weighting system was given by Sheiham A and Striffler DF in 1970 in Table 3.3.

Table 3.3: Weighting system used for the modified PDI and the PDI

Modified PDI	PDI (original)
0–3 mm = 5	0–3 mm = 4
3–6 mm = 6	3–6 mm = 5
over 6 mm = 7	over 6 mm = 6

Calculation

The PDI score for the individual is obtained by totaling all the scores and dividing by number of teeth examined. Whether or not the periodontal support has been lost because of Periodontitis or atrophy is not considered in the PDI index.

It ranges from 0 to 6. If some of the teeth which were scheduled to be examined were missing or unerupted so they could not be examined, then individual scores for each of the examined teeth should be added and divided by the number of teeth examined and there should be no substitution for absent teeth.

Advantages

1. It provides an average value for gingivitis of entire mouth.
2. It provides data needed for assessment of prevalence of both gingivitis and periodontitis, besides measuring its severity.
3. It provides data to assess total need of periodontal treatment for individual and population.
4. It establishes an accurate record of level of periodontal support at the time of indexing.
5. It is useful for clinical research concerning pathogenesis of periodontal disease and irritation as it provides data regarding pocket formation and loss of attachment.

Disadvantages

The index does not differentiate loss of periodontal support by periodontitis or by atrophy.

Calculus examination: Subgingival calculus apparently is much more important in the pathogenesis of periodontitis than supragingival calculus and consequently it has been given a higher score than supragingival calculus (Table 3.4). Subgingival calculus is located with a #17 probe if there is uncertainty when probing with the University of Michigan # 0 probe.

Plaque examination: Scoring of plaque is done after staining with Bismarck brown solution based on the scoring criteria described in Table 3.4.

The scoring of the calculus and plaque does not constitute a part of the PDI index, but since an extremely high correlation has been established between periodontal disease and the presence of plaque and calculus it is usually included in total assessment of periodontal status.

Calculation

Plaque or calculus score: Total plaque or calculus score/number of teeth examined.

Bibliography

1. Ramfjord SP. Indices for prevalence and incidence of periodontal disease. J Periodontol 1959;30: 51–9.
2. Ramfjord SP. The periodontal disease index. J Periodontol 1967;38(6):602–10.
3. Sheiham A, Striffler DF. A comparison of four epidemiological methods of assessing periodontal disease. 1. Population findings. J Periodontal Res 1970;5:148–154.

3A.3 Periodontal Disease Rate Index

This was proposed by Sandler and Stahl in 1959. PDR is a simple index where the number of diseased teeth are counted and then divided by the total number of teeth present in the mouth. It is expressed as a percentage. The criteria used to indicate whether tooth is affected by periodontal disease or not were:

- Gingival necrosis, hypertrophy or inflammation encircling the teeth or a purulent exudate from the gingival crevice.
- A gingival crevice depth of 3 mm or more
- Tooth mobility greater than 1 mm in any direction
- Radiographic evidence of resorption of alveolar bone extending more than 3 mm apically from the CEJ.

Bibliography

1. Sandler HC and Stahl SS. The measurement of periodontal disease prevalence. JADA 1959;58: 93–97.

3A.4 Gingival Periodontal Index (GPI)

It was developed by O' Leary TV, Gibson WA, Shannon IL Schuessler CF and Nabers CL in

	Table 3.4: Calculus and plaque component of PDI	
	Criteria	*Score*
Calculus	None	0
	Supragingival calculus extending only slightly below the free gingival margin (not more than 1 mm)	1
	Moderate amount of supra and subgingival calculus or subgingival calculus alone	2
	An abundance of supra and subgingival calculus	3
Plaque	None	0
	Present on some but not on all interproximal buccal and lingual surfaces of tooth	1
	Plaque present on all of the interproximal buccal and lingual surfaces but covering less than half of these surfaces	2
	Plaques extends over all interproximal buccal and lingual surfaces and covering more than one half of these surfaces	3

1963 as part of Periodontal Screening Examination for the needs of military dental service.

This index evaluates gingival health and status of supporting alveolar bone. The periodontal screening examination also consists of Irritant Index (II). Since time required for probing all surfaces is impractical, probing of only the mesial surface of each tooth was done [as it resulted in 94% correct diagnosis].

To permit the clinician to localize the areas requiring treatment, the mouth is divided into six segments.

The highest score found for any one tooth in a segment is recorded as score for the segment. The highest gingival and/or periodontal score is used to compute the GPI. The highest score for plaque and other local factors is used to calculate the irritant score of the segment.

Gingival and Periodontal Status

Each segment is dried with compressed air and evaluated for gingival status based on scoring criteria described in Table 3.5. Periodontal status is assessed by probing the mesiofacial line angle using a Merritt type probe. Probing is similar to PDI.

Rules in Scoring

- The distance from the gingival margin to the CE junction is noted. Then the probe is advanced to the depth of the pocket and the depth from the gingival margin is noted. Subtracting the first reading (from the gingival margin to CEJ) from the reading taken at the depth of the pocket gives the amount of loss of periodontal attachment.
- The recording is at the mesial-facial or buccal line angle with the probe directed to long axis of the tooth.
- Orientation of the CEJ is necessary. In the posterior segments, the CEJ is approximately same level on mesial surfaces as it is on facial or lingual surface. In the anterior segments, the CEJ on the proximal surface curves incisally as much as 2.5 mm. At mesial-facial line angle of anterior teeth the

Table 3.5: Criteria for GPI

	Score	Criteria
Gingival status	0	Gingiva tightly adapted to teeth, firm consistency with a physiologic architecture
	1	Slight to moderate inflammatory changes are present. One or combination of the following involving one or more teeth in the segment but not completely surrounding the teeth. Change in color, loss of normal consistency as evidenced by retraction of the gingival margin from the tooth surface when the tissue is dried with firm blast of compressed air, blunting and enlargement of marginal or papillary gingiva
	2	Above changes, singly or in combination, are found completely encircling one or more teeth in the segment
	3	Marked inflammation or gingival contour changes which include: acute gingival inflammation, as loss of surface continuity [ulceration], spontaneous hemorrhage, loss of faciolingual continuity or interdental papilla, marked deviation from normal contour (gross thickening of the marginal tissue enlargement or gingival tissue covering more than 1/3rd of the anatomic crown; loss of continuity of inter-dental papilla; clefts).
Periodontal status	0	Probe does not extend 1 mm apical to CEJ and there is no exposure of CEJ on any surface of any teeth
	4	Probe extends up to 3 mm apical to CEJ of any tooth in a segment
	5	Probe extends from 3 – 6 mm, apical to CEJ any tooth a segment
	6	Probe extends more than 6 mm of any tooth in a segment

CEJ is approximately 1 mm more incisal than it is on the facial surface.

- To ensure uniformity in scoring, the probe tip is directed along the crown towards the CEJ at a 45° angle until the junction is located. Then if pocketing is present, the angle of the probe is decreased so that the probe may reach the depth of the pocket.
- When CEJ is exposed on any surface on any tooth in a segment by recession, the appropriate periodontal score (4, 5 or 6) is determined by measuring from the exposed CEJ to the depth of gingival crevice.

The highest score [gingival or periodontal] found for each dentulous segment is recorded and the sum divided by number of segments gives GPI score for individual.

Bibliography

1. O'Leary TJ. The periodontal screening examination. J Periodontol 1967 38: 617–624.

3A.5 Gingival-Bone Count Index

It was developed by Dunning JM and Leach LB in 1960.

It records gingival condition and level of crest of alveolar bone. Subjective measurement of gingivitis is made on a 0–3 scale for each tooth, and proportional measurement of bone loss is made on a 0–5 scale. Bone level is assessed by clinical examination but radiographs are recommended for greater accuracy.

The gingival score (Gc) was ascertained clinically by mirror and no. 17 explorer and clinical bone score (Bc) was obtained by probing with an explorer to determine the amount of bone loss surrounding each tooth. Whole mouth mean scores are then added together to obtain a GB count. This count weights gingivitis and bone loss on a 3–5 basis: an arbitrary relationship, realistic only to the extent that bone loss makes a greater threat to the usefulness of the tooth than gingivitis. As the whole mouth means for gingiva and bone are separately recorded, the conditions making up the GB count can always be known. No attempt is made to evaluate the missing teeth in the mouth. The scoring system used is applicable whether explorer examination, bite-wing X-ray examination, full X-ray survey, or a combination of these methods is used.

Scoring criteria for gingivitis and bone loss are scored as per criteria are given in Table 3.6.

Gingival score: One score is assigned to each tooth studied. A mean is then computed for the whole mouth.

Table 3.6: Gingival-bone count index

	Score	Criteria
Gingival score	0	Negative
	1	Mild gingivitis involving free gingiva (margin, papilla or both).
	2	Moderate gingivitis involving free and attached gingiva
	3	Severe gingivitis with hypertrophy and easy hemorrhage.
Bone loss score	0	No bone loss
	1	Incipient bone loss
	2	Bone loss approximating ¼ of roots length or pocket formations one side not over ½ root length.
	3	Bone loss approximately ½ of root length or pocket formation one side not over ¾ root length. Mobility – slight*
	4	Bone loss approximately ¾ of root length or pocket formation one side to apex. Mobility – moderate*
	5	Bone loss completed. Mobility – marked*

* If mobility or impairment of masticatory function varies considerably from that to be expected with bone loss seen, the score may be altered up or down one point.
Maximum possible GB count per person is 8.

Bone loss: One score is assigned to each tooth studied. A mean is then computed for the whole mouth.

The Gc and Bc score are added to get GB score of person.

Bibliography

1. Dunning JM, Leach LB. Gingival bone count: a method for epidemiological study of periodontal disease. J Dent Res 1960 39:506–13.

3A.6 Community Periodontal Index of Treatment Needs (CPITN)

The PI and simplified OHI were the two preferred methods for data collection after the initiation of WHO global oral health data bank. It became clear that these were not satisfactory to estimate the magnitude and severity of periodontal condition. Hence a WHO scientific group meeting was convened in Moscow in 1977 to seek and consider a more realistic system of PD measurement. The Moscow Stomatological Institute was the venue and it produced a prototype index— "TRS 621 method" and conducted with a recommendation to consider the above.

A joint working group [4 members of FDI and four of WHO] was established is as recommended in WHO tested the CPITN prototype, series [TRS 621, 1978] for its appropriateness and acceptance. After field trials, the CPITN was agreed at meeting of joint FDI, WHO working group 1 in Rio de Janeiro in September 1981.

This index is primarily designed to assess the periodontal treatment needs rather than periodontal status. Primarily it is a screening procedure for identifying actual and potential problems posed by periodontal disease both in the community and by the individual with this information appropriate oral care services can be planned for population and for individual.

Procedure

The dentition is divided into six parts [sextants]: each sextant is given a score. For epidemiologic purpose, only specific index teeth are scored while for clinical practice, the highest score in each sextant is recorded after examining all teeth.

The mouth is divided into six sextants as: 17–14; 13–23; 24–27; 47–44; 43–33; 34–37. The third molars are not included except when they are functioning in place of second molar. The treatment need is recorded only when 2 or more teeth are present in a sextant and not indicated) for extraction. When only one tooth is present in a sextant, it is included in adjoining sextant.

Use of Index Teeth

For epidemiological survey for adults aged 20 years and above, index teeth are 17/16, 11, 26/27, 47/46, 31, 36/37.

These ten teeth have been identified as the best estimators of the worst periodontal condition of the mouth. Though molars are examined in pairs, only one score, highest is recorded. For young people up to 19 years, only six index teeth are considered. The second molar are excluded because of high frequency of false (non-inflammatory associated with tooth eruptions) pockets. The six index teeth are 16, 11, 26, 46, 31, 36.

In children less than 15 years, pockets are not recorded although probing for bleeding and calculus are carried out. For screening and monitoring in dental practice all teeth in a sextant are examined for adults over age 19 years. Only one score which is highest is recorded for each sextant.

The CPITN Probe

The recommended probe for use with CPITN was first established in WHO 621 report (1978) and later reported in detail by Emslie (1980) which was designed by Jukka Ainamo. The probe has the following specifications.

1. It should be of metal with knurled handle of diameter 3.5 mm and a maximum weight of 4.5 grams.

2. It should have at the working tip a sphere of 0.5 mm diameter; the probe has a minimum diameter of 0.25 mm at the neck where sphere is attached.
3. It should have a black band between 3.5 and 5.5 mm from the end of the probe.

This probe is designed for gentle manipulation of very sensitive soft tissues around the teeth; as such it is different from probes for dental caries and most other oral care instruments. The ball tip of the probe allows easy detection of sub-gingival calculus. This feature combined with light weight facilitates identification of base of pocket correctly and decreases tendency for false over measurements. This new type of tactile probing or sensing instrument should be considered to be an extension of examiners fingers. A variant of this probe has two additional lines at 8.5 mm and 11.5 mm from the working tip which is used for recording of deep pockets.

Validity of CPITN Probe

Wilson et al conducted a study to determine the validity of the WHO periodontal probe in assessing pocket depths defined by CPITN. It was concluded that WHO probe is less accurate is assessing pockets of 3.5–5.5 mm. It was also suggested to incorporate a measure of gingival recession in epidemiological studies involving CPITN.

Probing Procedure

The sensing force is used both to determine pocket depth and to detect sub-gingival calculus. It should correspond to 20 g or less. The probe is inserted between the tooth and gingiva and the sulcus depth or pocket depth sensed and read against the color code or measuring lines. The direction of the probe during insertion should, whenever possible, be in the same plane as the long axis of the tooth. The ball end should be in contact with root surface. Pain to the patient during probing is an indication of a too heavy sensing force.

For practical purposes the following training methods are suggested: practice on gingival sulcus of your own front teeth, or use the fingernail test by identifying a pressure which allows gentle insertion of the probe under a fingernail without causing pain or discomfort or use a pressure sensitive device of similar dimensions. To enhance both the fine control of the movement of the probe and accuracy of the sensing of small movements of the tip of the probe in the gingival sulcus a light not a firm grip of the instrument is recommended.

The scoring of the teeth is based on the criteria described in Table 3.7 and Fig. 3.1.

Table 3.7: CPITN	
Code	Criteria
X	When only one or no tooth is present in a sextant. Third molars are excluded unless they function in place of second molars
4	Pathological pocket of 6 mm or more i.e., black band of the CPITN probe is not visible [if designated tooth or teeth are found to have a 6 mm or deeper pocket in the sextant being examined, a code of is given to the sextant. Recording of code 4 makes further examination of that sextant unnecessary]
3	Pathological pocket of 4 – 5 mm present, i.e. gingival margin is on black band of the probe [once code 3 is recorded there is no need to examine for bleeding and calculus]
2	Calculus or other plaque retentive factors such as ill-fitting crowns or poorly adopted edges of restorations are seen or felt during probing [it is unnecessary to examine for gingival bleeding]
1	Bleeding observed during or after probing. Gingiva of the designated tooth or teeth should be inspected for bleeding before the subject is allowed to swallow or close his mouth. At times bleeding may become evident only 10–30 seconds after probing.
0	Healthy tissue

Examination procedure: The aim is to determine the highest score applicable to each sextant. First decide whether the sextant can be validly scored. The requirement is that more than one functional tooth is present. If no, then score X and move to next sextant. If yes, examine index teeth or all teeth only in the order for presence of 6 mm or deeper pockets, 4 or 5 mm pockets, calculus or tooth plaque retentive factor, bleeding. Determine appropriate highest score for each sextant. As soon as the highest scored criterion has been determined there is no need to examine for the presence of lower score criteria.

Recommended sites for probing are mesial, midline and distal on both facial and lingual/palatal surfaces. The probing may be done by withdrawing the probe between each probing or alternatively, with the probe tip remaining in the sulcus, the probe may be walked around the tooth. Sites in addition to the recommended ones should be probed if there is suspicion that a higher scoring condition is present.

Excluded teeth: Index and substitute teeth are excluded from CPITN seeing when the decision has been may to extract for any causes.

Classification of Treatment Needs (TN)

Population group or individuals are allocated to appropriate treatment need (TN) as given in Table 3.8.

Rules for substitutions for excluded and missing index teeth:

1. Two or more functioning teeth must be present in a sextant to quantify for scoring.
2. In posterior sextant, if one of the two index teeth is not present or excluded, recording is based on examination of remaining index tooth.
3. If both index teeth in post sextant are absent or excluded, all remaining teeth highest score recorded.
4. In anterior max sextant, if 11 is excluded, substitute 21. If 21 is also excluded, identify the worst score for remaining teeth. Similarly substitute if 31 is missing / excluded.
5. If subject is under 20 years, and if molar is not present, the nearest adjacent premolar is examined.
6. If all teeth in a sextant are missing or only one functional tooth remains, sextant is coded as missing.
7. A single tooth in a sextant is considered as a tooth in the adjacent sextant and subject to rules for that sextant. If the single tooth is an index tooth, the worst index tooth score is recorded.

Advantages

1. Scoring is simple
2. Minimal equipment required.
3. Scoring of 10 index teeth can be done in less than 10 min.
4. International uniformity, as few, simple basic rules.
5. Measurable and widely understandable periodontal goals can be set.

Table 3.8: TN criteria	
TN Code	
0	Code 0 (healthy) or X (missing) for all sextants indicates no need for treatment
1	A code of 1 or higher indicates a need for improving personal oral hygiene of that individual
2	a. A code of 2 or higher – Need for professional cleaning of teeth and removal of plaque retentive factors
	b. Shallow to moderate pocketing (4 or 5 mm-code 3)
3	A sextant scoring code 4 (6mm or deeper pockets) may or may not be successfully treated by deep scaling code 4 is therefore assigned as 'Complex Treatment' which can involve deep scaling, root planning and more complex surgical procedures.

6. It is widely accepted for use in surveys, clinical settings, health projects, etc.
7. It records common treatable conditions like periodontal pockets, gingival inflammation, dental calculus and other plaque retentive factors.

Disadvantages

1. Reproducibility/validity: Score 1 is difficult to reproduce.
2. Debate on partial and complete recording exists.
3. It does not record irreversible changes such as recession or other factors of periodontal health like tooth mobility. Hence it is not a diagnostic tool and cannot be used for planning of specific clinical treatment of individual patients.
4. No distinction is made between supra- and subgingival calculus despite the fact that the removal of subgingival calculus is both more difficult and more time-consuming than the removal of supragingival calculus.
5. No distinction is made between the presence of calculus with and without associated bleeding.

Uses

1. Measure TN for population groups, thus helping in public health planning.
2. Used in descriptive studies of periodontal disease.
3. Can be used to measure periodontal conditions over time.
4. Screening of individuals for manifestation of periodontal disease.
5. Generation of data for health promotion.
6. Used as tool in analytical epidemiology identify risk factors and their association.

Limitations

Baelum and Papapanou listed several of its short comings, i.e. the hierarchical principles underlying the use of the CPITN not being universally valid; the partial recording approach of the CPITN leading to gross underestimation of prevalence of deep pockets and giving distorted estimates of severity of periodontal destruction in a given population.

Tabulation of Results

- Percentage distribution of dentate subjects according to the highest score recorded
- Mean number of sextants affected per person scoring 0, 1, 2, 3, 4 or X on a cumulative basis [i.e. 1 or higher score, 2 or higher score, etc.] (WHO preferred cumulative tabulation).
- Mean number per dentate person with score 0, 1, 2, 3, 4 or X respectively

Takahashi Modification of CPITN

Sextants given a scoring code of 2 were subdivided into a code of 2 + when calculus was associated with gingival bleeding and a code of 2 – when calculus was present without any associated bleeding. The worst finding for each sextant was recorded.

Bibliography

1. Ainamo J, Barmes D, Beagrie G, Cutress T, Martin J, Sardo-Infirri J. Development of the World Health Organization (WHO) community periodontal index of treatment needs (CPITN). International Dental Journal 1982;32, 281–91.
2. Baelum V, Papapanou PN. CPITN and the epidemiology of periodontal disease. Community Dent Oral Epidemiol 1996;24(6):367–8.
3. Takahashi Y, Kamijyo H, Kawanishi S, Takaesu Y. Presence and absence of bleeding in association with calculus in segments given code 2 in the Community Periodontal Index of Treatment Needs (CPITN). Community Dent Oral Epidemiol 1988; 16; 109–11.

3A.7 Community Periodontal Index

A specially designed light weight CPI probe with a 0.5 mm ball tip is used, with a black band between 3.5 and 5.5 mm and ring at 8.5 and 11.5 mm from the ball tip is used. The mouth is divided into 6 sextants similar to CPITN. A sextant is examined only if there are two or more teeth present which are not indicated for extraction based on the scoring criteria specified in Table 3.9 and Fig. 3.1. Index teeth and probing are similar to CPITN.

Table 3.9: Scoring criteria for CPI	
Code	Criteria
0	Healthy
1	Bleeding observed, directly or by using a mouth mirror, after probing.
2	Calculus, detected during probing, but all black band of probe visible.
3	Pocket of 4–5 mm (gingival margin within the black band)
4	Pocket 6 mm or more (black band not visible)
X	Excluded sextant
9	Not recorded

Loss of Attachment (LOA)

Information on loss of attachment is recorded to obtain an estimate of lifetime accumulated destruction of periodontal attachment. It is recorded immediately after CPI score for that particular sextant based on the criteria presented in Table 3.10 and illustrated in Fig. 3.2. The highest CPI and loss of attachment score may not be necessarily found in same tooth. It is not recorded in children under 15 years.

Bibliography

1. World Health Organization. Oral health surveys— Basic methods. 4th edition, Geneva: World Health Organization; 1997.

Table 3.10: LOA scoring criteria	
Score	Criteria
0	Loss of attachment 0–3 mm (CEJ not visible and CPI score 0–3)
	If the CEJ is not visible and the CPI score is 4, or if the CEJ is visible
1	Loss of attachment is 4–5 mm (CEJ within the black band)
2	Loss of attachment is 6–8 mm (CEJ between the upper limit of the black band and the 8.5 mm)
3	Loss of attachment 9–12 mm (CEJ between the 8.5 mm and 11.5 mm rings)
4	Loss of attachment 12 mm or more (CEJ beyond 11.5 mm rings)
X	Excluded sextant (less than two teeth present)
9	Not recorded (CEJ neither visible nor detectable)

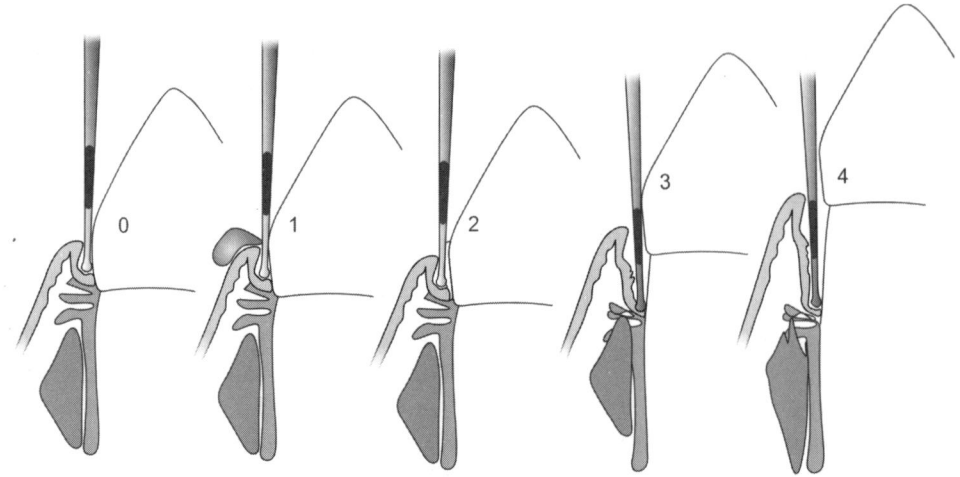

Fig. 3.1: Scoring criteria for CPI

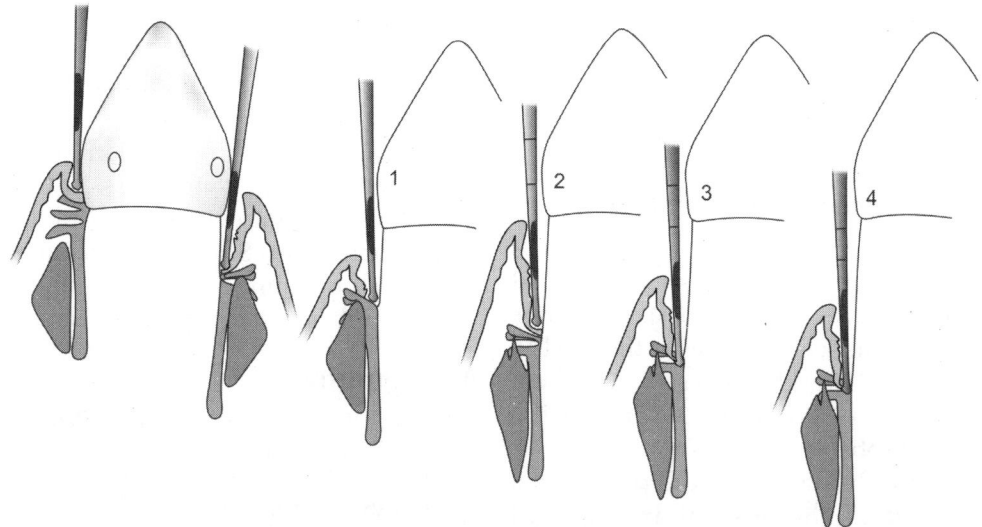

Fig. 3.2: Scoring criteria for LOA

3A.8 Dutch Periodontal Screening Index (DPSI)

It was introduced in 1998 by the Dutch Society of Periodontology as a component of periodontal diagnosis and treatment protocol. A procedure that functions as an initial evaluation to determine the level of additional periodontal examination and subsequently, the treatment needs of patients with differing disease levels. This index is also a modification of the CPITN and aims to screen for subjects with minor, moderate and severe periodontal disease. To achieve this, the original CPITN codes 0, 1, 2 remained unchanged, i.e. written as DPSI 0, 1, 2, respectively (Table 3.11).

The "Dutch perio-protocol" recognizes three categories of patients:

1. Patients that require only oral hygiene instruction and calculus removal (DPSI 1: bleeding pockets ≤ 3 mm; DPSI 2: supra- or subgingival calculus),
2. Patients that require a limited periodontal examination in order to be able to make a proper treatment plan (DPSI 3) and
3. Patients that require an extensive periodontal examination in order to be able to make a proper treatment plan (DPSI 4 and DPSI 5).

Table 3.11: Clinical criteria per score of the Dutch periodontal screening index (DPSI), to apply per sextant based on the site with the highest score

Score	Clinical criteria for the score per sextant
0	No pockets >3 mm in depth, no calculus, no overhanging restorations and no bleeding on probing to the bottom of the pocket
1	No pockets >3 mm in depth, no calculus, no overhangs of restorations, but presence of bleeding on probing to the bottom of the pocket
2	No pockets >3 mm in depth, presence of bleeding on probing to the bottom of the pocket, and presence of calculus or overhanging restorations
3	Presence of pathological pockets of 4–5 mm without gingival recession
4	Presence of pathological pockets of 4–5 mm with gingival recession
5	Presence of pathological pockets ≥ 6 mm

Bibliography

1. van der Velden U. The Dutch periodontal screening index validation and its application in The Netherlands. J Clin Periodontol 2009; 36: 1018–24.

3A.9 Basic Periodontal Examination

A basic periodontal examination (BPE) was recommended by the British Society of Periodontology (BSP) (1986, 2001). This index includes the same scoring codes as the CPITN, but the symbol * is added to a sextant if there is attachment loss at any site ≥ 7 mm or if a furcation is probable.

The asterisk denotes that a full periodontal examination of the sextant is required regardless of the BPE score.

Management of Sextants

- Sextants of the mouth for which code 0 are recorded do not require treatment;
- Sextants scoring code 1 can be treated by oral hygiene instruction and prophylaxis;
- Sextants scoring code 2 can be treated as for sextants scoring code 1 with the addition of supra and subgingival scaling at selected sites. Patients whose BPE scores for all sextants are codes 0, 1 or 2 should be screened again after an interval of 1 year.

When patients have sextants scoring Code 3 further data will have to be collected at completion of treatment. Plaque distribution and gingival inflammation are recorded and, in addition, probing depths are taken in the sextants scoring

- Treatment of sextants scoring Code 3 will be the same as those scoring Code 2 but a longer time will be required for completion.

Patients with BPE score 3 for one or more sextants should have pocket depth measurements taken in those sextants at not more than yearly intervals in addition to the BPE screening of the other sextants.

- Patients with sextants scoring Code 4 or * will require extensive periodontal assessment both at the outset and duration of treatment.

Following initial treatment, which will be as for sextants scoring Code 2, some resolution can be expected. Full probing depth charts will then be required for all sextants scoring Code 4 or *, together with evaluation of furcation involvements, root concavities and grooves, and other relevant details using radiographs when appropriate. Subsequent treatment may include root planing and periodontal surgery, whilst emphasis on plaque control is sustained.

Bibliography

1. British Society of Periodontology. Periodontology in general practice. A first policy statement. British Society of Periodontology 1986.
2. British Society of Periodontology. Periodontology in general practice in the United Kingdom. A policy statement. British Society of Periodontology. (2001)

3A.10 Periodontal Screening and Recording (PSR) Index

The American Dental Association (ADA) with the endorsement of the American Academy of Peridontology (AAP) introduced the periodontal screening and recording index as the system recommended for the early detection of periodontal disease in the US on October 6, 1993. PSR was derived from Basic Periodontal Examination [BPE] which was developed from simplified periodontal examination [SPE] which was developed in New Zealand [1984–87]. It was revised into BPE during 1989–90.

PSR Method

PSR was derived from the Basic Periodontal Examination (BPE) which was itself a development of the Simplified Periodontal Examination (SPE) which was developed and used in New Zealand 1984–1987. It was revised and updated to become the basic periodontal examination during 1989–1990. Periodontal screening and recording (PSR) was adopted in the United States by the American Dental Association (ADA) and the American Academy of Periodontology (AAP).

The PSR index divides the mouth into 6 segments (sextants) and the greatest probe depth in each sextant of the mouth is determined and recorded. Probing is accomplished by a plastic PSR probe that has a 0.5 mm diameter ball tip and a color-coded band extending 3.5 mm to 5.5 mm from the tip. The probe is gently inserted into the gingival sulcus until resistance is met and then explored by "walking" around the tooth or implant.

Recording sites: Six areas in each tooth or implant should be examined: mesiofacial, midfacial, distofacial, and the corresponding lingual/palatal areas.

Apart from one difference [asterisk code] PSR is identical to CPITN. In addition to CPITN scores, PSR index provides a detailed picture of periodontal status by recording the presence of furcation involvement, mucogingival problems and gingival recession exceeding 3.5 mm. When at least one of the above condition is present, an asterisk [*] is recorded with the PSR score of the sextant (Table 3.12).

Bibliography

1. Landry RG and Jean M. Periodontal Screening and Recording (PSR) Index : precursors, utility and limitations in a clinical setting. Int Dent J. 2002;52:35–40.

3A.11 Periodontal Index for Treatment (PIT)

The Periodontal Index for Treatment (PIT) was developed between 1981 and 1985 for use in the UK Armed Forces.

The major factors influencing the design of this index was

- Predominantly young population (mean age 25 years);
- The need for universal acceptability
- Limited time available for initial dental examination of recruits

Index teeth: All first molars and the maxillary right and mandibular left central incisors are assessed with a specially designed periodontal probe (the PIT probe) and the use of bitewing radiography. (PIT probe has markings at 4, 6, 8 and 11 mm and a 0.5 mm ball tip).

Technique: Maxillary sites are probed using a palatal approach, inserting the PIT probe into the gingival sulcus/pocket at the most disto-palatal point and walking the probe gently around the palatal aspect to the most mesio-palatal point, without removing it from the sulcus/pocket. Mandibular sites are probed in a similar manner, but with a buccal approach, from the most disto-buccal to the most mesio-

Code	Clinical signs	Treatment plan
0	Absent	Not required
1	Bleeding on probing	Oral hygiene instructions
2	Supra and/sub-Gingival calculus and/defective margins	Removal of calculus and correction of plaque retentive margins
3	Periodontal pocket 4–5.5 mm deep (colored band partially visible)	Removal of calculus, root planning, detailed periodontal examination of sextant or entire mouth if more than two sextants have code 3 score
4	Periodontal pocket 6 mm deep (colored band not visible)	Detailed periodontal examination of entire mouth, complex treatment
*	Periodontal abnormalities present	Detailed periodontal examination of affected sextant
X	Sextant absent or fewer than 2 teeth	

Table 3.12: PSR codes and treatment plan

The periodontal examinations recommended for codes 3, 4 and * should include radiographs preferably bite wings of the affected regions and detailed measurement of the following parameters

1. Actual probing depth 2. Gingival recession 3. Attachment levels
4. Mucogingival problems 5. Tooth mobility 6. Furcation involvement

buccal points based on the scoring criteria described in Table 3.13. Access to these sites is usually easy and the tongue does not interfere. A probing force of 0.25 N is recommended (as in the CPITN technique). Only six insertions of the probe are required at sites usually free from supragingival calculus deposits, thus increasing reliability.

The choice of maxillary palatal and mandibular buccal probing sites in the design of the PIT examination was intended to reduce the confusion which supragingival deposits may introduce into such probing sites, particularly around the maxillary molars buccally and lingual to the mandibular incisors. Unlike CPITN the level of deposits is not recorded in the PIT examination, which is intended to stress the presence of gingival inflammation, pockets and/or bone loss in its assessment of disease.

The radiographs are ideally viewed when the periodontal screening technique is carried out, enabling posterior teeth to be examined for interdental bone loss. If the clinician concerned considers bone loss to be evident radiographically at either "PIT" or "non-PIT" sites, then the patient may be re-categorized accordingly. The PIT technique when used in conjunction with bitewing radiography provides simple, rapid and reliable periodontal screening.

Bibliography

1. Eaton KA, 'Woodman A,T: Evaluation of simple periodontal screening technique currently used in the TJK armed forces. Community Dent Oral Epidemiol 1989; 17:190–5.

3A.12 Extent and Severity Index

This index was introduced by James P Carlos, Mary D Wolfe and Albert Kingman in 1986.

The ESI was developed because of lack of satisfaction with the previous indices and because of a newer conceptual model of periodontal disease by Socransky et al. In the ESI, the measurements are estimates of the level of attachment of the periodontal tissue, determined by subtracting the probing distance (mm) from the gingival crest to the cementoenamel junction (CEJ), from the distance measured from the gingival crest to the bottom of the sulcus. When the gingival crest is located apically to the CEJ, the first measurement is recorded as a negative value (Ramfjord 1974).

The ESI is a bivariate statistic which expresses the percentage of sites exhibit disease (E) and measures mean attachment Loss in Millimeters(S). Disease is defined arbitrarily as any site with more than 1 mm of attachment loss. Unlike the other indices this index describes the distribution of disease.

Method: The ESI uses a periodontal probe to determine attachment levels. It is based on probe measurements of Mesio-buccal and Mid-buccal locations at 14 sites in one maxillary quadrant and 14 sites in contralateral mandibular quadrant.

Bibliography

1. Carlos JP, Wolfe MD, Kingman A. The extent and severity index: a simple method for use in epidemiologic studies of periodontal disease. J Clin Periodontol 1986;13:500–5.

Table 3.13: PIT scoring criteria

Pit score	Clinical observation	Diagnostic implications
0	No pocketing of more than 4 mm or gingival bleeding	Health
1	No pocketing of more than 4 mm but gingival bleeding within 20 seconds or probing	Gingivitis
2	Pockets of 4–5 mm present [indicating a full pocket]	Possible early periodontitis
3	Pockets of 6 mm or more present [depth chart to be necessary]	Established periodontitis

The overall patient score ("PIT score") is recorded as the highest score of the six test teeth.

3A.13 Navy Periodontal Disease Index

It was introduced by Grossman F.D and Fedi P.F in 1974 as a part of their navy Periodontal screening examination.

It has two parts

1. A gingival score which assess the inflammation as determined by color, consistency, density, enlargement and bleeding.
2. A pocket score which measures tissue destruction as determined by pocket depth.

Method

The gingival and pocket score is done on six selected teeth (16, 21, 24, 36, 41 and 44). The gingival scores are determined by examining the gingival tissues and the pocket scores by probing sulcular or pocket depth based on the criteria in Table 3.14. The gingival examination is for color, consistency, contour and bleeding. Pocket is measured by periodontal probe on mesial, middle and distal areas of both facial and lingual surfaces. The greatest single measurement determines the pocket score for the tooth. If any of the selected posterior teeth is missing, substitute the next most posterior tooth and if the central incisor is missing substitute the nearest incisor of the same arch.

Calculation: The gingival and pocket scores of all teeth are added to obtain NPDI score for the individual.

Treatment recommendations were also laid down.

0–2 = Oral prophylaxis, plaque control instruction

5–7 = Complete oral examination, periodontal treatment, plaque control instruction.

8–10 = Complete oral examination, periodontal treatment initiated by general practitioner, with possible referral to periodontist.

Bibliography

1. Grossman FD, Fedi PF. Navy periodontal screening examination. J Am Soc Prev Dent 1974 3:41–45.
2. Hancock EB, Wirthlin MR. An evaluation of the Navy periodontal screening examination. J Periodontol 1977 48: 63–6.

3A.14 Periodontal Treatment Need System

It was proposed by Johansen JR, Gjermo P and Bellini HT in 1973. It can be used to determine the periodontal therapeutic needs in a population. It can be used to estimate the manpower and costs needed to address the problems found on examination.

The system is based on an evaluation of the need for 1) motivation and oral hygiene instruction (OH); 2) scaling and elimination of overhangs (Sc); 3) surgery (Su) and on the

Table 3.14: Navy periodontal disease index	
Score	*Criteria*
Gingival score	
0	Gingival tissue is of normal color, has firm consistency and no exudates is present
1	Inflammatory changes are present and do not completely encircle the tooth, changes may include, any color change, loss of normal consistency, slight enlargement, and blunting of papilla and tendency to bleed on palpation.
2	Inflammatory changes listed above encircling the tooth
Pocket score	
0	Probing reveals pocket depth not over 3 mm
5	Probing reveals pocket depth greater than 3 mm but less than 5 mm
8	Probing reveals pocket depth greater than 5 mm

time needed to perform the various types of treatment.

Classification

Class 0 – No treatment needed

Class A – Motivation and oral hygiene instructions

Class B – Scaling and removal of overhangs

Class C – Surgery

In class A, only one classification is needed for the whole mouth and can be given alone or together with the other classes.

For classes B and C, each quadrant in the mouth is scored separately. A quadrant is defined as a segment containing 4–8 teeth. Less than 8 teeth in one jaw is considered as one quadrant. Four teeth or less in the mouth are recorded as one quadrant.

Criteria for Classification (Table 3.15)

Class 0: Patients with no clinical signs of inflammation. The location of the gingival margin is disregarded.

Class A: All patients needing any kind of periodontal treatment are grouped here. In the presence of gingivitis and supragingival plaque only (no calculus nor overhangs), the patient is classified only in this class.

Class B: In this class each quadrant with one or more pathologic pockets.

5 mm deep or less, is included. The registration of one quadrant in this class implies that class A must be added.

Class C: In this class each quadrant with one or more pathologic pockets deeper than 5 mm is recorded. Any quadrant classified as C will also require class A and class B treatment.

Patient Assessment

Classes 0 and A are assigned based on assessment of the entire mouth.

Classes B and C are assigned based on oral quadrants.

Normally the mouth is divided into 4 quadrants (left maxillary, right maxillary, left mandibular, right mandibular).

- If less than 8 teeth are present on the maxilla or mandible, then this is taken as one quadrant.
- If 4 teeth or less are in the mouth as a whole, then the mouth is considered to have one quadrant.

Scoring: A periodontal probe and mouth mirror are used. Probing should start from the most distal tooth in the upper right. Each tooth is probed on all surfaces. If a pocket deeper than 5 mm is found, then the whole quadrant is scored as C. In case there is no such pockets, give score A in the presence of plaque and gingivitis and score B in the presence of calculus and/or overhangs. A pocket deeper than 5 mm mesially to the central incisors is not scored as C, if it is the only C pocket in that quadrant, and if the other quadrant on the same jaw has been scored as C. Only true pockets (pockets due to loss of attachment) on the distal surface of last molars give the score C for the quadrant. A pocket deeper than 5 mm mesially to the central incisors does not give score C when it represents the only C pocket in the quadrant, provided C is scored for the other quadrant in the jaw.

Time scoring: Time was measured from the moment the dentist started to wash his hands till the treatment procedure was ended.

Table 3.15: Criteria for PTNS classification

Plaque	Calculus and/or overhang	Inflammation	Pocket depth	Class
No	No	No	Not applicable	0
Yes	No	Yes	≤ 5 mm	A
Yes	Yes	Yes	≥ 5 mm	B
Yes	Yes	Yes	> 5 mm	C

Class	Treatment	Time to complete
	Table 3.16: Treatment plan	
0	No treatment needed	0
A	Oral hygiene instructions	60 minutes
B	Scaling and removal of calculus and overhangs	30 minutes per quadrant for scaling
C	Surgery	60 minutes per quadrant for surgery

Preparations of the equipment, of the instruments and the appointments, were made by the chair side assistant and the time was not considered as treatment time. The time for each procedure (OH, Sc and Su) was recorded in each session. For OH the time was recorded for each individual and for Sc and Su the time recording was for each quadrant (Table 3.16).

A patient with Class B disease also requires Class A management. A patient with Class C disease also requires Class A and Class B management. The maximum time estimates for a person with all teeth present and severe periodontal disease involving all quadrants would be 7 hours (1 hour for each quadrant for surgery, 30 minutes for each quadrant for cleaning, and 1 hour for training, or 4 + 2 + 1). Limitations: The time estimates seem overly generous except for the surgery on severely affected areas.

Bibliography

1. Johansen JR, Gjermo P, Bellini HT. A system to classify the need for periodontal treatment. Acta Odont Scand 1973;31:297–305.

3A.15 Periodontitis Severity Index (PSI)

It was developed by Adams RA and Nystorm GP in 1985. At any location, periodontitis is considered to be present when there is concurrent tooth-supporting tissue loss and clinically apparent inflammation. Loss of tooth supporting tissue is determined by measuring either the reduction in alveolar bone height or the extent of detachment of the periodontium from cementum. Typically, gingival inflammation is diagnosed when any of the following signs are detected in the marginal gingiva: edema, suppuration, bleeding upon provocation, increased crevicular fluid flow or color deviation. The absence of all clinical signs of inflammation renders a diagnosis of health (Table 3.17).

While gingival inflammation must be present for a diagnosis of periodontitis to be made at an area with supporting tissue loss, there is no evidence that the supposed degree of gingival inflammation has any bearing on the severity of the ongoing periodontitis. When the gingiva is not clinically inflamed, it is considered healthy. This holds true for the reduced periodontium. A reduced but clinically inflammation-free periodontium typically follows successful therapy.

Score	Criteria
	Table 3.17: Periodontitis severity index
0	Absence of inflammation in the marginal area of gingiva
1	Presence of inflammation in the marginal area of the gingiva

A full mouth series of periapical radiographs is taken for the patient using long cone technique. A modified Schei ruler is used to measure the radiographs. The rules are changed from that originally described in that it acknowledges the enamel junction in ideal health and is divided into tenths, permitting analysis of the percentage of bone loss in 10% increments (Table 3.18). At each mesial and distal tooth surfaces, a whole number, bone loss score is determined using the ruler.

Calculation: PSI = CIS*BLS
Interpretations

- No inflammation, CIS = 0 the PSI = 0, regardless of extent of bone loss, reflecting the reduced but healthy periodontium.

Table 3.18: Bone loss score	
Bone loss in percent	*Bone loss score*
0	0
1–10%	1
10–20%	2
20–30%	3
30–40%	4
40–50%	5
50–60%	6
60–70%	7
70–80%	8
80–90%	9
90–100%	10

- When the inflammation is detected, CIS = 1, the PSI is directly proportional to BLS
- No bone loss in the presence of inflammation (gingivitis) results in a PSI of '0'
- The PSI can range from '0'–'10', depending upon the amount of bone loss and health status of the patient.

Advantages

Healthy sites can be distinguished from diseased sites, ratio data can be produced, arbitrarily weighted clinical observations can be largely avoided, and direct measurements of periodontitis severity can be made.

Disadvantage

In order to recalculate the PSI over time, further radiographs are necessary and also, radiographs do not permit buccal or lingual PSI calculations. Due to these limitations the PSI is limited to longitudinal studies and lacks validation.

Bibliography

1. Adams RA, Nystrom GP. A periodontis severity index. J Periodontol 1986 57: 176–9.

3A.16 Gingivitis Periodontitis Missing Teeth Index

It was developed by Peter Gaengler in 1983 which represents full mouth periodontal recordings.

Method: Full mouth examination is done for gingival bleeding, periodontal pocketing, the presence of supragingival or subgingival calculus and for recession. A standardized Morita Probe is used and a six point checking is done on the buccal and lingual of each tooth with the exception of third molars based on the criteria specified in Table 3.19.

Scoring Criteria

Calculation: The periodontal status of an individual is expressed as the ratio of Gingivitis: Periodontitis: Missing teeth, i.e. is G: P: MT.

Table 3.19: Gingivitis periodontitis missing teeth index		
	Score	*Criteria*
Calculus	0	Absence of calculus
	1	Presence of supragingival calculus
	2	Presence of subgingival calculus
Bleeding	0	No bleeding
	1	Bleeding on probing
Pocketing	0	Pocket depth of less than 3.5 mm
	1	Pocket depth between 3.5 mm and 5.5 mm
	2	Pocket depth greater than 5.5 mm
Recession	0	Recession less than 3.5 mm
	1	Recession between 3.5 mm and 5.5 mm
	2	Recession greater than 5.5 mm

3A.17 Probing Depth and LOA/CAL

Probing Periodontal Depth is the distance from the gingival margin to the base of the pocket.

Probing Attachment level or clinical attachment level or loss of attachment is the distance from a fixed reproducible point and the pocket base. The ideal fixed reference point is the CEJ but alternatives are the occlusal surface or a fixed point on a stent precisely located on the teeth to be recorded.

PD and CAL are measured using a manual or controlled force probe with a precision of 1 mm. In epidemiologic studies, measurements of CAL and PD have been taken on all teeth, all teeth in two randomly selected quadrants (one maxillary and one mandibular), the single site with the most advanced disease in each sextant, and on selected index teeth; measurements have been made at six, four, two, and one location per tooth. PD and CAL measurements are considered to be accurate to within 1 mm 90% of the time when made by trained and experienced examiners.

The periodontal probe must be fine enough to enter a narrow periodontal pocket but must have a blunt end so that it reduces the likelihood of penetration of the tissues at the base of the pocket. The probe should be inserted into the pocket as near as possible to the long axis of the tooth. However, it is necessary to slightly angulate the probe to pass under the contact areas of molar and premolar tooth to reach the deepest point of interproximal pockets. The angulation may be compensated by a slight reduction of recorded depth usually 1 mm for a molar tooth. Care should be taken to manipulate the probe to reach the base of the pocket without penetrating the tissue.

The accuracy of probing depends on:

- Size of the probe
- Angulation of the probe
- Probing force used
- Inflammatory state of the tissues
- Contour of tooth and root surface

CAL is accepted as the gold standard for periodontitis and is considered to be a measure of past, in contrast to current, disease activity. Thus, CAL is considered to be a more accurate measure of history of disease and disease progression than PD. Table 3.20 enlists working definitions proposed by CDC for surveillance of periodontitis. Table 3.21 lists some case definitions related to probing depth and loss of attachment used in previous studies.

Bibliography

1. Page RC and Eke PI. Case definitions for use in population based surveillance of periodontitis. J Periodontol 2007;78:1387–99.
2. Savage Amir, Eaton KA, Moles DR, Needleman I. A systematic review of definitions of periodontitis and methods that have been used to identify this disease. J Clin Periodontol 2009; 36: 458–67.

3A.18 Periodontitis Index

Albandar et al. described the periodontitis index to measure the prevalence and severity of periodontitis in the US population. This index classifies each person as having mild, moderate or advanced periodontitis, or with no periodontitis, based on the number (or percentages) of teeth showing certain thresholds of probing depth and attachment loss.

Because this index does not combine parameters of different diseases, it does not endure some of the validity limitations found in the other periodontal indices. In the absence of periodontal inflammation and pocketing, the Periodontitis index does not regard the presence of attachment loss alone as a measure of periodontitis

Table 3.20: Clinical case definitions proposed by the CDC working group for use in population-based surveillance of periodontitis*

Periodontitis Category	Clinical definition		
	CAL		PD
Severe	≥ 2 interproximal sites with CAL ≥ 6 mm (not on same tooth)	and	≥ 1 interproximal site with PD ≥ 5 mm
Moderate	≥ 2 interproximal sites with CAL ≥ 4 mm (not on same tooth)	or	≥ 2 interproximal sites with PD ≥ 5 mm (not on same tooth)
No or mild	Neither "moderate" nor "severe" periodontitis		

*Third molars excluded

Table 3.21: Case definitions related to probing depth and loss of attachment

	≥ 2 mm	≤ 2 mm	≤ 3 mm	≤ 4 mm	≤ 5 mm	≤ 6 mm
CAL study Timmerman et al. (1998) (no or minor periodontitis) at one or more sites		Agerholm and Ashley (1996) at one or two approximal sites	Craig et al. (2001) at 4 sites	Borrell et al. (2005) at 3 sites	Timmerman et al. (1998) (advanced periodontitis) at one or more sites	Anagnou-Vareltzides et al. (1996) (severe periodontitis) at mean sites
			Timmerman et al. (1998) (moderate periodontitis) at one or more sites	Agerholm and Ashley (1996) at one or two approximal sites		Holmgren et al. (1994) at mean sites
		Chiappe et al. (1997) at one site	Agerholm and Ashley (1996) at one or two approximal sites			Machtei et al. (1992) at two or more teeth
PPD study			Borrell et al. (2005) at 2 sites	Querna et al. (1994) (early) worst individual score at sextant.	Querna et al. (1994) (moderate–advanced) at the highest score per sextant	Anagnou-Vareltzides et al. (1996) (severe periodontitis) at mean sites
			Craig et al. (2001) at 4 sites Peng et al. (1990) (3.5 mm CPITN) worst individual score at sextant	Brown et al. (1989) (modified Russell index) at one site	Machtei et al. (1992) at one or more teeth Peng et al. (1990) (5.5 mm CPITN) worst individual score at sextant	Brown et al. (1989) advanced periodontitis (modified Russell index) at one site

Procedure: The distance from the cemento-enamel junction (CEJ) to the free gingival margin (FGM) and the distance from the FGM to the bottom of the pocket/sulcus were assessed at the mesiobuccal and midbuccal surfaces. The measurements were made in millimeters and were rounded to the lowest whole millimeter. The assessment was made by using the NIDR periodontal probe.

Assessment of furcation involvement was made on 5 posterior teeth. The assessments were made at the mesial, buccal, and distal furcations of maxillary first and second molars, the mesial and distal furcations of maxillary second premolars, and the buccal and lingual furcations of mandibular first and second molars. Explorer #17 was used for maxillary molars and premolars, and explorer #3 for mandibular molars.

- Partial furcation involvement (grade I) was scored in sites where the explorer was definitely catching into but did not pass through the furcation.
- Total furcation involvement (grade II) was used when the explorer could be passed between the roots and through the entire furcation

Individuals with less than 6 teeth present (out of a maximum of 28 teeth) were not included in the classification for severity of periodontal disease. The individuals were classified according to extent and severity of periodontal disease using the following criteria:

Advanced periodontitis
- Two or more teeth (or 30% or more of the teeth examined) having ≥ 5 mm probing depth, or
- Four or more teeth (or 60% or more of the teeth examined) having ≥ 4 mm probing depth, or
- One or more posterior teeth with grade II furcation involvement.

Moderate periodontitis
- One or more teeth with ≥ 5 mm probing depth, or
- Two or more teeth (or 30% or more of the teeth examined) having ≥ 5 mm probing depth, or
- One or more posterior teeth with grade I furcation involvement and accompanied with ≥ 3 mm probing depth.

Mild periodontitis
- One or more teeth with ≥ 3 mm probing depth, or
- One or more posterior teeth with grade I furcation involvement.

No periodontitis: persons with 6 or more teeth who did not fulfill any of the above criteria were regarded as not having detectable levels of periodontitis.

Each person was assigned a given classification if he/she fulfilled one or more of the criteria of that classification, and was given the most advanced classification.

Bibliography

1. Albandar JM, Brunelle JA, Kingman A. Destructive periodontal disease in adult of 30 years of age and older in the United States, 1988–1994. J Periodontol 1999;70:13–29.
2. Albandar JM. Periodontal diseases in North America. Periodontol 2000 2002 29: 31–69.

3B Some New Derived Measures for Periodontal Disease

3B.1 Derived Community Periodontal Index (dCPI)

A person's dCPI score was based on WHO scoring criteria and was derived from the worst tooth condition observed for each quadrant using the CPIs inherent hierarchical assumptions. For instance, if a tooth had any evidence of bleeding, but no calculus or probing depths of 4 mm or more, then that tooth was scored a "1". If a tooth had any probing depths of 6 mm or more, then that tooth was scored a "4". The dCPI scoring guidelines used were probing depth measurements as specified by Ainamo in 1994 for CPITN (Ainamo and Ainamo 1994) and by WHO for CPI (WHO 1997). A dCPI subject-level score was determined by the selection of the worse of the two quadrant scores (Table 3.22).

3B.2 Attachment Loss Extent Index (ALEI)

For the ALEI score, the number of dental sites per person affected by clinical AL was summed, divided by the number of dental sites evaluated, and multiplied by 100. This percentage was categorized into five groups: 0–4% of sites affected, 5–24% of sites affected, 25–49% of sites affected, 50–74% of sites affected; and 75% or more of sites affected (Table 3.22).

3B.3 Attachment Loss (AL)

Clinical AL, as an indicator of past periodontal disease, was defined as a minimum of 2 mm of measured loss. These criteria were established to reflect a previously published AL extent and severity index (Carlos et al. 1986). For the AL score, clinical AL measured in millimetres at each dental site was summed and divided by the number of sites examined to produce a mean clinical AL score. This score was categorized into five groups: 0–1 mm of average clinical AL, 1.1–1.5 mm of average clinical AL, 1.6–2.0 mm clinical AL, 2.1–2.5 mm of average clinical AL, and 2.6 mm or more average clinical AL (Table 3.22).

3B.4 Periodontal Status Measure (PSM)

A person's PSM score was derived based on the worst tooth condition observed for each quadrant. Then the overall PSM score was

Table 3.22: Description of clinical presentation for derived periodontal status measures

Measure	ALEI	AL	dCPI	PSM
0	0–4% of sites with 2 mm or more of clinical AL	0–1 mm average amount of clinical AL	Healthy (no bleeding, calculus, probing depth ≥ 4 mm)	Healthy (no bleeding or clinical or AL)
1	5–24% of sites with 2 mm or more of clinical AL	1.1–1.5 mm average amount of clinical AL	Bleeding with probing is present	Gingivitis (bleeding is present, probing depth <3 mm, clinical AL ≤ 1mm)
2	25–49% of sites with 2 mm or more of clinical AL	1.6–2.0 mm average amount of clinical AL	Calculus is present (supra or sub gingival)	Mild periodontitis (at least one site with a probing depth 3–4 mm, clinical AL 2–3 mm, no furcations)
3	50–74% of sites with 2 mm or more of clinical AL	2.1–2.5 mm average amount of clinical AL	At least one site with a probing depth 4–5 mm	Moderate periodontitis (at least one site with a probing depth 5–6 mm, clinical AL 4–5 mm, may have a class I furcation)
4	75–100% of sites with 2 mm or more of clinical AL	2.61 mm average amount of clinical AL	At least one site with a probing depth 6 mm or more	Advance periodontitis (at least one site with a probing depth > 6 mm, clinical AL >5 mm, may have a class I or II furcation)

ALEI: attachment loss extent index; AL: attachment loss; dCPI: derived community periodontal index; PSM: periodontal status measure.

determined by the selection of the worse of the two quadrant scores. The PSM scoring range of 0–4 is similar to CPI, but unlike the CPI, the PSM incorporates clinical AL and dental furcation status into the index (Table 3.22).

Research goals and analytical plans need to account for limitations incurred by a specific periodontal measure; investigators should choose outcome measures for periodontal disease appropriate to the specific objectives of the study. For instance, if the research aim is to assess the influence of an intervention activity on reducing periodontal disease by utilizing mechanisms that increases the number of dental visits among a population at risk for disease, then a better primary outcome measure may be an index employing probing depth measures (such as dCPI or possibly PSM) with ALEI or AL as a less favorable choice.

The structure of these four measures also represents differing processes in the use of periodontal data to describe the periodontal condition. The dCPI and PSM identify the worst periodontal site assessed to derive a subject level score whereas ALEI and AL identify a summary measure representing a proportion of all sites. Another process involves the combination of information detailing various conditions of the periodontium such as bleeding or clinical AL. The presence of bleeding contributes information only to the dCPI and PSM indices whereas clinical AL is incorporated into three of the four indices. Consequently, these four measures present a broad yet contrasting picture of a population's periodontal status.

Bibliography

1. Dye BA, Selwitz RH. The relationship between selected measures of periodontal status and demographic and behavioural risk factors. J Clin Periodontol 2005; 32: 798–808.

3B.5 Periodontal Inflamed Surface Area—Quantification of Inflammatory Burden

The biological model for the plausibility of periodontitis as a risk factor for other diseases holds that periodontitis causes an inflammatory burden by eliciting bacteraemia leading to systemic inflammatory responses. This inflammatory burden in turn causes damage to the human body far beyond the oral cavity. Following this biological model, the larger the amount of inflamed periodontal tissue has higher chances of periodontitis eliciting bacteremia, systemic inflammatory responses or cross-reactivity. Therefore, any classification of periodontitis as a risk factor for other diseases should quantify the amount of inflamed periodontal tissue in order to quantify the inflammatory burden.

Many studies express periodontitis as a non-continuous variable. These studies use cut-off points to classify patients as being either unaffected or affected by mild, moderate or severe periodontitis. By definition, these classifications do not quantify the amount of inflamed periodontal tissue.

Some studies linking periodontitis to other diseases do quantify periodontitis as a continuous variable, i.e. using mean probing pocket depth (PPD) or mean clinical attachment level. Although these are continuous variables, this does not necessarily mean that these outcome measures quantify the amount of inflamed periodontal tissue. Thus, none of the classifications currently used expresses periodontitis as a continuous variable that is a measure of the amount of inflamed periodontal tissue. Hence these classifications may not quantify the inflammatory burden posed by periodontitis.

A classification that quantified the total surface area of attachment loss was reported by Hujoel et al. 2001), which would be named as attachment loss surface area (ALSA). To calculate the ALSA, formulas were generated whereby linear probing measurements, from the cementoenamel junction (CEJ) to the bottom of the pocket (i.e. CAL), around a particular tooth are transformed into the ALSA for that particular tooth (Despeignes 1979, Hujoel 1994, Hujoel et al. 2001).

The ALSA quantifies the root surface area that has become exposed due to attachment loss. However, the ALSA cannot be used to quantify the amount of inflamed periodontal tissue. ALSA does not quantify the periodontal epithelial surface area (PESA), because CAL instead of PPD measurements are used to calculate ALSA. To calculate the PESA, the recession surface area (RSA) has to be subtracted from ALSA. Since ALSA = PE – SA + RSA, it can be deducted that ALSA – RSA = PESA. To calculate the PESA there are three arithmetical possibilities, depending on the location of the gingival margin (LGM):

1. The LGM is below the CEJ so the RSA > 0. In this case, PPD < CAL and thus PESA < ALSA. Therefore PESA = ALSA – RSA.
2. The LGM is exactly at the CEJ. In this case, PPD = CAL, RSA = 0. Therefore, PESA = ALSA.
3. The LGM is above the CEJ. Since PPD > CAL, PESA > ALSA. Using CAL will lead to an underestimation of PESA. Calculating the PESA is only possible by using PPD instead of CAL, i.e. entering PPD as CAL in the formula transforming linear measurements to surface area. This will still lead to an underestimation of PESA.

Thus, PESA accurately quantifies the surface area of pocket epithelium if LGM is at or below the CEJ. However, PESA does still not quantify the surface area of inflamed pocket epithelium. After all, the PESA also includes healthy pocket epithelium. Healthy pocket epithelium contains relatively few inflammatory cells and may pose an effective barrier against bacteria trying to enter the circulation. Therefore, part of the PESA that consists of healthy epithelium may not contribute to the inflammatory burden. The inflamed part of the PESA on the other hand, does theoretically pose an inflammatory burden. To calculate the inflamed part of the PESA, assessment of the PESA that is affected by BOP is considered since BOP reflects decreased collagen density, increased blood vessel density and fragility and a reduction of epithelial thickness and epithelial integrity. Thus, the bleeding surface area, the periodontal inflamed surface area (PISA), may be thought of as the main contributor to any systemic inflammatory burden posed by periodontitis. Therefore, the PISA is proposed as a classification of periodontitis that quantifies the amount of inflamed periodontal tissue and as such, quantifies the systemic inflammatory burden.

Limitations: Although PISA is thought to be the best tool for assessment of the amount of periodontal inflamed tissue that is currently available, for several reasons PISA might not precisely quantify the amount of inflamed tissue.

- CAL, recession and BOP measurements used for the calculation of PISA always include measurement errors related to observer, instrument, teeth patients and their interactions.
- The formulas transforming CAL and recession to surface area, use population-based mean values of both root surface areas and root lengths.
- Individual variations in root surface area and root length are not taken into account when calculating PISA.
- PISA quantifies the amount of inflamed periodontal tissue in two dimensions, whereas in fact periodontitis is a three dimensional inflammatory process, i.e. extending into the connective tissue around the root.

For the above reasons, PISA may not precisely quantify the amount of inflammatory tissue. However, PISA likely quantifies the amount of inflamed periodontal tissue for each individual patient more accurately than any classification currently used.

PISA is, however, unable to accurately quantify the amount of inflamed periodontal tissue in case of pseudo pockets or gingival overgrowth, i.e. when the gingival margin is located above the CEJ. Fortunately, cases of gingival overgrowth are relatively rare, and often due to usage of medication (e.g. antiepileptic drugs, immune suppressive drugs, calcium blockers) or presence of certain diseases (e.g. leukaemia). These cases are not representative for the general population. Therefore, PISA can be used in the majority of cases, i.e. when the gingival margin is located at or below the CEJ.

Finally, PISA might not adequately predict the probability of periodontitis to cause other diseases, even if it would be possible to measure precisely the amount of inflamed periodontal tissue. For example, the type of inflammation might be more important in causing other diseases than the amount of inflammation. It also does not take into account the type of microbiological flora. Certain oral microorganisms might play a key role in causing other diseases, e.g. *Campylobacter rectus, Prevotella intermedia, Porphyromonas gingivalis* and *Peptostreptococcus micros*.

Although the PISA still has shortcomings, theoretically it appears to be a far better classification of periodontitis as a risk factor for other diseases than any classification currently used.

Bibliography

1. Nesse W, Abbas F, van der Ploeg I, Spijkervet FKL, Dijkstra PU, Vissink A. Periodontal inflamed surface area: quantifying inflammatory burden. J Clin Periodontol 2008; 35: 668–673.

3C Indices to Assess Gingival Recession

3C.1 Sullivan and Atkins (1968)

Sullivan and Atkins classified recession involving mandibular incisor teeth which used descriptive terms like "narrow", "wide", "shallow" and "deep" to classify recession into 4 groups.

3C.2 Mlinek et al, 1973

Mlinek et al, classified defects as "shallow-narrow" clefts as being <3 mm both dimensions, and "deep wide" defects as being >3 mm in both dimensions.

3C.3 Miller (1985)

Miller proposed 4 classes of marginal tissue recession based on both the level of the underlying alveolar bone and degree of involvement of the mucogingival junction.

Based on the above criteria Miller classified the gingival recession defects into four classes and also took prognosis into account as specified in Table 3.23.

3C.4 Mahajan's Modification of Miller Index

An outline of classification system:
- **Class I:** GRD (Gingival recession defects) not extending to the MGJ (Mucoginigival junction).
- **Class II:** GRD extending to the MGJ/ beyond it.
- **Class III:** GRD with bone or soft-tissue loss in the interdental area up to cervical 1/3 of the root surface and/or malpositioning of the teeth.

- **Class IV:** GRD with severe bone or soft tissue loss in the interdental area greater than cervical 1/3rd of the root surface and or severe malpositioning of the teeth.

Prognosis

- **BEST:** Class I and Class II with thick gingival profile.
- **GOOD:** Class I and Class II with thin gingival profile.
- **FAIR:** Class III with thick gingival profile.
- **POOR:** Class III and Class IV with thin gingival profile.

Bibliography

1. Mahajan A. Mahajan's modification of the Miller's classification for gingival recession. Dental Hypotheses 2010;1(2):45–50.

3C.5 Index of Recession (IR)

This index is proposed by Smith RG in 1997. The IR consists of two digits separated by a dash (e.g. F2- 4*). The first digit denotes the horizontal and the second the vertical component of a site of recession, with the prefixed letter (F or L) denoting whether the recession is on the facial or lingual aspects of the tooth, and an asterisk (*) denoting involvement of the Mucogingival junction.

Class	Symptoms	Treatment	Success
Table 3.23: Millers classification for gingival recession			
I	Narrow or wide localized classical recession isolated to facial surface, with papillae filling the interdental areas. The defects do not extend to the mucogingival line.	Complete root coverage is achievable	100%
II	Narrow and wide facially localized "classical recessions" which extend beyond the mucogingival line into the mobile mucosa. The papillae remain essentially intact.	Complete root coverage is achievable	100%
III	Broad recessions that extend beyond the mucogingival line into the mobile mucosa. The interdental papilla may be lost due to shrinkage and malpositioned teeth.	Only partial root coverage possible to the height of the contour of interproximal tissue.	50–70%
IV	Loss of periodontal hard and soft tissues around the entire tooth.	Root coverage is unpredictable and requires adjunctive treatment (i.e. orthodontics)	<10%

Table 3.24: Index of recession

Component	Score	Criteria
Horizontal	0	No clinical evidence of root exposure
	1	Similar to score 0, but a subjective awareness of dentinal hypersensitivity in response to a 1 second air blast is reported and/or there is clinically detectable exposure of the CEJ for up to 10% of the estimated MM-MD distance: a slit like defect
	2	Horizontal exposure of the CEJ >10% but not exceeding 25% of the estimated MM–MD distance
	3	Exposure of the CEJ >25% of the MM–MD distance but not exceeding
	4	Exposure of the CEJ >50% of the MM–MD distance but not exceeding 75%
	5	Exposure of the CEJ >75% of the MM–MD distance up to 100%
Vertical	0	No clinical evidence of root exposure
	1	Similar to score 0, but a subjective awareness of dentinal hypersensitivity is reported and/or there is clinically detectable exposure of the CEJ not extending >1 mm vertically to the gingival margin
	2–8	Root exposure 2–8 mm extending vertically from the CEJ to the base of the soft tissue defect
	9	Root exposure >8 mm from the CEJ to the base of the soft tissue defect.

The horizontal component — the first digit is expressed as a whole number value from the range 0–5 depending on what proportion of the CEJ is exposed, on either the facial or lingual aspects of the tooth, between the mesial and distal midpoints (MM–MD distance) approximally (Table 3.24).

Allocation of these codes does not imply that the extent of recession is equally dispersed about the facial or lingual midpoints of the area of exposed roots. The second digit of the IR gives the vertical extent of recession measured in whole mm on a range 0–9 (Table 3.24).

An asterisk is a fixed to the second digit whenever the vertical component of the soft tissue defect encroaches into the MGJ or extends beyond it into alveolar mucosa. The absence of an asterisk thus implies either absence of MGJ at the indexed site or its non-involvement in the soft tissue defect. Thus, an IR of F2–4*, as quoted earlier, will denote a zone of recession on the facial aspect of a tooth 4 mm deep involving the MGJ, but not extending more than 25% horizontally at the level of the CEJ towards the approximal midpoints.

When a tooth has recession on both facial and lingual aspects of a root, each site will receive a separate IR. Thus, for example, a tooth being scored F5–4/L5–2 has complete exposure of the CEJ, with vertical sites of recession of 4 mm and 2 mm on facial and lingual aspects respectively, neither involving the MGJ.

In instances of extensive vertical recession, consideration may be given to allotting a further horizontal component of the IR at a specified intermediate level between the CEJ and the base of the soft tissue defect. If a molar tooth is being assessed, it may be appropriate to allocate separate values to each exposed root. This IR is now in use in cross-sectional and longitudinal studies relating to gingival recession prevalence, incidence, severity and etiology.

Bibliography

1. Smith RG. Gingival recession. Reappraisal of an enigmatic condition and a new index for monitoring. J Clin Periodontol 1997;24:201–5.

3D. Radiographic Bone Criteria/Indices

3D.1 Sheppard (1936)

Sheppard graded the degree of bone resorption from zero to ten. "The number 'one' signifies just enough loss to be visible on the radiograph. Thus 'five' indicates the loss of half the alveolar bone, while 'ten' implies complete loss of alveolar support. Intermediate numbers denote corresponding degrees of bone loss". They evaluated radiographically six regions of the dental arches and gave the average of these six region values as the index of the particular case.

3D.2 Miller and Seidler (1940)

Miller and Seidler used essentially the same system. The dental arches were divided into four segments. "The extreme amounts of periodontal experience for each of the four segments were recorded as 0 to 5. An index of 0 was ascribed to a segment when there was no bone dissolution evident; 5 units were given when the bone was destroyed to the apices of the teeth. An index of 3 was recorded when half the bone in a segment had disappeared. Units of 1, 2, and 4 were estimated as fractions of 3 and 5."

3D.3 Alveolar Bone Loss Index

Alveolar Bone loss Index was given by Marshall Day and Shourie K.L in 1949. Alveolar bone loss can be quantified using radiographs. Scoring is done from 0–10. The number 10 is assigned to full root length of a given tooth. The degree of bone resorption is then measured in lengths from '0' (no bone loss) to '10' (complete bone loss). The scores for bone loss are summed up to give the area total and then averaged to give a "resorption" figure for the individual patient.

3D.4 Sheiham A and Striffler DF

Sheiham A and Striffler DF developed a Radiographic index (XI) in 1970. The criteria uses radiographs (Table 3.25).

Table 3.25: Radiographic index (XI)

Score	Criteria
0	Normal
4	Lack of continuity of cortical plate at the crest of interdental bone, with possible widening of periodontal membrane
5	Up to 1/3 of supporting bone lost
6	More than 1/3 and up to 2/3 supporting bone lost
7	More than 2/3 of supporting bone lost

Bibliography

1. Sheiham A, Striffler DF. A comparison of four epidemiological methods of assessing periodontal disease. 1. Population findings. J Periodontal Res 1970;5:148–54.

3D.5 Hull PS, Hillam DG and Beal JF (1975)

Radiographic evidence of periodontitis was recorded as present or absent for the following interproximal spaces of mesial and distal to each of the upper and lower first permanent molars. Where either or both of the teeth were absent or if the inter-proximal space was obscured, then this was categorized as unreadable.

Periodontitis was considered to be present when the alveolar crest was irregular with loss of continuity of its surface. Further evidence of periodontitis was considered to be present when there was widening of the periodontal ligament space at its alveolar crest and when the bone crest was greater than 3 mm from the CEJ. Areas in which the evidence was questionable were considered to be negative. Bone loss was considered to be absent when:

- The bone crest was approximately 1.5 mm from the cementoenamel junction (CEJ)
- The alveolar crest was flat, regular and parallel to a line drawn from the CEJ of one tooth to that of the adjacent tooth

Bibliography

1. Hull PS, Hillam DG, Beal JF. A radiographic study of the prevalence of chronic periodontitis in 14-year-old English school children. J Clin Periodontol 1975;2:203–10.

3D.6 Blankenstein R, Murray JJ and Lind OP (1978)

The radiographic technique was standardized according to the principles advanced by Moller (1966) using stationary X-ray units. Disposable bitewing holders were used; the radiographs were developed immediately after exposure. All the radiographs were examined without magnification using a standard transilluminator with a uniform source of light. The interproximal alveolar crests of 17–16; 16–15; 47–46; 46–45; 25–26; 26–27; 35–36; and 36–37 were examined for the following features:

a. **Irregularity and notching of the alveolar crest:** Absence of the radiopaque "white line" on the crest of the interdental septum was not considered as an irregular surface.

b. **Linear distance greater than 3 mm between the cementoenamel junction and the bone crest:** Measured directly from the radiograph with dividers.

c. **Widening of the periodontal ligament space at its alveolar crest:** This space was considered in the first instance as having an increased width by comparing it visually with the periodontal ligament space on the opposite side of the tooth, and with the ligament spaces of the other teeth on the radiograph.

The radiograph was then placed in a X-ray film enlarger, with a 13-fold magnification, and the distance from the inner surface of the alveolar crest to the cementum was measured with dividers. Where the outline of the alveolar crest was obscured due to overlap or malpositioning of the film, it was recorded as a non-readable surface. Where the second premolar was still erupting, the interdental crest was recorded as being normal. When the first permanent molar had been extracted, the second permanent molar was not substituted, even though this tooth may have drifted mesially.

Bibliography

1. Blankenstein R, Murray JJ and Lind OP. Prevalence of chronic periodontitis in 13–15-year-old children — a radiographic study. J Clin Periodontol 1978;5:285–92.

4

Indices used to Assess Gingival Diseases

INTRODUCTION

Gingivitis, which is prevalent in a large proportion of children and adults, is an inflammatory lesion of gingival tissues which has been shown to be reversible (Löe et al. 1965). The clinical signs of this pathology include changes in gingival color (redness), alteration of normal contour (edema), loss of stippling, increased gingival crevicular fluid flow, engorgement, bleeding and in some cases, ulceration of gingival tissues.

Gingival indices are used to describe the relative status of the degree of either health, disease, or both, of the gingival tissues. Most of the indices incorporate a graduated scale with definite upper and lower limits. All gingival indices rely on one or more of the following criteria: (1) color, (2) contour, (3) bleeding, (4) extent of involvement and (5) crevicular fluid flow. Some indices have shown a correlation between the various criteria used and histologic signs of inflammation, particularly in the case of bleeding and visual signs of inflammation.

In the selection of a gingival index, the researcher must consider the precision, accuracy, reliability and the validity of the measurements produced with the use of the index. Many of the indices utilize an ordinal scale to assign numbers from 0 to 3 or 4 to record the status of gingival health under a given set of circumstances. Such data can also be treated as a dichotomous scale with inflammation present or absent. When used as an ordinal scale, it is common practice to treat the data as individual mean mouth scores or to pool the individual scores and calculate group mean score. These scores can be utilized to make statistical comparisons among groups of subjects.

Ainsworth and Young (1925) first attempted to differentiate between children with no gingivitis and children with gingivitis. They also classified gingivitis as slight, medium and severe, but made no serious attempts to employ a quantitative method. King (1945), and Schour and Massler (1947) attempted to define mild, moderate and severe types of gingivitis in a more precise and objective manner. The gingiva was for the first time divided into gingival units, and the papillary gingiva, marginal gingiva and attached gingiva were clearly differentiated. The PMA index is probably the first successful attempt to design a numerical system for recording gingival health. The PMA index has been modified and used for a variety of studies over the years (Massler et al., 1950, Parfitt, 1957). Its major purpose has been in the evaluation of gingival inflammation in children. An epochal contribution was made by the introduction of the gingival index of Löe and Silness (1963). This was followed by development of many gingival indices.

A number of gingival indices and their modifications exist in the literature because of which a single index for universal application or acceptance becomes impossible. Chilton pointed that a universal index is not possible and the appropriate indices must be utilized for the various entities tested. This chapter helps the researcher gain knowledge about the various gingival indices which existed in literature and also helps to choose the appropriate index for the research.

Bibliography

1. Ciancio SG. Current status of indices of gingivitis. J Clin Periodontol 1986;13:375–8.

4.1 Papillary Marginal Attached (PMA) Index

It was developed by Maury Massler and Schour in 1944 and probably the first successful attempt to design a numerical system for recording gingival health. The number of gingival units is counted rather than the severity of inflammation.

The gingival unit was divided into three component parts: Interdental papilla (P), marginal gingiva (M) and attached gingiva (A). Since the various types of gingivitis are not clearly defined during that era, it was decided to adopt a classification of severity which would avoid ambiguity and would be based on naked-eye appearance. The severity of inflammation was, therefore, graded numerically in successive degrees according to increasing intensity and extent.

Method of recording: Each examination started from the lower left arch and was carried out to the lower right side and similarly in the upper arch. The gingival papilla between second and third molars was counted as 7 and between first and second molars as 6 and so on. All the papillae were recorded, including those between the central incisors. The scoring criteria are discussed in Table 4.1.

Bibliography

1. Barnes GP, Parker WA, Lyon TC, Fultz RP. Indices used to evaluate signs, symptoms and etiologic factors associated with diseases of the periodontium. J Periodontol 1986;57:643–51.

2. Massler M. The P-M-A index for the assessment of gingivitis. J Periodontol 1967;38(6):S592–601.

Site	Code	Criteria
P	0	Normal; no inflammation
	1+	Mild papillary engorgement; slight increase in size
	2+	Obvious increase in size of papilla; bleeding on pressure
	3+	Excessive increase in size with spontaneous bleeding
	4+	Necrotic papilla
	5+	Atropy and loss of papilla
M	0	Normal; no inflammation
	1+	Engorgement; slight increase in size
	2+	Obvious increase in size; bleeding on pressure
	3+	Swollen collar, spontaneous bleeding, beginning infiltration into attached gingivae
	4+	Necrotic gingivitis
	5+	Recession of the marginal gingivae below the CEJ due to inflammatory changes
A	0	Normal; pale rose, stippled
	1+	Slight engorgement with loss of stippling; change of color may or may not be present
	2+	Obvious engorgement of attached gingivae with marked increase in redness. Pocket formation present.
	3+	Advanced periodontitis. Deep pockets evident

Table 4.1: PMA scoring criteria

4.2 Papillary Marginal (PM) Index

It was developed by Muhlemann and Mazor in 1958 as a modification of papillary marginal attachment (PMA) index (Table 4.2).

	Table 4.2
Score	Criteria
0	No inflammation
1	Bleeding from gingival sulcus on gentle probing. Tissue otherwise appears normal
2	Bleeding on probing plus a change in color due to inflammation. No oedema
3	Bleeding plus a change of color and oedematous swelling.
4	Ulceration or additional symptoms

Bibliography

1. Hazen SP. Indices for the measurement of gingival inflammation in clinical studies of oral hygiene and periodontal disease. J Periodontal Res. 1974;9; Suppl 14:61–77.
2. Muhlemann HR, Mazor ZS. Gingivitis in Zurich school children. Helv Odont Acta 1958;1:3.

4.3 Gingival Index

Gingival index (GI) was developed by Löe H and Silness J in 1963 to describe the clinical severity of gingival inflammation as well as its location (Table 4.3).

Teeth examined: 16, 12, 24, 36, 32 and 44

Surfaces examined on each tooth: Each gingival unit (buccal, lingual, mesial and distal) of the individual tooth is given a score from 0–3, called the GI for the area. The scores from the four areas of the tooth are added and divided by four to give the GI for the tooth.

The scores of the individual teeth (incisors, premolars and molars) may be grouped to designate the GI for the group of teeth. Finally, by adding the indices for the teeth and dividing by six the GI for the patient is obtained. The index for the patient is thus an average score for the areas examined (Table 4.4). Before examination for GI, the gingivae were dried either by a blast of air and/or cotton rolls.

Table 4.4: Categories of GI	
Average GI	Interpretation
2.1 – 3.0	Severe inflammation
1.1 – 2.0	Moderate inflammation
0.1 – 1.0	Mild inflammation

Löe H in 1967, described plaque and gingival index in detail. It may be used as all surfaces of all or selected teeth, or for selected areas of all or selected teeth. When only one of the interproximal surfaces are examined instead of both (current examinations have been restricted to buccal, mesial and lingual aspects of the teeth), the score for the one interproximal surface should be doubled and the total score for the tooth divided by four.

Bibliography

1. Löe H, Silness J. Periodontal disease in pregnancy. I. Prevalence and severity. Acta Odontol Scand. 1963;21:533–51.
2. Löe, H. The gingival index, the plaque index and the retention index systems. J Periodontol 1967;38:610.

Table 4.3: Scoring criteria for Gingival index			
Appearance	Bleeding	Inflammation	Score
Normal	No bleeding	None	0
Slight change in color and little change in texture	No bleeding	Mild	1
Moderate glazing, redness, oedema and hypertrophy	Bleeding on pressure	Moderate	2
Marked redness, and hypertrophy, ulceration	Spontaneous bleeding	Severe	3

4.4 An Index to Evaluate Gingival Health

Williams NB, Parfitt GJ and Richards MD in 1964 proposed an index to evaluate gingival health.

Examination: All patients were examined with good light, bright natural light being preferred. The lips and cheeks were retracted and the gingiva examined for color, texture, contour, ease of bleeding, height on tooth surface and tonus of the free margin. The areas of the mouth to be sampled were evaluated as to state of gingival health. The specific description for each assessment was given in Table 4.5.

Grading

0–6: very good
7–12: fair
13–18: poor
19–24: extremely poor

Bibliography

1. Williams NB, Parfitt GJ and Richards MD. A Preliminary Study of Microbial Smears as an Aid in Diagnosis of Gingival Health. Journal of Periodontology 1964;35(3):197–201.

Fischman and co-workers (Fischman et al. 1973) introduced an "end point" method of assessing gingivitis. Their rationale was that the time it took for a subject with pre-existing gingivitis to reach an arbitrary level of gingivitis would be a measure of the efficacy of a preventive agent. This arbitrary level of gingivitis could be defined in terms of the Loe Index. It could be clinically distinct from the baseline level of gingivitis, but less severe than the level of undesirable, irrevocable tissue damage. The authors felt that this system would permit the evaluation of potential therapeutic agents in groups with pre-existing gingivitis. One of the criticisms of this system is that it measures the deterioration in gingival health and not an improvement, although the criteria could be reversed in terms of the "end point".

An advantage of this index is that it permits the evaluation of agents without the need to empirically search for an optimum time period to evaluate a drug's effect.

Bibliography

1. Fischman S, Cancro L, Podur M, Bolton S, and Picozzi A. A new method for assessing inhibition of gingivitis by potential therapeutic agents. J Periodontology 1973;44:535–9.

4.5 Modified Gingival Index (MGI)

MGI was developed by Lobene RR, Weatherford T, NM Ross, Lamm RA, and Menaker L in 1986 as modification of Loe and Silness gingival index.

Unlike the GI, the MGI has a non-invasive approach. Determining the severity of gingivitis is strictly based on visual observation. The reason for developing this index is to increase the sensitivity in the low region of the scale and there is no gentle probing to possibly provoke bleeding on pressure.

Score	Criteria
	Table 4.5: Scoring criteria for gingival health
0	Indicates no clinical evidence of inflammation in the area.
1	Indicates a detectable hyperemia in the papilla, margin or attached mucosa. This level of change might not be recognized in clinical practice as requiring treatment.
2	Denotes, in addition to score 1, a loss of stippling, easily visualized hyperemia, swelling, or bleeding on pressure. This level is recognized in clinical practice.
3	Denotes such severity that patient claims symptoms such as bleeding sensitivity, itching sensation or tenderness.
4	Represents severe hyperemia, obvious swelling or spontaneous hemorrhage from touch of fingers, food or toothbrush. Severe gingival disease.

Method: The gingivae are segmented into marginal and papillary units. When used as full mouth examination with 28 teeth, a maximum number of 108 gingival units (56 marginal and 52 papillary). All the third molars are excluded. To obtain the MGI, the Labial or Facial and Lingual surfaces of the gingival margins and the interdental papilla of all erupted teeth or selected teeth are examined using the following criteria (Table 4.6).

Table 4.6: Scoring criteria for MGI

Appearance	Score
Normal/absence of inflammation	0
Mild inflammation (slight change in color, little change in texture) of any portion of the gingival unit	1
Mild inflammation of the entire gingival unit	2
Moderate inflammation (moderate, glazing, redness, edema and/or hypertrophy) of the gingival unit	3
Severe inflammation (marked redness and edema spontaneous bleeding) of the entire gingival unit	4

Bibliography

1. Lobene RR, Weatherford T, Ross NM, Lamm RA and Menaker L. A modified gingival index for use in clinical trials. Clin Prev Dent 1986;8(1)3–6.

4.6 The Columbia Gingival Index (GI) for Gingivitis

Chilton et al. reported this index to evaluate patients with gingivitis. This can help diagnose patients with gingivitis and monitor the response to interventions. The evaluation can be performed either on a subset of 6 teeth or all the teeth in the mouth.

The authors demonstrated that the findings from testing 6 teeth were comparable to that of the whole mouth.16, 21, 24, 36, 41 and 44 are the index teeth. 6 sites on each tooth are scored: mesiobuccal, buccal, distobuccal, mesiolingual, lingual and distolingual. Each site is scored based on the gross evidence of gingivitis as described in Table 4.7.

Bibliography

1. Chilton NW, Fertig JW, Talbott K. Partial and full mouth recording of gingivitis scores. Pharmacology and Therapeutics in Dentistry 1978;3:39–44.

Table 4.7: Scoring criteria for Columbia gingival index

Color	Appearance	Points
Pink	Firm, knife like gingival margin; interdental papilla triangular	0
No or slight color change discreet areas of redness along most coronal surfaces of the free gingival margin	Gingival margin slightly swollen and no longer knifelike and firm	1
		2
Obviously red	No bleeding on gentle finger pressure	3
Obviously red	Bleeds on gentle finger pressure	4

4.7 Glass Index for Assessment of Gingival Changes

Table 4.8: Scoring criteria for glass index

Score	Criteria
0	Normal gingiva – may have some loss of stippling
1	Norma gingival architecture - no gingival enlargement – minimal detectable color change
2	Slight enlargement limited to the papilla. Color changes may or may not be present.
3	Slight enlargement of the papilla and margin – the extention of score no 2, which starts in the papilla
4	Any more severe involvement

Bibliography

1. Glass RL. A clinical study of hand and electric brushing. J Periodontol 1965;36:322–327.

4.8 Gingival Assessment Index

It was developed by John D Suomi and Joseph P Barbano in 1968.

Method: Assessment of gingival conditions was done on all teeth, using a plane mouth mirror and a number 23 explorer using the criteria described in Table 4.9. The gingival margins and papillae surrounding each tooth are examined from both the lingual and facial aspects. Each quadrant of the mouth is divided into three segments: molar, premolar and anterior teeth creating 12 segments. The papillae between the first molar and second premolar and canine and first premolar are arbitrarily assigned to the premolar region.

Calculation: Mean gingivitis score is obtained by adding the scores of units of the segment and dividing by the number of units examined.

Bibliography

1. Suomi JD and Barbano JP. Patterns of gingivitis. Journal of Periodontology 1968;39:71–74.

4.9 Dental Health Centre Index

It is developed by John D Suomi, John C Greene, Jack R Vermillion, Jacquelline J Chang and Ernest C Leatherwood in 1969. The index is assessed on 8 index teeth (all first permanent molars, upper right central incisor, upper left first premolar, lower left central incisor and lower right first premolar). Substitution of teeth is not done except for using the adjacent central incisor when the incisor of choice is missing, crowned or otherwise unsuitable for scoring. The facial and lingual gingival tissues of the eight designated teeth were scored separately for gingival inflammation using the criteria described in Table 4.10.

Bibliography

1. Suomi JD, Greene JC, Vermillion JR, Chang JJ, Leatherwood EC. The effect of controlled oral hygiene procedures on the progression of periodontal disease in adults: results after two years. J Periodontol 1969;40(7):416–20.

Table 4.9: Criteria for gingival assessment index

Score	Criteria
0	Absence of inflammation — gingiva is pale pink in color and firm in texture. Swelling is not evident and stippling can usually be noted
1	Presence of inflammation — a distinct color change to red or magenta is evident. There may be swelling and loss of swelling. The gingiva may be spongy in texture
2	Presence of severe inflammation — a distinct color change to red or magenta is evident. There is swelling, loss of swelling and a spongy consistency. There is either gingival bleeding upon gentle probing with the side of an explorer or the inflammation has spread to the attached gingiva.

Table 4.10: Criteria for dental health centre index

Score	Criteria
0	No inflammation — gingiva adjacent to the tooth surface being examined in pale pink in color and firm in texture. Swelling is not evident and stippling can usually be noted (hypertrophy, recession or change in gingival contour in the absence of color change was not considered inflammation)
1	Inflammation not encompassing all tissue adjacent to the tooth surface (including papillae), gingiva is a definite red or magenta color
2	Inflammation encompassing all tissue adjacent to the tooth surface (including papillae)

4.10 Papillary Marginal Gingivitis Index (PMGI)

It was introduced by de la Rosa and Sturzenberger OP in 1976. It is combination of PMA Index of Massler and Schour and Gingival Index of Loe and Silness.

Method

All facial and lingual gingival papillae and gingival margins of all natural teeth were examined. To provide uniformity in this assessment, each papilla was considered the gingival structure distal to a tooth. Exceptions were the papillae between the central incisors. Since they are not distal to a tooth, they are labeled the "midline papillae". Identification of the margins presents no problem because each one is readily relatable to a specific tooth.

Before the start of methodical grading of gingivitis, the examiner records missing teeth. Examination should begin at the maxillary right posterior facial tissue and proceeds across the midline around the arch to the left. From there he continues on the lingual from left to right. Next, the mandibular facial gingiva are examined from right to left.

Finally, the lower lingual is examined from left to right. The examination is limited to the 28 natural teeth of the dentition and does not consider third molars. A maximum of 60 gingival papillae (including 4 midline papillae) and a maximum of 56 gingival margins, or a maximum of 116 units in total, are therefore considered for scoring (Table 4.11).

Calculation

Sum of all inflammation scores divided by the number of papillary and marginal units examined per subject.

Bibliography

1. de la Rosa M and Sturzenberger OP. Clinical reduction of gingivitis through the use of a mouthwash containing two quaternary ammonium compounds. J Periodontol 1976;47: 535–7.

4.11 Gingival Tissue Index

It was developed by Garg Subhash, Kapoor KK, Mehrotra KK and Dixit Jaya in 1979. It was based on inflammatory hyperplastic states of gingival units (each gingival units included one papillary or one marginal

Table 4.11: Criteria for papillary marginal gingivitis index	
Score	Criteria
0	No Inflammation/Normal gingiva
1	Mild inflammation, slight change in color and little change in texture
2	Moderate inflammation, moderate glazing, redness, edema and enlargement; bleeding on pressure with a blunt instrument.
3	Severe inflammation, marked redness and enlargement; tendency for spontaneous bleeding

Table 4.12: Criteria for gingival tissue index		
Compartments	Score	Criteria
Inflammatory hyperplastic	3	Severely inflammatory hyperplastic, deformed and spongy gingival unit
	3A	Moderately inflammatory- hyperplastic and spongy gingival unit
	3B	Mild inflammatory- hyperplastic, deformed soft and edematous gingival unit
Non- Inflammatory hyperplastic	2	Non-inflammatory severely hyperplastic, deformed and slightly firm gingival unit

Contd.

Table 4.12 *(Contd.)*

Compartments	Score	Criteria
	2A	Non-inflammatory-moderately hyperplastic deformed and slightly firm gingival unit
	2B	Non-inflammatory-mildly hyperplastic, deformed and slightly firm gingival unit
	1	Non-inflammatory-moderately hyperplastic deformed and moderately firm gingival unit
	1A	Non-inflammatory-mildly hyperplastic, deformed and moderately firm gingival unit
	1B	Substantial regression in non-inflammatory-mildly hyperplastic state and nearly firm gingival unit
Non- inflammatory non-hyperplastic	0	Physiologic architecture gingival unit; pink, firm, resilient, stippled, and knife edged

gingiva from facial aspect). It has a range of ten scores with 3 components (Table 4.12).

Bibliography

1. Garg S, Kapoor KK, Mehrotra KK, Dixit J. Periodontal treatment systems - A clinical assessment and gingival tissue index, gingival pain index and tooth hypersensitivity index. J Indian Dent Asso.1986;58:513–26.

4A Gingival Indices for Special Groups

4A.1 The Gingival Overgrowth Index (GOI)

Seymour et al developed a Gingival Overgrowth Index (GOI) for assessing gingival hyperplasia. This can be useful for monitoring a patient taking a medication or disease that can cause gingival hyperplasia. Seymour divided the teeth into gingival units, with each unit extending from the midpoint of 1 tooth to the midpoint of the adjacent tooth. The midpoint of the unit is the inter-dental space. This is flanked on either side by one half of

each tooth. 20 gingival units involving the anterior upper and lower teeth are examined (10 mandibular, 10 maxillary).

Parameters

➤ Vertical extent (extent of gingival encroachment on adjacent teeth)
➤ Horizontal extent (gingival thickening along the labial or lingual aspect)

The horizontal extent of the gingiva anteriorly (along labial aspect) normally does not extend beyond a plane connecting the midline of the 2 teeth in the gingival unit. The horizontal extent of the gingiva posteriorly (along the lingual aspect) is harder to measure since the normal extent is a curved plane connecting the posterior midlines of the 2 teeth in the gingival unit with the apex indented towards the teeth (concave) (Fig. 4.1). For vertical extent, each of the tooth halves in the gingival unit is divided vertically into thirds adjacent to interdental space, middle and

Table 4.13: Criteria for gingival overgrowth index

Horizontal gingival thickening (labio-lingual)	Vertical (extent of gingival encroachment on adjacent teeth)	Grade
Normal width	no encroachment	0
0.1 to 2 mm of thickening	up to 1/6th of labial surface of tooth crown encroached	1
> 2 mm thickening	1/6th to 2/6th of labial surface of crown encroached	2
–	encroachment over the labial surface of the crown to midpoint (2/6th to 3/6th)	3

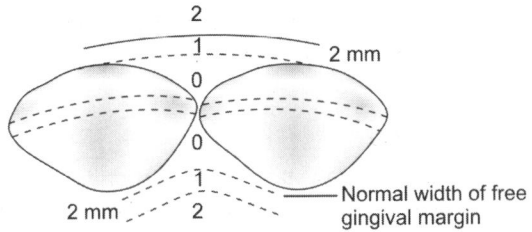

Fig. 4.1: Assessment of horizontal gingival thickening (labio-lingual)

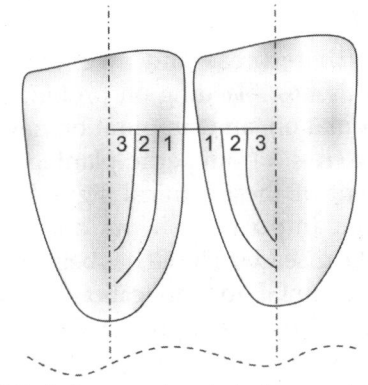

Criteria for assessing gingival encroachment on adjacent tooth surfaces for a gingival unit

Fig. 4.2: Assessment of vertical extent of gingival encroachment on adjacent teeth

adjacent to midline of tooth (Fig. 4.2). Since half of a tooth is divided into thirds, each of these vertical segments is 1/6th of the tooth width.

Bibliography

1. Seymour RA, Smith DG, Turnbull DN. The effects of phenytoin and sodium valproate on the periodontal health of adult epileptic patients. J Clin Periodontology 1985; 12: 413–9.
2. Varga E, Lennon MA, Mair LH. Pretransplant gingival hyperplasia predicts severe cyclosporin induced gingival overgrowth in renal transplant patients. J Clin Periodontology 1998;25: 225–30.

4A.2 Gingival Inflammation Index for Frail Elders (GIIFE)

The most commonly used method of assessing gingivitis is bleeding on probing in a dental clinic setting. In some cases, where the gingiva appears inflamed bleeding does not occur. This may be due to variance of probing force,

depth and angulations between and within examiners which create greater problem among frail elders in institutions since the oral assessments usually take place within the facility. Because these individuals have limited mobility, most oral assessments are performed while subjects are sitting up in wheelchairs, often with no head support. Lack of head support makes it difficult to keep the head from moving during the assessment, which can be dangerous to the resident or examiner when an instrument such as a periodontal probe is being used. Considering all the factors, Donnelly, Wyatt and Brondani (2010) proposed an index for frail elders.

The GIIFE is a simple dichotomous assessment of six areas of the tooth/root/implant surface namely, mesial buccal, mid-buccal, distal buccal, distal lingual, mid-lingual and mesial lingual:

  0 - no visual sign of redness or swelling
  1 - visual signs of redness or swelling

The instruments needed to perform the assessment are a mirror and light or an illuminated mirror as it provides superior vision and light to an overhead lamp or flashlight. This index is easy for the examiner to perform and for the subject to tolerate since it is only a visual assessment. The examination can be quick increasing participant tolerance and examiner comfort. Head support is not required reducing the risk of injury from sudden movement since only a mirror will be in the resident's mouth. The visual characteristics are simple and easily distinguishable from each other. In order to reduce the subjectivity, thus increasing examiner reliability, the degree to which the gingiva is red or swollen does not quantify.

Depending on the stage of the gingivitis, edema or fibrosis of the gingiva may be present. Therefore to simplify further the criteria, swelling was chosen to describe change in tissue contour, consistency, and texture. All intact teeth, fractured teeth, and root tips present will be examined, thereby minimizing potential areas of gingival inflammation being excluded from the assessment. All areas of the gingiva will be assessed to ensure that sites more or less prone to gingivitis are given equal representation. By excluding a bleeding on probing assessment this index eliminates the need for antibiotic prophylaxis, and can be applied to all who are dentate. The exclusion of probing should also decrease the time per examination (Table 4.14).

Limitations

- Subjectivity of redness and swelling can still be susceptible to examiner variability.
- Medical conditions such as arthritis treated with anti-inflammatory medications may mask some visual signs of inflammation.
- Some residents may still not be able to tolerate the full assessment.

Table 4.14: Specific criteria of the GIIFE

1. All teeth, including fractured teeth, root tips and implants are to be assessed.
2. Each tooth is assessed at 6 areas of the gingiva (MB, B, DB, ML, L, DL).
3. Redness defined as any area of the gingival unit no longer appearing coral pink.
4. Swelling defined as loss of scalloping, knife edge or stippling of any of the gingival unit.
5. Overall gingivitis score calculated by summing all scores and dividing by the number of surfaces.
6. Overall score will determine extent or percentage of gingival inflammation.
   Average score: 0.00 – 0.33 = minimal; 0.34 – 0.66 = moderate; 0.67 – 1.00 = extensive

---

- In the absence of good lighting, certain areas of the gingiva and early signs of gingivitis may be missed.

Bibliography

1. Donnelly LR, Wyatt CCCL and Brondani MM. A potential Gingival Inflammation Index for Frail Elders. Can J Dent Hygiene 2010;44:118–123.

4A.3 Indices used to Assess Marginal Mucosal Conditions Around Oral Implants

Along with redness and swelling of the marginal tissues, bleeding on probing (BOP), pocket formation, and suppuration have been reported to result from periimplant infections. Assessment of these clinical signs has been considered important in the diagnosis of periodontal diseases. The GI has been modified and adapted (mGI) for application around oral implants, while a simplified GI has been proposed by Apse and associates (Table 4.15).

Bibliography

1. Apse P, Zarb GA, Schmitt A, Lewis DW. The longitudinal effectiveness of osseointegrated dental implants. The Toronto study: Periimplant mucosal response. Int J Periodontics Restorative Dent 1991;11:95–111.
2. Mombelli A, Van Oosten MAC, Schürch E, Lang NP. The microbiota associated with successful or failing osseointegrated titanium implants. Oral Microbiol Immunol 1987;2:145–51.
3. Salvi GE, Lang NP. Diagnostic parameters for monitoring peri-implant conditions. Int J Oral Maxillofac Implants. 2004;19 Suppl:116–27.

Table 4.15: Criterias for gingivitis around implants

Score	Mombelli et al (mGI)	Apse et al
0	No bleeding when a periodontal probe is passed along the mucosal margin adjacent to the implant	Normal mucosa
1	Isolated bleeding spots visible	Minimal inflammation with color change and minor edema
2	Blood forms a confluent red line on mucosal margin	Moderate inflammation with redness, edema, and glazing
3	Heavy or profuse bleeding	Severe inflammation with redness, edema, ulceration, and spontaneous bleeding without probing

5

Indices used to Assess Gingival Bleeding

Introduction

Gingival bleeding is an objective sign of inflammation in the gingival connective tissues. Bleeding occurs because of frequent microulcerations in the epithelium that lines the soft-tissue wall of a periodontal pocket. Gingival bleeding is not a diagnosis; it does not distinguish between different forms of periodontal diseases and is not pathogno-monic of any one form of the disease. Indeed, gingival bleeding is associated with various forms of periodontal diseases including gingivitis, acute necrotizing ulcerative gingivitis, juvenile periodontitis, adult periodontitis, rapidly progressive periodontitis, and refractory periodontitis.

A bleeding index can fulfill several very different purposes. Epidemiologists have used it as one measure of periodontal disease prevalence and also to estimate treatment needs and costs in a population. Researchers have used it as one way to measure the effectiveness of anti-plaque and anti-gingivitis agents, to compare responses to various treatment modalities (e.g. scaling and root planning/periodontal surgery), and to correlate bleeding to disease activity. Clinicians have used bleeding on probing in their diagnosis and treatment of periodontal diseases to record baseline data related to disease, to identify problem sites that require additional treatment, to screen patients before deciding on need for periodontal treatment, and to motivate patients to improve oral hygiene.

Clearly, the purpose can determine the most appropriate type of index to use. For epide-miological surveys, partial recording of selected teeth or sites may suffice. For research and for therapeutic purposes, a quantitative measurement of bleeding is more informative than a dichotomous index of presence or absence of bleeding on provocation. For patient education and motivation, a dichotomous index will suffice.

5.1 Sulcus Bleeding Index (SBI)

It was developed by Mühlemann HR and Son S 1971. This index is a modification of PM index. The purpose of this index is to locate areas of gingival sulcus bleeding upon gentle probing and thus to recognize and record the presence of early inflammatory gingival disease. Probing should be done under proper illumination. Probe should be held parallel with long axis of the tooth for marginal units and direct the probe towards the col area for Papillary units. After probing wait for 30 seconds before scoring healthy gingival bleeding. Tooth should be dried gently to observe color changes clearly.

Four gingival areas are scored which are labial and lingual marginal gingivae (M units) mesial and distal papillary gingivae (P units) using the following criteria (Table 5.1).

Table 5.1: Criteria for SBI

Score	Criteria
0	Healthy appearance of P and M, no bleeding upon probing
1	Bleeding on probing, no color change, no swelling of P and M
2	Bleeding on probing, change in color, no swelling of P and M
3	Bleeding on probing, change in color, slight swelling of P and M
4	Bleeding on probing, change in color, obvious swelling of P and M
5	Spontaneous bleeding, change in color, marked swelling with or without ulceration

Calculation: Each of the four units (M and P) is scored from 0–5. The scores are totaled and divided by four to obtain the SBI for the tooth. By totaling the scores for individual teeth and dividing by number of teeth individual SBI score is determined.

Bibliography

1. Benamghar L, Penaud J, Kaminsky P, Abt F and Martin J. Comparison of gingival index and sulcus bleeding index as indicators of perio-dontal status. Bulletin of the World Health Organization 1982;60:147–51.
2. Mühlemann H, Son S. Gingival sulcus bleeding — a leading symptom in initial gingivitis. Helv Odontol Acta 1971;15:107–13.

5.2 Papilla Bleeding Index (PBI)

It was developed by Saxer UP and Muhlemann HR in 1975. The sulcus is swept with a blunt periodontal probe and the amount of papillary bleeding is recorded 20–30 seconds after each quadrant has been probed. The amount of bleeding is scored from 1 to 4 as described in Table 5.2. The PBI is the average bleeding score across all papillae examined.

Calculation: Each papilla is scored according to the criteria. The scores are totaled and divided by the number of papilla examined to obtain individual score.

Table 5.2: Criteria for PBI

Score	Criteria
0	No bleeding after probing
1	A single discreet bleeding point appears after probing
2	Several isolated bleeding points or a single fine line of blood appears
3	Inter-dental triangle fills with blood after probing
4	Profuse bleeding occurs after probing; blood flows into the gingival sulcus

Bibliography

1. Cited in Marks RG, Magnusson I, Taylor M. Clouser B, Maruniak J and Clark WB. Evaluation of reliability and reproducibility of dental indices. J Clin Periodontol 1993;20:54–8.
2. Saxer U, Turconi B, Elsässer C. Patient motivation with the papillary bleeding index. J Prev Dent 1977;4:20–22.

5.2A Modification of the PBI (Saxer et al. 1977)

Table 5.3

Score	Criteria
1	Single bleeding point 20–30 seconds after probing
2	A fine line of blood or several bleeding points
3	Blood fills interdental triangle soon after probing
4	Immediate bleeding profuse bleeding, fills interdental areas, flows over tooth and gingiva

Bibliography

1. Saxer U, Turconi B, Elsässer C. Patient motivation with the papillary bleeding index. J Prev Dent 1977;4:20–22.

5.2B Modified Papillary Bleeding Index (Barnett ML et al. 1980)

Table 5.4

Score	Criteria
0	No bleeding within 30 seconds of probing
1	Bleeding between 3 and 30 seconds of probing
2	Bleeding within 2 seconds of probing
3	Bleeding immediately after probe placement

Bibliography

1. Barnett ML Ciancio S, Mather M. The modified Papillary Bleeding Index: comparison with Gingival Index during the resolution of gingivitis. J Prev Dent 1980;6:135–8.

5.3 Bleeding Time Index

This was given by Nowicki et al. in 1981. A Michigan "0" probe was inserted in the sulcus until slight resistance was felt and the gingiva was stroked back and forth once over an area of approximately 2 mm. The probe was removed and the time for bleeding to occur was recorded. If no bleeding was recorded evident for 15 seconds, the stroking procedure was repeated and bleeding time recorded up to an additional 15 seconds. Scoring was given as per the following criteria shown in Table 5.5.

Table 5.5: Criteria for bleeding time index	
Score	Criteria
0	No bleeding within 15 seconds of twice probing (i.e. 30 seconds total time)
1	Bleeding within 6–15 seconds of second probing
2	Bleeding within 11–15 seconds of first probing or 5 seconds after second probing
3	Bleeding within 10 seconds after initial probing
4	Spontaneous bleeding occurred prior to stimulation

Bibliography

1. Nowicki D, Vogel R, Melcer S, Deasy M. The gingival bleeding time index. J Periodontol 1981;52:260–2.

5.4 Gingival Bleeding Index

It was developed by Carter HG and Barnes GP in 1974 to record the presence or absence of gingival inflammation as determined by bleeding from interproximal gingival sulci. All interproximal areas having mesial and distal sulcus component are considered to be risk areas. Each inter proximal area has two sulci which can be scored as one or scored individually. A full complement of teeth has 30 proximal areas. Areas involving third molars are not scored because of variations in arch position, access and vision. Other areas may also be classified as non-scoreable when tooth position, diastema or other factors compromise the desirable interproximal relationship.

Procedure: Unwaxed dental floss is alternately passed interproximally into the gingival sulcus on both sides of the interdental papillae. With the floss extended as far as possible towards the buccal and lingual, the floss is carried to the bottom of the sulcus. The floss is then moved in an inciso-gingival motion for one double stroke. Care is taken not to cause laceration of the papillae. A new length of clean floss is used for each interproximal unit. Bleeding is generally immediately evident in the area or on the floss, but 30 seconds are allowed for re-inspection of each segment. If bleeding is copious, the patient should rinse between segments.

The mouth is divided into six segments and flossed in the following order; upper right, upper anterior, upper left, lower left, lower anterior and lower right.

Bleeding assessment

1. No attempt is made to quantify the degree of bleeding
2. Bleeding is assessed only as present or absent

Total scoreable areas = 26 – (number of nonscoreable areas)

Gingival bleeding score = total bleeding areas

Advantages are simple and readily available armamentarium.

Good validity, reliability and sensitivity.

Bibliography

1. Carter HG, Barnes GP. The Gingival Bleeding Index. J Periodontol 1974 Nov;45(11):801–5.

5.5 Gingival Bleeding Index

This was proposed by Ainamo J and Bay I in 1975. A blunt probe is used for gentle probing of the orifice of the gingival crevice. No pain should be caused by the probing. If bleeding occurs within 10 seconds after probing, a positive finding is recorded. The number of positive findings is then expressed as percentage of the number of gingival margins examined.

Bibliography

1. Ainamo J, Bay I. Problems and proposals for recording gingivitis and plaque. International Dental Journal 1975;24:229–35.

5.6 Periodontal Pocket Bleeding Index

van der Veiden U proposed a new index for assessment of bleeding using a constant pressure of 0.75N. The criteria were: 0 = no bleeding of the pocket after probing with a force of 0.75N, 1-bleeding of the pocket within 30 sec after probing with a force of 0.75N.

Bibliography

1. van der Veiden U. Probing force and the relationship of the probe tip to the periodontal tissues. J Clin Periodontol 1979;6:106–114.

5.7 Modified Sulcular Bleeding Index

It was developed by A Mombelli, MA van Oosten, E Schürch Jr and NP Land in 1987 to determine the severity of gingival bleeding. It is also known as modified sulcus bleeding index (mSBI).

Method: Periodontal probe is passed along the gingival margin to provoke bleeding and clinical findings are recorded according to the following criteria (Table 5.6).

Table 5.6: Criteria for mSBI

Score	Criteria
0	No bleeding when a periodontal probe is passed along the gingival margin
1	Isolated bleeding spots visible
2	Blood forms confluent red line on margin
3	Heavy or profuse bleeding

Bibliography

1. Mombelli A, van Oosten MAC, Schürch E, Lang NP. The microbiota associated with successful or failing implants. Oral Microbiol Immunol 1987;2:145–151.

5.8 Eastman Interdental Bleeding Index (EIBI)

It was developed by Abrams K, Caton J and Polson A in 1984 to assess the inflammation in the interdental area through the presence or absence of bleeding. A triangular wooden interdental cleaner is used which is gently inserted into each interdental area and removed quickly in such a way to depress the papilla about 1–2 mm. The path of insertion is parallel to occlusal surface taking care not angle the point apically. The insertion is done four times and then moved to the next proximal area. Bleeding should be recorded within 15 seconds. No. of bleeding sites is totaled.

EIBI = number of bleeding areas × 100 / total number of areas examined.

Bibliography

1. Caton J, Polson A. The Interdental Bleeding index. The Compendium of Continuing Education in Dentistry (1985) 6,88–92.

5.9 The Bleeding Index (BI) of Edwards

Edwards developed a Bleeding Index (BI) for measuring the mesial and distal interproximal sulcus health of 6 designated teeth (16, 21, 24, 36, 41 and 44) based on their tendency to bleed after a standard stimulus. Monitoring the index over time can help determine if a plaque control program is effective. Both the mesial and distal interproximal sulcus of each selected tooth is tested, for a total of 12 sites (6 × 2).

Method: Dental tape is placed against the tooth surface in a buccolingual manner and inserted to the base of the intersulcular gingival crevice. An apical-coronal movement is made with tape twice. The tape is then removed and the site is observed for 15 seconds for onset of bleeding (Table 5.7).

Table 5.7: Criteria for bleeding index

Status at end of 15 seconds	Points
No bleeding	0
Bleeding	1

Bibliography

1. Edwards RC. Bleeding index— a new indicator in personal plaque control. J Am Soc Prev Dent. 1975;5:20–37.

5.10 Gingival Status Index

It was developed by Hancock EB, Cray RJ and O Leary TJ in 1979.

Method: The gingival status of the facial surfaces of the teeth are recorded. Each area is evaluated for edema, retractibility and bleeding tendency following probing, using a university of Michigan 0 probe, and were assigned scores according to the following score (Table 5.8).

Bibliography

1. Hancock EB, Cray RJ, O'Leary TJ. The Relationship Between Gingival Crevicular Fluid and Gingival Inflammation A Clinical and Histologie Study. J Periodontol. 1979;50:13–19.

5.11 Papillary Bleeding Score

It was developed by Walter J Loesche in1979. A wooden interdental cleanser (stim-u-dent) is inserted inter-proximally on all papillae anterior to the second molars. The gingival bleeding from these inter-proximal areas are noted. The readings from the buccal and lingual gingival margins are omitted as these sites are rarely involved in the initial stages of gingivitis, and low scores derived from them in most clinical scoring systems dilute the more meaningful data that can be obtained from the data.

The PBS expands the score 2 of the gingival index by Loe and Silness, into three easily recognised clinical conditions, thereby increasing the sensitivity of the clinical observations concerned with gingival bleeding (Table 5.9).

Bibliography

1. Loesche W. Clinical and microbiological aspects of chemotherapeutic agents used according to the specific plaque hypothesis. J Dent Res 1979;58:2404–12."

Table 5.8: Criteria for gingival status index

Score	Classification	Criteria
0	Healthy	No bleeding probing. Tissues firm and slightly adapted to tooth
1	Slight gingivitis	Delayed bleeding on probing after 10 seconds but within 30 seconds. Slight edema or slight retractability present
2	Moderate gingivitis	Bleeding on probing within 10 sec but not continuous bleeding. Slight to moderate edema and retractability present
3	Severe gingivitis	Immediate and continuous bleeding or tendency to spontaneous bleeding. The tissue is edematous and easily retractable with air

Table 5.9: Criteria for papillary bleeding score

PBS = 0	Healthy gingiva; no bleeding upon insertion of stim-u-dent inter-proximally	GI = 0
PBS = 1	Edematous, reddened gingiva; no bleeding upon insertion of stim-u-dent inter-proximally	GI=1
PBS = 2	Bleeding without flow upon insertion of stim-u-dent inter-proximally	GI=2
PBS=3	Bleeding with flow along gingival margin upon insertion of stim-u-dent inter-proximally	GI=2
PBS = 4	Copious bleeding upon insertion of stim-u-dent inter-proximally	GI=2
PBS = 5	Severe inflammation, marked redness and edema; tendency to spontaneous bleeding	GI=3

5.12 Quantitative Gingival Bleeding Index

It was developed by Garg S and Kapoor KK in 1985. This index takes into consideration, the magnitude of blood stains covering toothbrush bristles on brushing and squeezing gingival tissue units in a segment. Only one score is assigned for entire one segment (canine to canine, or left or right premolars and molars in maxillary and mandibular arches), (six segments in all).

Bleeding is generally evident on the bristles of the brush; however 30 seconds were allowed for reinspection of the each segment. This index has good reproducibility, reliability, objectivity, simplicity of use, recording instrument is very simple and recording is helpful as a part of treatment, instead of unneccessary hurting the already inflammed and tensed tissue as according to other recodring systems.

Table 5.10: Criteria for quantitative gingival bleeding index

Score	Criteria
0	No bleeding on brushing; bristles free from blood stains
1	Slight bleeding on brushing; bristle tips stained with blood
2	Moderate bleeding on brushing; about half of bristle length from tip, downwards stained with blood
3	Severe bleeding on brushing, entire bristle length of all bristles including head covered with blood

Bibliography

1. Garg S, Kapoor KK. The quantitative bleeding index. J Indian Dent Assoc 1985;57:112–3.

5.13 Bleeding and Inflammation Index

Bleeding tendency was assessed after air drying by inserting the probe into the gingival crevice to a depth of approximately 1 mm and moving it around the crevice, at an angle of approximately 60° to the long axis of the tooth, stroking the inner surface of the sulcular epithelium. Bleeding detected within 30s of probing was recorded. A score of 1 or 0 was assigned according to Loe (1967) to define a score of 1. A further score of 1 or 0 was assigned according to whether the site exhibited bleeding on probing. By collecting data in this way, two indices could be formed to express the state of gingival health. The data was combined to form a version of the gingival index (GI) and an inflammation index (II).

The difference between the indices was that, in the Inflammation Index, sites which bled on probing but were without visual symptoms of inflammation were considered to be inflamed. The gingival index created was a simplified version of the original (Loe H, 1967), being weighted towards bleeding tendency between scores 1 and 2. The clinical assessments were performed on the mesial, buccal, distal and lingual aspects.

The presence or absence of erythema and bleeding tendency were recorded separately and were recombined to form two indices by which gingival health could be expressed. Inspection of the data clearly revealed that the "gingival index" in comparison with the Inflammation Index would have underestimated the severity of gingivitis by overestimating the proportion of "healthy" sites.

Bibliography

1. Saxton C, van der Ouderara FGJ. The effect of a dentifrice containing zinc citrate & triclosan on developing gingivitis. J Perio Res 1989 24: 75.

5.14 Parallel and Angulated Bleeding Index

Based on the differences in the angulation of the probe in relation to the tooth surface, 2 variations were proposed to assess by van der Weijden for bleeding assessment (Fig. 5.1).

Parallel bleeding index (ParBI): In this technique, the probe is run along the marginal gingiva and is held parallel to the longitudinal axis of the tooth (van der Weijden, 1993).

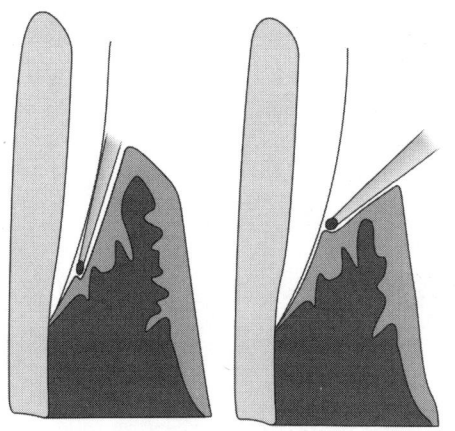

Parallel bleeding index   Angulated bleeding index

Fig. 5.1: Parallel and angulated bleeding index

Angulated bleeding index (AngBI): In this technique, the probe is run along the marginal gingiva and it is held at an angle of approximately 60° to the longitudinal axis of the tooth (van der Weijden, 1993, Saxton & van der Ouderaa, 1989).

Bibliography

1. van der Weijden GA, Timmerman MF, Nijboer A, Reijerse E, van der Velden U. Comparison of different approaches to assess bleeding on probing as indicators of gingivitis. J Clin Periodontol 1994:21:589–94.

5.15 Bleeding on Interdental Brushing Index

Hofer et al. 2011 developed the bleeding on interdental brushing index. This index is scored by passing through a light interdental brush placed buccally, just under the contact point and guided between the teeth with a jiggling motion, taking care not to exert force. If the brush met any resistance, a smaller brush was substituted and the insertion procedure is repeated. Bleeding was scored as either present or absent, for each interdental site within each quadrant after 30s. The advantages of using an interdental brush to test for bleeding include atraumatic manipulation of the papilla, ease of application, integration into existing oral hygiene instruction and motivating patients to monitor their own progress at home, while at the same time performing a beneficial oral hygiene procedure and removing any interdental plaque that may be present.

Bibliography

1. Hofer D, Sahrmann P, Attin T, Schmidlin PR. Comparison of marginal bleeding using a periodontal probe or an interdental brush as indicators of gingivitis. Int J Dent Hygiene 2011; 9:211–5.

6

Indices used for Assessment of Plaque

Dental plaque is an essential precursor of the two main oral diseases, dental caries and periodontal disease. Plaque indices were developed originally for the use in epidemiological studies correlating local factors to periodontal disease. The epidemiological indices (Ramfjord, 1959) were characterized mainly by their simple scoring criteria; the maximum score for evaluating the total smooth tooth surface for plaque coverage was usually 3, with very little or no attempt at all to concentrate on the gingival or proximal plaque.

Once the association between oral hygiene and periodontal disease had been demonstrated epidemiologically, an increasing interest in experimental research and clinical trials developed. In most cases the objective of such trials was to evaluate various oral hygiene measures. Therefore more sensitive indices which discriminate between high and low plaque scores were required. Increasing the sensitivity or the discriminatory power of plaque indices has been accomplished mainly by increasing the number of scores and emphasizing the gingival and/or the embrasure areas of the surface by giving those sites the highest scores.

This led to the development of more sensitive indices which include: a maximum score of 5, of which 3 were given to the gingival third (Quigley and Hein, 1962); a score of 7, of which 5 were given to the gingival third (Bastiaan, 1984); a score of 9, of which 6 were given to the gingival third (Grossman and Fedi, 1973); a score of 15, all of them at the gingival and proximal areas (Benson et al., 1993), and finally a score of 25, of which 24 were given to the proximal and gingival borders of the surface (Fischman et al., 1987). The following section provides a collection of various plaque indices which will guide the researcher/clinician in choosing the best index to achieve the desired objectives.

6.1 Plaque Index

It is developed by Silness and Löe in 1964. Plaque index is unique because it assesses only the thickness of plaque at the gingival area of the tooth and ignores the coronal extent of plaque.

Method

Six index teeth selected were 16, 12, 24, 36, 32, 44. Only the plaque of cervical third of the tooth is evaluated with no attention to plaque that has extended to the middle or occlusal thirds. Prior to examination the gingivae and the teeth were dried by a blast of air. No cotton was used in order not to interfere with the soft deposits. For the assessment of plaque it was found that running an explorer along the surfaces of the teeth both supra and subgingivally gave better results than the use of disclosing solution and was, therefore, the method of choice. Surfaces examined were distal, facial, mesial and lingual surface using the criteria described below.

Table 6.1: Criteria for plaque index

Score	Criteria
0	No plaque
1	A film of plaque adhering to the free gingival margin and adjacent area of tooth. The plaque may be seen in situ only after application of disclosing solution or by using probe on tooth surface
2	Moderate accumulation of soft deposits within the gingival pocket, or the tooth and gingival margin which can be seen with the naked eye
3	Abundance of soft matter within the gingival pocket and/or on the tooth and gingival margin

Calculation: Each of the four surfaces of the teeth (buccal, lingual, mesial and distal) is given a score from 0–3, the plaque index for the area. The scores from the four areas of the tooth are added and divided by four in order to give the plaque or calculus index for the tooth (Table 6.1). The indices for the teeth (incisors, premolars and molars) may be grouped to designate the index for the group of teeth. By adding the indices for the teeth and dividing by six the index for the patient is obtained. The index for the patient is thus an average score of the number of areas examined.

Limitation: Subjective interpretation in estimating the plaque which can be overcomed by performing measurements by single trained examiner throughout.

Bibliography

1. Silness J, Löe H. Periodontal Disease in Pregnancy II. Correlation between oral hygiene and periodontal condition. Acta Odontologica Scandinavica 1964;22:121–35.

6.1A Modification of Plaque Index

Löe H, in 1967 described plaque and gingival index in detail. A typical examination of all surfaces of all teeth usually starts with the right upper second molar, is continued over the midline to the upper left second molar. On the teeth of the right side the sequence will be: distal surface, buccal surface, mesial surface and on those of the left side: mesial surface, buccal surface and distal surface. When these three surfaces of all teeth have been assessed, the palatal surfaces of all maxillary teeth are assessed beginning with the upper left second molar. Examination of the lower jaw starts with the lower left second molar and is carried through to the lower right second molar. On the teeth of the left side the sequence will be: distal surface, buccal surface, mesial surface and on those of the right side: mesial surface, buccal surface and distal surface. Finally, all lingual surfaces are scored beginning with the lower left second molar. It may be used as all surfaces of all or selected teeth, or for selected areas of all or selected teeth.

Thus, the plaque index scores consider only differences as to thickness of the soft deposit in the gingival area of the tooth surfaces, and no attention is paid to the coronal extension of the plaque. The assessment of plaque is made on top of calculus deposits, on fillings and crowns. When both GI and PI are to be used, assessment of PI should always precede that of GI.

The method involved in PI relies on estimated measurements of plaque and may be used on a whole mouth or selected mouth basis. It has been applied to studies in children as well as adults and is a reliable technique for evaluating both mechanical antiplaque procedures and chemical agents.

Table 6.2: Grades for plaque index

Average PI	Score
Excellent	0
Good	0.1–0.9
Fair	1.0–1.9
Poor	2.0–3.0

Bibliography

1. Löe H. The gingival index, the plaque index and the retention index systems. J Periodontol 1967;38:610.

6.1B van der Weijden GA et al (1993)

Introduced a modification for Silness and Löe (1964) plaque index (MSLPI). 6 surfaces of each tooth were scored: the buccal and lingual surfaces and the mesial and distal surfaces examined from both the buccal and lingual aspect. The index system was slightly modified to increase the weight upon the interproximal surfaces.

Bibliography

1. van der Weijden GA, Danser MM, Nijboer A, Timmerman MF, van der Velden U. The plaque removing efficacy of an oscillating/rotating toothbrush. A short-term study. J Clin Periodontol 1993;20:273–8.

6.2 Quigley-Hein Index

Quigley G and Hein J in 1962 reported a plaque measurement that focused on gingival third. They examined only the gingival third of facial surfaces of anterior teeth using basic fuschin mouth wash as a disclosing agent. Numerical scoring system of 0–5 was used as shown in Table 6.3 and Fig. 6.1.

6.2A Turesky S, Gilmore ND and Glickman I in 1970 Modified the Quigley-Hein Index

➢ By adding labial/buccal and lingual surfaces
➢ By redefining the scores, estimate the area of tooth covered by plaque

This technique of scoring plaque on the labial, buccal and lingual surfaces provides a comprehensive method for evaluating anti-plaque procedures such as tooth brushing and flossing, as well as chemical anti-plaque agents.

Calculation

Index = Total score/the no. of surfaces examined

Table 6.3: Scoring criteria for Quigley-Hein index

Score	Criteria
0	No plaque
1	Separate flecks of plaque at the cervical margin
2	A thin continuous band of plaque (up to 1 mm) at the cervical margin
3	A band of plaque wider than 1 mm but covering less than 1/3rd of crown
4	Plaque covering at least 1/3rd but less than 2/3rds of the crown
5	Plaque covering 2/3rds or more of the crown surface

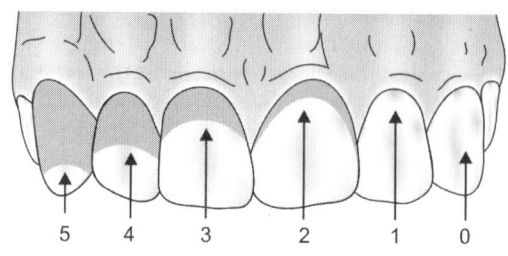

Plaque

Fig. 6.1

Bibliography

1. Fischman SL. Current status of indices of plaque. J Clin Periodontol 1986;13:371–4.
2. Turesky S, Gilmore ND, Glickman I. Reduced plaque formation by the chloromethyl analogue of Victamine C. J Periodontol 1970;41:41–3.
3. Quigley GA, Hein JW. Comparative cleansing efficiency of manual and power brushing. J Am Dent Assoc 1962;65:26–9.

6.2B Bastiaan Modification of Quigley and Hein Plaque Index

Bastiaan slightly modified the Quigley and Hein plaque index (Table 6.4).

Bibliography

1. Bastiaan RJ. Comparison of the clinical effectiveness of a single and a double headed toothbrush. Journal of Clin Periodontol 1984;11:331–9.

6.2C Shaver and Schiff Modification of Quigley and Hein Plaque index (1970)

Plaque was disclosed using disclosing agent (FD and C red no 3). The stained area was

Table 6.4: Criteria for Bastiaan modification

Score	Criteria
0	No plaque
1	Separate flecks of plaque at the cervical margins of the tooth.
2	Plaque 1 mm in width on either the mesial, cervical or distal margin.
3	Plaque up to 1 mm in width on either the mesial and distal or mesial and cervical or cervical and distal margins.
4	Plaque up to 1 mm in width in a continuous band from the mesial to the distal margin.
5	A band of cervical plaque wider than 1 mm but covering less than 1/3rd of the crown.
6	Plaque covering at least 1/3rd but less than 2/3rd of the crown.
7	Plaque covering 2/3rd or more of the crown

numerically estimated by a scoring procedure which allowed a maximum number of 12 per tooth. Each tooth was evaluated as three vertical segments (Table 6.5).

Table 6.5: Criteria for Shaver and Schiff modification

Score	Criteria
1	A trace of deposit
2	Deposit falling within the gingival quarter of the segment
3	Deposit falling within the gingival half of the segment
4	Deposit extending into the incisal half of the segment

The buccal surfaces of all the existing teeth from the first molar forward in all four quadrants were scored for a possible maximum score of 288 (Table 6.6).

Bibliography

1. Shaver KJ, Schiff T. Oral clinical functionality of enzyme AP used as a mouthwash. J Periodontology 1970;41:333–6.

6.2D McCracken Modification of Quigley-Hein Index

Dental plaque was disclosed and scored using a WHO probe (Fig. 6.2) and the following modification of the original Quigley and Hein (1962) index.

Table 6.6: Criteria for the Mc Cracken modification

Score	Criteria
0	No sub- or supragingival plaque present
1	No supragingival deposits; subgingival plaque after sweeping ball tip along subgingival surface
2	Discrete deposits of supragingival plaque laterally along surface at the gingival margin
3	Continuous deposits of supragingival plaque extending less than 3 mm from the free gingival margin
4	Supragingival plaque extending coronally beyond 3 mm from the free gingival margin
5	Supragingival plaque extending coronally beyond 5 mm from the free gingival margin, or extending to the occlusal surface/marginal ridge irrespective of the height from the gingival margin.

Plaque was recorded on 6 surfaces (mesio-buccal, mesiolingual, buccal, lingual, disto-buccal, distolingual) of all teeth and a full mouth score calculated for each subject.

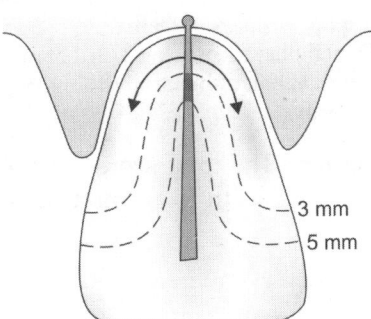

Fig. 6.2: Modified version of the original Quigley and Hein (1962) plaque index. The WHO probe is placed perpendicular to the free gingival margin with the ball tip being just subgingival. The edges of the black band therefore denotes boundaries at 3 and 5 mm from the gingival margin as the probe is swept around the tooth's circumference. When no supragingival plaque is evident the ball tip is swept subgingivally at the site to identify subgingival deposits

Bibliography

1. McCracken GI, Heasman L, Stacey F, Steen N, de Jager M, Heasman PA. Testing the efficacy of 2 prototype brush heads for a powered toothbrush: refining the model. J Clin Periodontol 2002; 29: 42–7.

6.3 Shick and Ash Modification of Plaque Criteria

The original criteria of the plaque component of PDI index of Ramfjord's were modified by Shick RA and Ash MM (1961).

Method: It consists of examining six selected tooth by excluding consideration of interproximal areas of the teeth and restricting the scoring plaque to the gingival half of the facial and lingual surfaces of the 6 index teeth (Ramfjord's teeth).

Table 6.7: Criteria for Shick and Ash modification of plaque index

Code	Criteria
0	Absence of dental plaque
1	Dental plaque in the interproximal areas or at the gingival margin covering less than 1/3rd of the gingival half of the facial or lingual surface
2	Dental plaque covering more than 1/3rd but less than 2/3rd of gingival half of facial or lingual surfaces of teeth
3	Dental plaque covering 2/3rd or more of the gingival half of he facial or lingual surfaces of teeth

Calculation: The total score is divided by the number of teeth examined to derive a mean score.

Bibliography

1. Fischman SL. Current status of indices of plaque. J Clin Periodontol 1986;13:371–374.
2. Shick RA, Ash MM. Evaluation of the vertical method of toothbrushing. J Periodontol 32: 46, 1961.

6.4 Global Plaque Index

It is the index which evaluates the extent of erythrosin-stained deposits in 5% increments (0–100%) on the facial and lingual surfaces of the teeth. This index scores plaque on the total visible tooth surface and has proven more sensitive than the Turesky et al modification of the Quigley and Hein and less fatiguing (and less error prone) than the Shaver and Schiff modification. It also offers the advantage of relating directly to the amount of plaque present or removed rather than relating it to a subjective, unitless score. Its disadvantage is that it does not specify the location of plaque. This estimate gives a reading equivalent to a 21 point scale and it is more sensitive than often used 4 point scale.

The facial and lingual surfaces of all teeth except third molars were evaluated for plaque coverage. This index has the advantage of being able to evaluate small disperse and unconnected areas of plaque (Fig. 6.3).

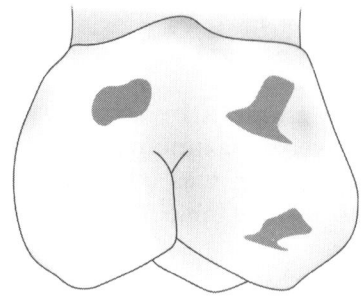

Fig. 6.3: Disperse plaque areas on facial and lingual surfaces are scored as a percent of total surface area covered in 5% increments from 0 to 95%

Bibliography

1. Meckel AH. Plaque grading in human clinical tests (abstract 662). Journal of Dental Researeh 1973;52, 224.
2. Finkelstein P, Grossman E. The clinical quantitative assessment of the mechanical cleaning efficiency of tooth brushes. Clin Prevent Dent 1984;5;7–12.
3. BJ Benson, G Henyon, E Grossman, S Mankodi, NC Sharma. Development and Verification of the Proximal/Marginal Plaque Index. J Clin Dent 1993;4:14–20.

6.5 Navy Plaque Index

It was developed by Elliot JR et al. 1972.

Method: It is obtained by scoring the amount of plaque in six index teeth by using a disclosing agent.

Teeth examined: 16, 21, 24, 36, 41, and 44.

Each tooth surface is divided horizontally into a gingival, middle and incisal third. The gingival third is further divided horizontally, following the scalloped shape of the gingiva, into two halves. The lower half is immediately adjacent to the gingiva and does not exceed 1 mm in width. Both of the gingival halves are divided longitudinally into distal and mesial thirds. The middle third (horizontally) of the tooth is divided into a distal half and a mesial half, and the incisal third is coronal to the contact area and is not subdivided (Fig. 6.4).

This approach emphasizes the gingival 2/3rd of the tooth, with the gingival 3rd weighted twice as heavily (i.e. the plaque in the closest proximity to the gingival tissues is weighted more heavily because of its importance).

Calculation: The average total of all the nine subdivisions scores per tooth.

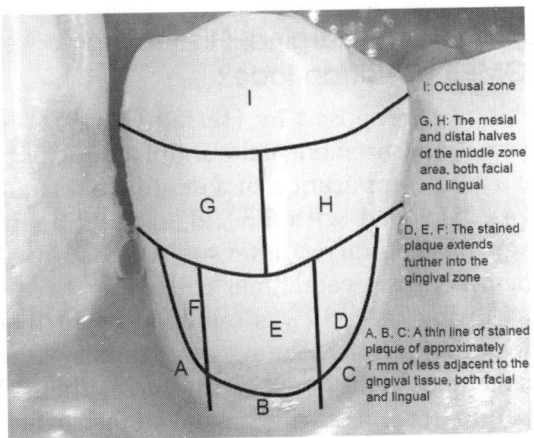

Fig. 6.4: Navy plaque index

Bibliography

1. Elliot JR, Bowers GM, Clemmer BA, Rovelstad GH. Evaluation of an oral physiotherapy center in the reduction of bacterial plaque and periodontal disease. J Periodontol 1972;43:221–4.
2. Fischman SL. Current status of indices of plaque. J Clin Periodontol 1986;13:371–4.

6.5A Rustogi Modification of Navy Plaque Index (1992)

Areas F and D were called as interproximal. Also the parts of I, H, G, C and A also contain parts of the proximal and interproximal areas, also, there was no occlusal embrasure and therefore no proximal surface above the contact. Both Navy index and Rustogi modifications have the additional problem in that they require an examiner to visually divide a facial or lingual surface into 9 parts (18 areas per tooth) with a score for each part. It is difficult to reproducibly divide a tooth into 9 areas, thereby might result in scoring errors (Fig. 6.5).

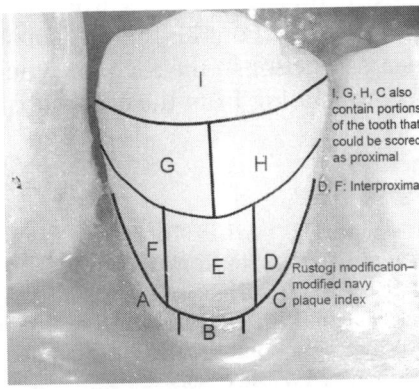

Fig. 6.5: Rustogi modification of navy plaque index

6.5B Modified Navy Plaque Index

It was developed by Grossman FD and Fedi PF to assess the plaque control status among naval personnel's and to measure any subsequent changes.

Method: It is obtained by scoring the amount of plaque in six index teeth by using a disclosing agent.

Teeth examined: 16, 21, 24, 36, 41, and 44

Facial and lingual surfaces are divided into three areas namely gingival area (G), mesial-proximal area (M) and distalproximal area (D). These areas are apical to an imaginary line connecting the contact area or height of contour depending on the presence or absence of adjacent teeth. The stained plaque in contact with the gingiva is scored as follows:

- Area M = 3
- Area G = 2
- Area D = 3

When plaque is found not in contact with gingival tissue but is found on any tooth surface, one point is added to the facial or lingual surface.

Calculation of the index: Highest score for any of the 6 teeth is the patient's NPI score. Scores of all teeth are added to give total NPI score.

Rules: If the designate tooth is missing, strike through indicated number and insert substitute tooth number beside it. If 16, 24, 36 or 44 were missing, substitute the next posterior tooth. If 21 or 41 is missing substitute with nearest incisor in the arch, or where all incisors are missing from the arch, substitute a cuspid.

Bibliography

1. Grossman FD, Fedi PF Jr. Navy Periodontal Screening Examination. J Am Soc Prevent Dentistry. 1974; 3: 41–5.
2. Hancock EB, Wirthlin MR Jr. An evaluation of the Navy periodontal screening examination. J Periodontol 1977;48:63–6.

6.6 Plaque Control Record

This was proposed by O'leary TJ, Drake RB and Naylor JE in 1972 to give the dental therapist, dental hygienist, or dental educator a simple method of recording the presence of plaque on individual tooth surfaces (mesial, distal, facial, lingual). The form also allows the patient to visualize his own progress in learning plaque control. This seems to have a motivating effect on patients.

At the initial control appointment a suitable disclosing solution such as Bismarck Brown is painted on all exposed tooth surfaces. After the patient has rinsed, the operator, using an explorer or the tip of a probe, examines each stained surface for soft accumulations at the dentogingival junction. When found, they were recorded by making a dash in the appropriate spaces in the record form. Those surfaces which have soft accumulations not at the dentogingival junction were not recorded. No attempt was made to differentiate between varying amounts of plaque on the tooth surfaces. Scoring the extent of accumulations require more decision making, prolongs the procedure and does not add appreciably to its clinical use. After all teeth were examined and scored, an index can be derived by dividing the number of plaque containing surfaces by the total number of available surfaces, the same procedure is carries out at subsequent appointments to determine the patient's progress in learning and carrying out the recommended procedures. The goal of such training procedures is to reduce plaque accumulations until they are found on 10% or less of the available tooth surfaces.

Bibliography

1. O'leary TJ, Drake RB, Naylor JE. Plaque Control Record. J Periodontol 1972;43:38–40.

6.7 Gingival Marginal Plaque Index (GMPI) or Harrap Index

This was proposed by Harrap GJ (1974) to permit measurement of the antiplaque activity of a single application of a dentifrice. Plaque was disclosed with 0.5% disclosing agent (aqueous neutral red) after subjects had rinsed their mouths several times with water. Excess disclosing reagent was removed by further rinsing with water. The examiner estimates the percentage of the length of the buccal gingival margin in contact with plaque on the surface of each tooth. The projection of the plaque on the lingual surface of the tooth and the thickness of the plaque were not considered. The buccal gingival margin was taken to extend into the interproximal region as far as could be seen when the adjacent teeth were in close proximity. When the next tooth was missing the measurement was made to the midpoint of the mesial (or distal) surface of the tooth. For high and low values of plaque (< 30 and > 70), the estimate was to the nearest 5. In the middle range the estimate was to the nearest 10. All teeth except the second and third molars in each quadrant were scored.

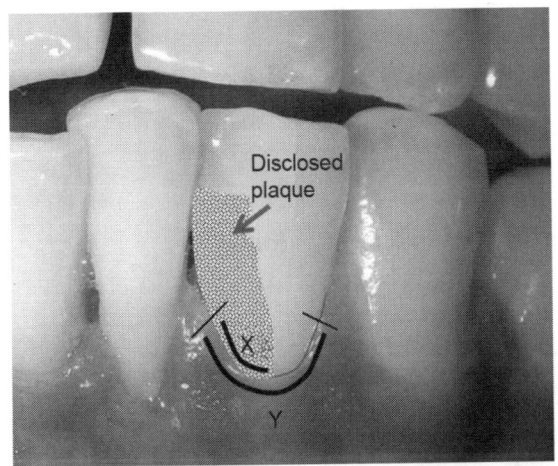

Fig. 6.6: Plaque score = (x/y)×100

Example of plaque scoring by the gingival margin plaque index. Gingival margin adjacent to disclosed dental plaque is expressed as percentage of the actual gingival margin distance

Results for each tooth were averaged to give a plaque score for the whole mouth (Fig. 6.6).

Bibliography

1. Harrap GJ. Assessment of the effect of dentifrices on the growth of dental plaque. J Clin Periodontol 1974;1:166–74.

6.8 Plaque Formation Rate Index

The plaque formation rate index (PFRI) of Axelsson describes the accumulation of dental plaque at 24 hours after a professional dental cleaning. This index can help identify patients at increased risk for caries, as described in Table 6.8.

Procedure

1. The teeth are cleaned by a professional dental hygienist.
2. The patient does not brush or clean the teeth for the next 24 hours.
3. 24 hours after the cleaning the teeth are examined for adherent plaque.

Surfaces examined on each tooth were mesiobuccal, buccal, distobuccal, mesiolingual, lingual and distolingual.

Calculation of PFRI = (total number of surfaces showing plaque) / [(number of teeth examined)× (6 surfaces examined)] × 100%

Table 6.8: Interpretation		
% of surfaces affected	*Level*	*Score*
0	None	0
1 – 10	Very low	1
11 – 20	Low	2
21 – 30	Moderate	3
31 – 40	High	4
> 40	Very high	5

Reference

1. Axelsson P. Diagnosis and risk prevention of dental caries, Volume 2. Quintessence Publishing Co, Inc. 2000. PP 7–9, 34–36.

6.9 Visible Plaque Index

This was proposed by Ainamo and Bay in 1975. The occurrence of clearly visible plaque on the mesial, buccal, lingual surfaces of all the teeth in the right quadrants of the jaws was recommended to be recorded. The plaque to be scored should be visible beyond doubt to all the examiners and preferably to the examined patient.

Bibliography

1. Ainamo J and Bay I. Problems and proposals in recording gingivitis and plaque. Int Dent J. 1975;25:229–5.

6.10 Cervical Plaque Index

This was proposed by Schmid MO and Curilovic Z (1975) (Table 6.9 and Fig 6.7).

Table 6.9: Criteria for cervical plaque index	
Grade	*Criteria*
0	No cervical plaque
1	Thin cervical band of plaque (up to 1 mm wide)
2	Thin cervical band of plaque (over 1 mm wide)
3	Thick cervical band of plaque (up to 1 mm wide)
4	Thick cervical band of plaque (over 1 mm wide)

Cervical plaque index

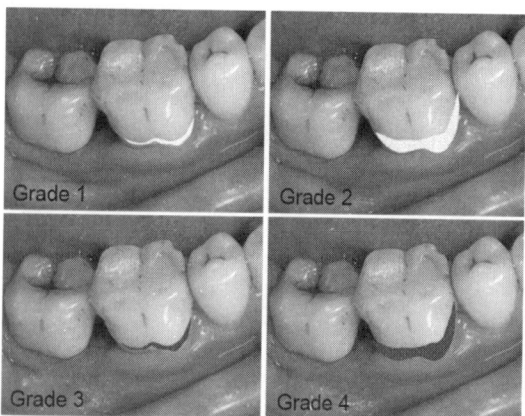

Grade 1   Grade 2
Grade 3   Grade 4

Scoring zone per tooth (1–6)

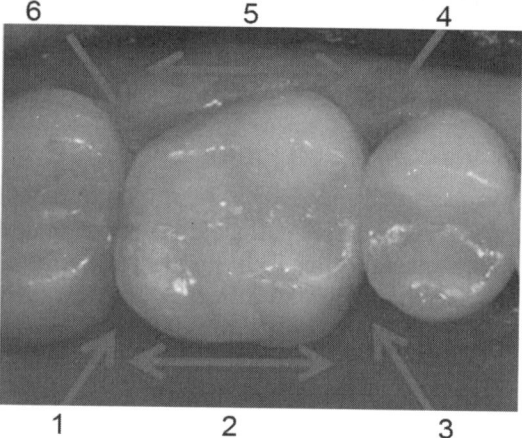

6   5   4

1   2   3

Fig. 6.7: Cervical plaque index

Table 6.10	
Code	Criteria
0	Absence of plaque
1	Plaque covering 1/3rd of the area
2	Plaque covering 2/3rd of the area
3	Plaque covering entire area

Area "R" is scored as follows:

Scoring criteria for proximal areas:

1 – presence of plaque

0 – absence of plaque

Calculation: Plaque scores can be represented as sums per tooth, per quadrant or per area of all teeth.

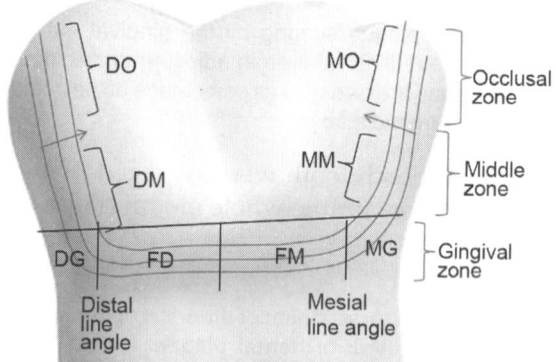

Fig. 6.8: Distal mesial plaque index

Bibliography

1. Cited in Schmid MO, Balmelli OP, Saxer UP. Plaque-removing effect of a toothbrush, dental floss, and a toothpick. J Clin Periodontol 1976;3(3):157–65.

6.11 Distal Mesial Plaque Index (DMPI)

It was described by Cancro L in 1983. DMPI places more emphasis on gingival or cervical portions as well as interproximal areas which are frequently missed by tooth brush and may be used to study the effects of the chemical agents brought to the tooth by such vehicles as paste or rinse without the interference by the mechanical action of brushing (Table 6.10 and Fig. 6.8).

Bibliography

1. Fischman S, Cancro LP, Pretara-Spanedda P and Jacobs D. Distal mesial plaque index: A technique for assessing dental plaque about the gingiva. Dental Hygiene 1987;61:404–9.
2. Fischman SL. Current status of indices of plaque. J Clin Periodontol 1986;13:371–4.

6.12 Proximal/Marginal Plaque Index (PMPI)

The facial and lingual surfaces are divided into three unequal segments. The three designated segments are: distal proximal, marginal and mesial proximal. All teeth, including the distal of the second molar are scored. For the mesial and distal areas. The surfaces scored were defined as follows: from the line angle toward the interdental area, under and above the contact area as far as visible. The surfaces scored border on the labial/buccal, lingual and incisal/occlusal embrasures. In the event that the entire interdental area is visible or there is no contact, the mid-line of the distal-mesial surface will determine the facial-lingual division. The marginal or middle segment is scored from the mesial line angle to the distal line angle, visualizing the area extending incisally/occlusally 3 mm from the marginal gingiva. Plaque in each segment is scored using the criteria described by Turesky et al (Table 6.11).

Table 6.11: Proximal/marginal plaque index (PMPI)	
Score	Criteria
0	No plaque
1	Separate flecks of plaque covering less than 1/3rd of the area
2	Discrete areas or bands of plaque covering less than 1/3rd of the area
3	Plaque covering 1/3rd of the area
4	Plaque covering more than 1/3rd but less than 2/3rd of the area
5	Plaque covering 2/3rd or more of the area

Both facial and lingual aspects of all natural teeth, excluding third molars are examined. All three areas can be scored and related as an average or these areas can be reported separately, i.e. proximal or marginal.

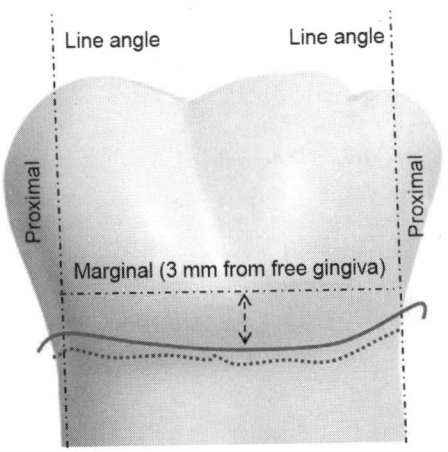

Fig. 6.9: Proximal/marginal plaque index

Bibliography

1. BJ Benson, G Henyon, E Grossman, S Mankodi, NC Sharma. Development and Verification of the Proximal/Marginal Plaque Index. J Clin Dent 1993;4:14–20.

6.13 New Method of Plaque Scoring (NMPS)

This method was devised to be simple but sensitive for use in clinical oral hygiene trials (Dababneh, 2002). The scoring system proposed for the NMPS is based on a numerical determination range from 0 to 10 representing the total stained plaque on the facial or lingual tooth surfaces, with the greatest weight of scores placed at the gingival and proximal regions of the surface. For scoring purposes, a horizontal boundary is imagined on the smooth facial or lingual tooth surfaces between the gingival third (A) and coronal two-thirds, the latter being subdivided vertically into thirds, mesial (B), middle (C) and distal (D). Depending on the extent of plaque coverage, whole number scores 0–3 are assigned to A, B and C and 0 or 1 to D (Table 6.12 and Fig 6.10).

Table 6.12: New method of plaque scoring	
Score	Criteria for zones A, B and C
0	No plaque
1	Up to one-third coverage
2	More than one-third and up to two-thirds coverage
3	More than two-thirds coverage
0/1	Absence/presence of plaque in zone D

Bibliography

1. Dababneh RH, Khouri AT, Smith RG, Addy M: A new method of plaque scoring: a laboratory comparison with other plaque indices. J Clin Periodontol 2002; 29: 832–7.
2. Dababneh RH, Khouri AT, Smith RG, Addy M. Correlation and examiner agreement between a new method of plaque scoring and a popular established plaque index, modelled in vitro. J Clin Periodontol 2002; 29: 1107–11.

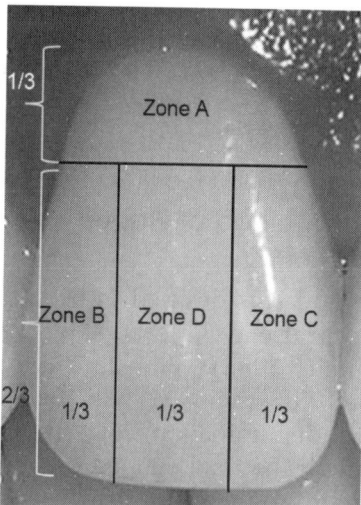

Fig. 6.10: The criteria for dividing the tooth surface according to the NMPS. Zone A: Gingival third, zone B: mesial third zone C: distal third and zone D: middle third

6.14 The Plaque Assessment Scoring System (PASS)

This was developed by Butler BL, Morejon O and Low SB. PASS allows an examiner to objectively record plaque accumulation on selected teeth in a time-efficient manner. It also records sub-gingival plaque accumulation, which is not evaluated by other indexes.

Method: To establish a PASS score, an examiner selects five teeth for examination (four first molars and one maxillary incisor). If one of these teeth is missing, then an adjacent distal tooth or, if that tooth is missing as well, a mesial tooth is considered. If no maxillary incisors are present, a mandibular incisor can be substituted. Each tooth selected is divided into four areas: mesial, distal, buccal and lingual. Using a periodontal probe, the examiner sweeps each quarter of the tooth approximately 1 mm into the sulcus to detect plaque. If plaque is visible on the probe, the surface is counted as positive for plaque accumulation. There are 20 possible plaque surfaces. The PASS score is the percentage of surfaces positive for plaque accumulation.

Bibliography

1. Butler BL, Morejon O, Low SB. An accurate time-efficient method to assess plaque accumulation. J Am Dent Assoc 1996;127:1763–6.

6.15 The Axial and Proximal Plaque Extension Indices

The axial plaque extension index (APEI) was recorded with a periodontal probe (PCP UNC 15) to measure the height of the accumulated plaque at the distal and mesial line angles and at the mid-surface of the buccal and lingual surfaces. The probe was held parallel to the long axis of the tooth. At the line angles, the height was measured, starting from the gingival margin to the contact area with the adjacent tooth. Estimates to the closest 0.5 mm were recorded.

The proximal plaque extension index (PPEI) was recorded at the mesial and distal part of the buccal and lingual tooth surfaces, starting from the gingival margin. The periodontal probe was kept parallel to an imaginary diagonal line running perpendicularly to the interdental papilla. Estimates to the closest 0.5 mm were recorded (Fig. 6.11).

Bibliography

1. Matthijs S, Moradi Sabzevar M, Adriaens PA. Intra-examiner reproducibility of 4 dental plaque indices. J Clin Periodontol 2001; 28: 250–4.

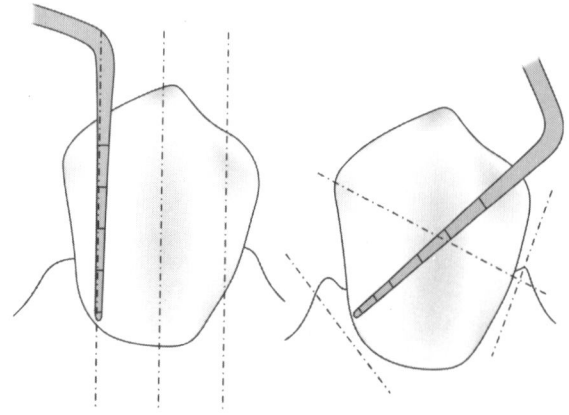

Fig. 6.11: Axial and proximal plaque extension indices

6.16 Topographic Plaque Index

Johansson et al. (2002) proposed an index to evaluate the plaque using a standard disclosing solution. The buccal surface of each maxillary anterior tooth was divided into five areas: (1) cervical, (2) mesioproximal, (3) distoproximal, (4) midbuccal, and (5) inciso-buccal, while the palatal surface was divided into three areas: (1) cervicoproximal, (2) midpalatal, and (3) incisopalatal. Each area was scored as 1 (plaque) or 0 (no plaque). Separate buccal and palatal TPI scores were calculated by adding all scores and dividing the sum by the number of teeth (i.e. 6). In this way, maximum TPI scores were 5 and 3 buccally and palatally, respectively (Fig. 6.12).

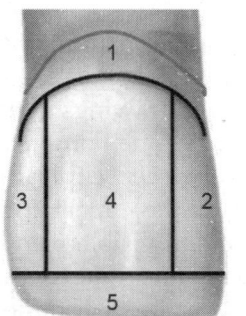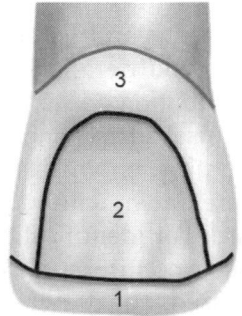

Fig. 6.12: Topographic plaque index: buccal and lingual surfaces are divided into five and three registration sites, Buccal surface: cervical, mesioproximal, distoproximal, midbuccal and incisobuccal and palatal/lingual surface: cervicoproximal, midpalatal, incisopalatal

Bibliography

1. Johansson AK, Lingstrom P, Birkhed D. Comparison of factors potentially related to the occurrence of dental erosion in high- and low-erosion groups. Eur J Oral Sci 2002; 110: 204–11.

6.17 Digital Estimation of Plaque Levels

This was developed by Aleksejuniene J, Scheie AA, Holst D.

Digital pictures were captured from right to left premolars after plaque was disclosed using a disclosing agent. The digital pictures of individuals who were lacking one or more premolars were taken to include first molars. The teeth were photographed with a Nikon camera using an artificial light from a dental unit. The camera was held perpendicular to the teeth being photographed. At the time of each clinical examination, the individual image was inspected and if necessary immediately retaken. After the image of baseline plaque levels was taken, all teeth were professionally cleaned. After a 24 h period, digital photographs were re-taken in order to obtain an estimate of the plaque formation rate. Subsequently images were analysed with the Adobe Photoshop program. The total labial tooth surface area was measured manually, using the drawing facility to outline the tooth boundaries on each image. To measure the plaque area, the 'pen tool' and 'make path' were used. Then all areas stained in red were marked and the number of pixels was recorded from the histogram option. The amount of plaque on the tooth was determined by summation of the number of plaque pixels. The number of plaque pixels was divided by the number of pixels corresponding to the total area examined and multiplied by 100. In this way, a 0% plaque score indicated an individual without plaque while a plaque score of 100% indicated an individual who had all buccal surfaces covered with plaque.

Bibliography

1. Aleksejuniene J, Scheie AA, Holst D. Inter-individual variation in the plaque formation rate of young individuals. Int J Dent Hygiene 4, 2006; 35–40.

6A Recent Advances in Computing Plaque Indices

6A.1 Planimetric Analysis of Plaque

It is a technique, usually based upon photographic images of the teeth, which can utilise an index known as the plaque percent index (PPI). The technique involves the disclosing of teeth, with subsequent photography of the tooth surfaces. These are then either traced by hand and an area calculated, or they are digitised and analysed by a computer. The use of the PPI permits plaque assessment on an interval scale, and thus permits greater resolution in the determination of plaque quantity.

6A.2 Computer-based Analysis of Dental Plaque

Staudt et al. described a computerized planimetric method. The images of the teeth were captured using a CCD-camera and specially designed positioner to ensure standardized images. A live representation of the image was available to the operator who determined when the image would be captured. A registration of the position of the camera was performed to ensure reproducible images. Using a modification of the plaque percentage index, PPI plaque area was calculated using proprietary software. In common with many other digital image techniques, the technique involves removing some colors while retaining others for measurement. With software manipulation the entire tooth area, and the tooth area without plaque were asked. These masks were then filled with new, specific colors, and the analysis software used to calculate the pixels contained within each of the areas. Plaque area was then expressed as a percentage of the total tooth area.

Other Novel Methods

Fluorescein disclosing and digital plaque image analysis (DPIA)

Plaque quantification using 3D co-ordinate data

Plaque detection with quantitative light-induced fluorescence (QLF)

Bibliography

1. Pretty IA, Edgar WM, Smith WM, Higham SM. Quantification of dental plaque in the research environment. J Dent 2005;33:193–207.

6B. Occlusal Site Specific Plaque Indices

6B.1 Plaque Assessment on Occlusal Surface of Molars

The occurrence and distribution of occlusal plaque was assessed at two levels. Visible plaque on the occlusal surface was recorded by means of the following score system as shown in Table 6.13.

Table 6.13: Criteria for occlusal site specific plaque indices

Score	Criteria
0	No visible plaque
1	Hardly detectable plaque, restricted to grooves and fossae
2	Plaque easily detectable in grooves and fossae
3	Occlusal surface partially or totally covered with heavy plaque accumulations.

The second level of plaque examination involved detailed mapping of the plaque distribution on standardized drawings of the occlusal surface morphology. The borders of the plaque, which could be seen clinically, were drawn with red ink on the morphology card. For identification of non-visible plaque on the occlusal surface, a plaque indicator can be used. The drawings of plaque distribution were transformed into numerical values as described in Table 6.14.

Table 6.14

Score	Criteria
0	No plaque
1	Thin plaque which was clinically visible only when the plaque indicator system was used
2	Thick plaque which was clinically visible.

Bibliography

1. Carvalho JC, Ekstrand KR, Thylstrup A. Dental plaque and caries on occlusal surfaces of first permanent molars in relation to stage of eruption. J Dent Res 1989;68:773–779.

6B.2 The Occlusal Fissure Plaque Index

The occlusal fissure plaque index was based on the absence or presence of disclosed plaque in the fissure pattern of premolar and molar teeth and the extension of plaque out of the fissures to cover the occlusal surface. The index is thus area based and can be scored using a numerical system with similarities to the Turesky et al (1970) modification of the Quigley and Hein (1962) plaque index. Alternatively, using schematic drawings of the occlusal surfaces for the appropriate teeth, the plaque can be recorded in units of area as described for smooth surface plaque in the Addy et al (1983) modification of the Shaw & Murray (1977) stain index (Table 6.15).

Table 6.15: The criteria for the numerical index (scored after disclosing teeth with an appropriate dye)

Score	Criteria
0	No disclosed plaque or discrete flecks in the fissure pattern
1	Line of plaque in fissure pattern but not outlining whole fissure system
2	Fissure system completely outlined by plaque
3	Plaque beginning to extend out of the fissure system at some sites with <1/3rd coverage
4	Plaque extending out of the fissure system with 1/3rd to 2/3rd of the coverage
5	Plaque extending to cover >2/3rd of the surface.

Area Index

The outline of the occlusal surface with the typical fissure pattern for upper and lower, left and right, premolars and molars was obtained from the tooth atlas (Wheeler, 1968) for the upper and lower arches. Following disclosing the clinical examiner draws an outline of the plaque as perceived onto the respective tooth grid. The area of these subjectively recorded plaque outlines is then accurately measured using a graphics tablet and pen attached to a microcomputer.

Advantages: The index could prove useful to demonstrate reduced oral function in sick or injured patients since mastication would in normal healthy individuals maintain low occlusal index scores. The occlusal surface plaque index proved easy to use, was highly repeatable and shown effective in detecting plaque removal. The index may have applications in clinical trials and depending on the restorative status of population could even be employed in epidemiological surveys.

Bibliography

1. Addy M, Renton-Harper P, Myatt G. A plaque index for occlusal surfaces and fissures. Measurement of repeatability and plaque removal. J Clin Periodontol 1998; 25: 164–8.

6B.3 Occlusal Site Specific Plaque Index

The index was designed for unrestored upper or lower premolars and molars. The occlusal surfaces are divided, by an imaginary grid, into 9 zones for molars, 6 zones for upper 1st and 2nd premolars and lower 2nd premolars and 4 zones for lower 1st premolars. Plaque within the zones was disclosed by erythrosin. The staining procedure involved air drying of surfaces followed by careful application of the erythrosin on cotton wool buds. After 3 min, the surfaces were air dried again and erythrosin reapplied. Plaque scoring was then performed as shown in Table 6.16 and Fig. 6.13.

Scoring was performed by examiners at 2.4 magnification using binocular loops.

Table 6.16: Criteria for occlusal site specific plaque index

Score	Criteria
0	0 = 0–2% coverage, stain retained by capillary action
1	1 = 3–10% coverage
2	2 = 11–33% coverage
3	3 = 34–65% coverage
4	4 = 66–100% coverage

Bibliography

1. Levinkind M, Owens J, Morea C, Addy M, Lang NP, Adair R, Baron I. The development and validation of an occlusal site-specific plaque index to evaluate the effects of cleaning by tooth brushes and chewing gum. J Clin Periodontol 1999; 26:177–82.

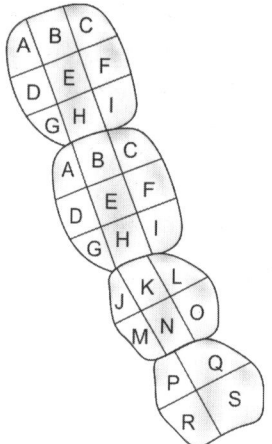

Fig. 6.13: Zones of occlusal surface

6C. Plaque Indices in Special Circumstances

6C.1 Plaque Indices for Implant Surfaces

Microbial biofilms have been shown to form on inert biomaterial surfaces in an aqueous environment. Implants placed in the oral cavity represent artificial surfaces colonized by bacteria from saliva and ecologic niches such as periodontal pockets, tonsils, and crypts of the tongue.

Several microbiologic features of the subgingival biofilm around implants have been correlated with the presence of clinically detectable plaque. Furthermore, periodontal pathogens from residual pockets of remaining teeth in patients treated for periodontal disease have been documented to colonize oral implants. Mombelli et al. modified the original plaque index introduced by Silness and Löe to assess biofilm formation in the marginal area around implants.

Lindquist and associates assessed oral hygiene levels according to a 3-point scale and reported a significant relationship between oral hygiene and peri-implant bone resorption. Therefore, it appears meaningful to monitor oral hygiene habits by quantifying plaque accumulation. The criteria for these methods are shown in Table 6.17.

Bibliography

1. Lindquist LW, Rocker B, Carlsson GE. Bone resorption around fixtures in edentulous patients treated with mandibular fixed tissue-integrated prostheses. J Prosthet Dent 1988;59:59–63.
2. Mombelli A, Van Oosten MAC, Schürch E, Lang NP. The microbiota associated with successful or failing osseointegrated titanium implants. Oral Microbiol Immunol 1987;2:145–51.

Plaque Indices for Orthodontic Subjects

Among subjects with fixed orthodontic appliances in place, the pattern of plaque accumulation is significantly affected by the presence of bonded attachments and arch wires. The suitability of routine plaque indices for bracketed orthodontic subjects must therefore be questionable. In relation to the occurrence and severity of gingivitis and periodontal disease, traditional indices may still be appropriate when orthodontic appliances are in place, but with regard to enamel decalcification, these indices are unlikely to satisfactorily reflect the pattern of plaque accumulation. Hence, special emphasis was placed on indices specially developed for plaque estimation among orthodontic population.

Score	Mombelli et al (mPI) criteria	Lindquist et al criteria
	Table 6.17: Criteria for plaque indices for implant surfaces	
0	No detection of plaque	No visible plaque
1	Plaque only recognized by running a probe across the smooth marginal surface of the implant	Local plaque accumulation
2	Plaque can be seen by the naked eye	General plaque accumulation greater than 25%
3	Abundance of soft matter	

6C.2 Plaque Along Wire Index (PLWI)

Artun proposed a system for assessment of plaque accumulation along the retainer wire in subjects wearing bonded lingual retainer following orthodontic treatment. The criteria are discussed in Table 6.18.

Table 6.18: Scoring criteria for PLWI

Score	Criteria
0	No plaque along wire.
1	No visible plaque along wire. Plaque may be recognized only by running a probe along the wire.
2	Moderate accumulation of plaque along wire. The deposit is visible to the naked eye.
3	Heavy accumulation of plaque along wire, the thickness of which fills out the niche produced by the wire and the tooth surface.

PlWI was scored both incisally and gingivally along the retainer wire in areas corresponding to all interproximal surfaces from the mesial aspect of one canine to the mesial aspect of the other canine and in areas corresponding to all lingual surfaces from canine to canine.

Bibliography

1. Artun J. Caries and periodontal reactions associated with long-term use of different types of bonded lingual retainers. Am J Orthod. 1984;86(2):112–8.

6C.3 Bonded Bracket Index (BBI)

Ciancio S, Cunat J, Mather M and Harvey DJ in 1984 developed BBI to overcome existing plaque indices that do not adequately reflect patterns of plaque accumulation over bonded and bracket teeth. They suggest this new index be used to evaluate bracket associated plaque which helps in assessing the plaque in orthodontic patients (Table 6.19).

Bibliography

1. Ciancio S, Cunat J, Mather M and Harvey DJ. A comparison of plaque accumulation in bonded vs. banded teeth (abstract 1664). Journal of Dental Research 1984;64:359.

Table 6.19: Scoring criteria for BBI

Score	Criteria
0	No plaque on bracket or tooth surface
1	Plaque on bracket only
2	Plaque on brackets and tooth, no extension to gingiva
3	Plaque on brackets and tooth, with extension to papilla
4	Plaque on brackets and tooth, with partial coverage to gingiva
5	Plaque on brackets and tooth, with full coverage to gingiva

2. Kilicoglu H, Yildirim M, Polater H. Comparison of the effectiveness of two types of toothbrushes on oral hygiene of patients undergoing orthodontic treatment with fixed appliances. Am J Orthod Dentofacial Orthop 1997;111:591–4.

6C.4 Ortho-Plaque Index

The Ortho-Plaque Index (OPI) was described by Heintze et al. Each bracketed tooth has three sites for measuring plaque: (i) cervical to the bracket toward the gingiva, (ii) the region of the "shadow" of the arch wire and mesial and distal to the bracket, and (iii) coronal to the bracket. This zoning of the tooth is very similar to zoning for the modified Silness and Loe index and similarly has much to recommend its use in orthodontic patients, because the gingival zone is appropriate for studies of gingivitis and the middle zone reflects the tendency for plaque to accumulate behind an arch wire. This index does not appear to have been used by other authors, possibly because of its relative complexity of calculation when compared, for example, with the modified Silness and Löe index.

Bibliography

1. Cited in Al-Anezi SA, Harradine NWT. Quantifying plaque during orthodontic treatment: A systematic review. Angle Orthod. 2012;82:748–53.

2. Heintze SD, Jost-Brinkmann PG, Finke C, Miethke RR. Oral Health for the Orthodontic Patient. 1st ed. Hanover Park, Ill: Quintessence Publishing Co.; 1998:67–70.

6C.5 Modification of the Silness and Loe Index

Williams et al. addressed the shortcomings of the Silness and Loe index for bracketed teeth by modifying it to take into account the pattern of plaque accumulation in orthodontic patients. In this index, the tooth is divided into mesial, distal, gingival and incisal regions in relation to the bracket. Plaque is then scored in each area based on the four codes used in the original Silness and Loe index, and values summed to obtain a total score, which can therefore range between 0 and 16 for each tooth. This index acknowledges the usual effects of orthodontic appliances on plaque distribution and has much greater categorical discrimination than the Silness and Loe index. These advantages must be viewed as substantial and as justifying discontinuation of the unmodified Silness and Loe index in orthodontic patients.

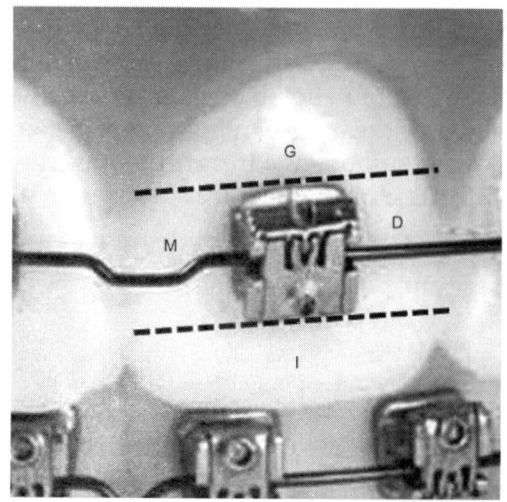

Fig. 6.14: Diagram showing modification of Silness and Löe index as described by Williams. The tooth is divided into mesial (M), distal (D), gingival (G) and incisal (I) regions for plaque measurement

Bibliography

1. Cited in Al-Anezi SA, Harradine NWT. Quantifying plaque during orthodontic treatment: A systematic review. Angle Orthod 2012;82:748–53.
2. Williams P, Clerehugh V, Worthington HV, Shaw WC. Comparison of two plaque indices for use in fixed orthodontic appliance patients. J Dent Res 1991;70:703. Abstract 276.

6C.6 Orthodontic Plaque Index

The orthodontic plaque index (OPI) was developed to accommodate the special circumstances in the evaluation of oral hygiene during orthodontic treatment. OPI helps in assessment of oral hygiene in addition to the caries and gingivitis risk of subjects using fixed orthodontic appliances. Furthermore, the OPI enables an estimation of the patient's need for prophylaxis, so that the appropriate preventive measures can be taken. Problematic oral hygiene sites can be pinpointed, and the patient's motivation to perform regular oral hygiene can be increased. The OPI visually documents the presence of plaque around the multibracket appliance by staining the teeth or surfaces with a plaque-disclosing solution (for instance, erythrosine). The evaluation includes only teeth or surfaces that bear an adhesively bonded bracket on the vestibular or oral (lingual/palatinal) aspect. Teeth bearing orthodontic bands are not included. The evaluation of the adjacent marginal gingivae for inflammation is a crucial component of the OPI and helps determine further prophylaxis need. In the clinical application of the OPI, the dentition is divided into sextants as it is for the Periodontal screening index (PSR), the successor of the community periodontal index of treatment needs (CPITN).

The degree of plaque accumulation on each aspect of the bracket base (mesial, distal, occlusal/incisal, and cervical) and the condition of the adjacent marginal gingivae are assessed. Score 0 indicates an absence of plaque and inflammation. Scores 1 to 3 refer severity of plaque deposits in the bracket vicinity and score 4 includes the inflammation status of the gingiva (Table 6.20).

The highest score found per sextant is recorded for that sextant. In addition, the highest

Table 6.20: Criteria for OPI	
Score	Criteria
0	No plaque deposits on the tooth surfaces surrounding the bracket base
1	Plaque deposits on one tooth surface at the bracket base
2	Plaque deposits on two tooth surfaces at the bracket base
3	Plaque deposits on three tooth surfaces at the bracket base
4	Plaque deposits on four tooth surfaces at the bracket base and/or gingival inflammation indicators (plaque deposits near the gingiva do not necessarily have to be present)

score per sextant represents the score for the dentition. The highest score of all sextants determines the current oral hygiene situation and identifies the patient's need for prophylactic treatment. An increased risk of caries and gingivitis is assumed as of score 3. The OPI can be used for both vestibular end lingual multibracket appliances. Depending on bracket placement, the index takes into consideration only the vestibular or lingual/palatal tooth surfaces. For this reason, the OPI is ideal for diagnostic application during the fixed treatment phase.

Bibliography

1. Beberhold K, Sachse-Kulp A, Schwestka-Polly R, Hornecker E, Ziebolz D. The Orthodontic Plaque Index: an oral hygiene index for patients with multibracket appliances. Orthodontics (Chic.) 2012;13:94–9.

6D. Indices for Denture Plaque Assessment and Cleanliness

6D.1 Budtz-Jorgensen E and Bertram U

Budtz-Jorgensen E and Bertram U proposed a method for examination of the denture cleanliness using a plaque detector to disclose the plaque on the fitting surface of the maxillary denture (Proflavine-monosulfate in 3% aqueous solution). According to the quantity of plaque on the denture base the patients could be divided into three groups

using the following index of denture cleanliness (Table 6.21).

Table 6.21	
Score	Criteria
Excellent	None or only few spots of plaque.
Fair	More extended plaque, less than half of the denture base covered by plaque
Poor	More than half of the denture base covered by plaque.

Bibliography

1. Budtz-Jorgensen E and Bertram U. Denture Stomatitis. I. The etiology in relation to trauma and infection. Acta Odontol Scand 1970;28:71–92.

6D.2 Budtz-Jorgensen E and Knudsen AM

Budtz-Jorgensen E and Knudsen AM proposed a classification for denture cleanliness of the fitting surface of the maxillary denture using a plaque detector (0.3% aqueous solution of proflavine monosulfate) and the denture was photographed. The amount of denture plaque was graded as showin in Table 6.22.

Table 6.22	
Code	Criteria
0	None visible
+	Less than 1/3 of the fitting surface of the denture
++	Covering 1/3rd to 2/3rd of the fitting surface
+++	Covering more than 2/3rd of the fitting surface

Bibliography

1. Budtz-Jorgensen E, Knudsen AM. Chlorhexidine gel and Steradent employed in cleaning dentures. Acta Odontol Scand 1978;36:83–7.

6D.3 An Additive Index for Denture Plaque Assessment

Ambjornsen E et al. 1982 developed an additive index for assessment of denture plaque based on plaque index introduced by Silness and Löe, 1964.

The plaque was recorded in five different areas, corresponding to: (1) the incisive papilla, (2) the most caudal areas of both maxillary tuberosities, and (3) two areas 1 cm lateral to the midline of the palate at the bisecting point between the impression of the superior labial frenum and the most posterior point on the median line of the maxillary denture. Each area was limited to a circle with a diameter of 1 cm. The localization of the five areas were considered to be representative for the fitting surface (Fig. 6.15).

Prior to the scoring procedure, the dentures were carefully rinsed in water and gently dried by air using a chip syringe. Each area was examined in good light. The five individual scores may be added. Used in this manner the plaque index values may range from 0 to 15 points for a denture.

The plaque index on complete maxillary dentures (Table 6.23).

Bibliography

1. Ambjornsen E, Valderhaug J, Norheim PW and Floystrand F. Assessment of an additive index for plaque on complete maxillary dentures. Acta Odontol Scad 1982, 40, 203–8.

6D.4 Ausberger and Elahi

Ausberger and Elahi (1982) suggested an index for scoring prosthesis for plaque accumulation. In this index the maxillary denture surface is divided into eight sites, four of which are on the labial and buccal surfaces, and four on the fitting (or palatal) surface. The mean plaque score is calculated from the sum of all eight sites. The index is scored as shown in Table 6.24 and Fig. 6.16.

Bibliography

1. Ausburger RH, Elahi JM. Evaluation of seven proprietary denture cleansers. Journal of Prosthetic Dentistry 1982;47: 356–9.

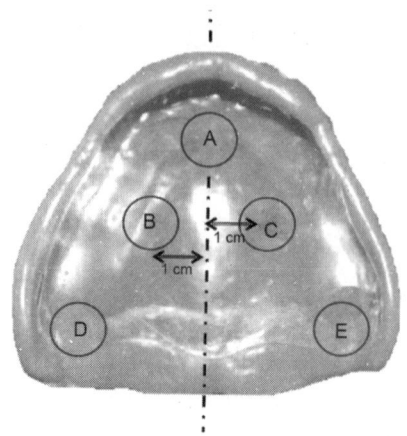

Fig. 6.15: Location of areas with a circle diameter of 1 cm on the fitting surface of the maxillary denture to record plaque accumulation. A = incisive papillar, B and C are 1 cm lateral to the midline of the palate, and D and E the most posterior areas of both maxillary tuberosities

Table 6.24: Scoring criteria

Score	Criteria
0	No plaque
1	Light plaque (1–25% of area covered)
2	Moderate plaque (26–50% of area covered)
3	Heavy plaque (51–75% of area covered)
4	Very heavy plaque (76–100% of area covered)

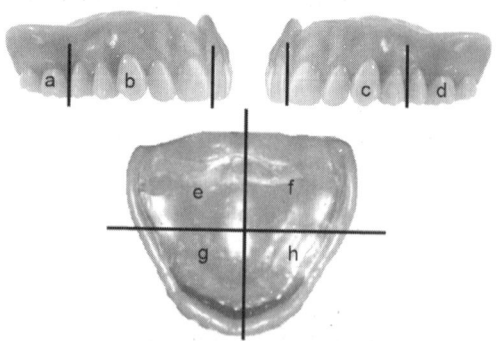

Fig. 6.16: Division for maxillary dentures

Table 6.23: Criteria for additive index

Score	Criteria	Descriptions
0	No plaque	No visible plaque could be seen when scraped with a blunt instrument
1	Plaque visible only by scraping with a blunt instrument	Plaque could be seen on the instrument
2	Moderate accumulation visible plaque	Areas plaque partly covered with visible
3	Abundance of plaque	Areas completely covered with visible plaque

7

Indices used for Assessment of Oral Hygiene

INTRODUCTION

Assessment of non-mineralized tooth deposits (plaque, materia alba, debris, pellicle and stain) is important in epidemiologic studies relating local factors to gingival and periodontal disease, the evaluation of oral hygiene status of individual patients and in studies assessing efficiency of oral hygiene procedures/products. In addition to naturally occurring deposits on teeth, food materials with special additives have been used to measure the ability of oral hygiene procedures or agents to "clear" the material from the oral cavity.

Some definitions for the terminology used for assessment of oral hygiene:

Materia alba is the loosely adherent, grayish-white to yellowish mass of bacteria and cellular debris which overlies the plaque, mainly along the gingival margins. It is unorganized and a product of mechanical accumulation. It can be removed by vigorous rinsing or water sprays.

Debris is particulate matter, mostly food particles, and unless mechanically trapped is readily dislodged by lip, tongue and cheek movements and rinsing, and is not part of plaque. When impacted and broken down by enzyme action it can contribute soluble materials for bacterial metabolic activity within the plaque.

Stains are products of chromogenic bacteria, tars and resin residues from tobacco, reaction of combinations of food components, medications, etc. A plaque may become stained — a stain is not a plaque.

Pellicles may be developmental (Nasmyth's membrane) or acquired. In functional teeth, the developmental pellicles are rare; the acquired are virtually ubiquitous. The acquired pellicle is a bacteria free film of glycoproteins and probably lipid derived from the saliva and/or gingival fluid and may cover the entire tooth surface. It often becomes stained, and in some areas may be colonized by bacteria. When covered by bacteria it becomes part of the plaque.

Plaques are not stains, pellicles (cuticles), materia alba or debris. Hence it is necessary to differentiate "plaque" which is a highly specific structural entity from the non-specific accumulations on the teeth. The following section is dealt with various indices designed specifically for assessing oral hygiene.

7.1 Oral Hygiene Index (OHI)

It was developed by John C. Greene and Jack R. Vermillion (1960) to classify and oral hygiene status. The OHI is composed of the combined Debris Index and Calculus Index. Each of these indexes in turn, is based on 12 numerical determinations representing the amounts of debris or calculus found on the buccal and lingual surfaces of each of the three segments of dental arch. They are the segment distal to the right cuspid, the segment distal to left cuspid and the segment mesial to the right and left first bicuspids. Separate recordings are made for the buccal and lingual surfaces in recognition of the difference in oral hygiene status that may exist between these surfaces.

Rules for Scoring

a. Only fully erupted permanent teeth are scored. Tooth is considered fully erupted when occlusal or incisal surface has reached the occlusal plane.
b. Third molars or incompletely erupted teeth are not scored because of the wide variations in heights of clinical crowns.
c. The buccal and lingual debris scores are both taken on the tooth in a segment having the greatest surface area covered by debris.
d. The buccal and lingual calculus scores are both taken on the tooth in a segment having the greatest surface area covered by supra-gingival and subgingival calculus.

Method: First the buccal and, second the lingual surfaces of the teeth in the upper right posterior segments are inspected and score for oral debris. Then the labial and lingual surfaces of the upper anterior teeth are classified. Finally, the buccal and lingual surfaces of the teeth in upper left posterior segment are examined and scored. The lower arch inspection proceeds in the same manner, but from left to right. This routine is repeated for calculus after the debris recordings have been completed.

The two debris scores assigned to a segment are based on the buccal surface and lingual surface having the greatest surface area covered by debris, the buccal score and lingual score for a segment need not be taken from the same tooth. The surface area covered by debris by running the side of a no 5 explorer along the buccal, labial and lingual surfaces. The occlusal or incisal extent of the debris and

calculus were recorded based on the criteria described in Tables 7.1 and 7.2.

Oral debris is defined as the soft foreign matter on the tooth surface of the teeth, consisting of mucin, bacteria and food, and varying in color form grayish white to green or orange.

Table 7.1 Oral hygiene index	
Score	Criteria for debris index
0	No debris or stain present
1	Soft debris covering not more than one-third of the tooth surface, or presence of extrinsic stains without other debris regardless of surface area covered
2	Soft debris covering more than one-third, but not more than two-thirds, of the exposed tooth surface.
3	Soft debris covering more than two-thirds of the exposed tooth surface.

Table 7.2 Oral hygiene index	
Score	Criteria for calculus index
0	No calculus present
1	Supragingival calculus covering not more than third of the exposed tooth surface.
2	Supragingival calculus covering more than one-third but not more than two-thirds of the exposed tooth surface or the presence of individual flecks of subgingival calculus around the cervical portion of the tooth or both.
3	Supragingival calculus covering more than two-third of the exposed tooth surface or a continuous heavy band of subgingival calculus around the cervical portion of the tooth or both.

According to the criteria, two scores are assigned to each segment having one or more fully erupted permanent teeth. The ratio of debris and calculus scores which make-up the OHI varies among population and no doubt differs in clinical significance. Therefore, both components indexes should always be given in conjunction with OHI.

Debris Index = (the total of the upper and lower buccal scores) + (the total of the upper and lower lingual scores)/(the number of segments scored).

Calculus Index = (the total of the upper and lower buccal scores) + (the total of the upper and lower lingual scores)/(the number of segments scored).

$$OHI = DI + CI$$

Bibliography

1. Greene JC, Vermillion JR. The oral hygiene index: a method for classifying oral hygiene status. J Am Dent Assoc 1960;61:172–9.

7.2 Simplified Oral Hygiene Index (OHI–S)

It was developed by John C. Greene and Jack R. Vermillion (1964) to reduce both the number of decisions required on the part of the examiner and time required for the inspection. It differs from the original OHI in the number of tooth surfaces scored (6 rather than 12), method of selecting the surfaces to be scored and scores which can be obtained. The criteria used for assigning scores to the tooth surfaces are same as those used for the OHI.

The six surfaces examined for the OHI-S are selected from the four posterior and two anterior teeth. In the posterior portion of the dentition, the fully erupted tooth distal to the second bicuspid, usually the first molar but sometimes the second or third molar, is examined on each side of the each arch. The buccal surfaces of the selected upper molars and the lingual surfaces of the selected lower molars are inspected. In the anterior portion of the mouth, the labial surfaces of the upper right and lower left central incisors are scored. In the absence of either of these anterior teeth, the central incisor on the opposite side of the mid-line is substituted.

For this procedure each surface, buccal or lingual, is considered half of the circumference of the tooth. For example, buccal surface of molar incudes half of the mesial and half of the distal surfaces.

Methods: Only fully erupted permanent teeth are considered. A tooth is considered fully erupted when the occlusal or incisal surface has reached the occlusal plane. Natural teeth with full crown restorations and surfaces reduced in height by caries or trauma are not scored. Instead an alternative tooth is examined. The surface area covered by debris is estimated by running the side of the no. 5 explorer along the surface being examined. The scoring criteria and calculations are same as OHI (*refer* Tables 7.1 and 7.2). At least two of the six possible surfaces must have been examined for an individual score to be calculated.

DI-S and CI-S

Good – 0.0 to 0.6

Fair – 0.7 to 1.8

Poor – 1.9 to 3.0

OHI-S

Good – 0.0 to 1.2

Fair – 1.3 to 3.0

Poor – 3.1 to 6.0

Bibliography

1. Greene JC, Vermillion JR. The Simplified Oral Hygiene Index. J Am Dent Assoc 1964;68:7–13.

7.3 Glass Index for Debris

It was developed by Glass RL in 1965. This index evaluates the presence and extent of debris accumulation, for evaluating tooth brushing efficacy.

Method: All the teeth are examined. The surfaces examined are facial and lingual surfaces which are scored as a unit based on the criteria described in Table 7.3. Third molars are excluded from consideration because of their variable appearance.

Calculation

Advantage of this index is it places more emphasis on gingival 3rd of the tooth than does the OHI-S and so helpful in clinical trials.

Table 7.3 Glass index	
Code	Criteria
0	No visible debris–tooth surface shiny — gingival crevice not obscured
1	Debris visible at gingival margin — but discontinuous – less than 1mm in height
2	Debris continuous at gingival margin — greater than 1 mm in height — entire gingival third not yet involved
3	Debris involving entire gingival third of tooth
4	Debris generally scattered over tooth surface

Bibliography

1. Glass RL. A clinical study of hand and electric brushing. J Periodontol 1965;36:322–7.

7.4 Patient Hygiene Performance (PHP) Index

It was developed by Podshadley AG and Haley JV in 1968.

The purpose of the index is to assess the extent of plaque and debris over a tooth surface. It is a simplified index and the assessments are based on six index teeth.

Procedure

A mouth mirror examination of selected teeth is made after the subject has been given an erythrosin disclosing wafer which stains the oral debris as dark pink. Oral debris is defined as the soft foreign material consisting of mucin, bacteria, and food that is loosely attached to the tooth surface. The patient is instructed to chew the disclosing wafer and to "swish" for 30 seconds. The subject may then expectorate but is not permitted to rinse the mouth until after the examination.

The examination is performed on the following teeth in this order: (a) maxillary right first molar, (b) maxillary right central incisor, (c) maxillary left first molar, (d) mandibular left first molar, (e) mandibular left central incisor and (f) mandibular right first molar. The tooth surfaces which are assessed are the buccal of the maxillary molars, the lingual of the mandibular molars, and the labial of the maxillary and mandibular incisors.

If the first molars are missing or less than three-fourths erupted or have full-crown restorations or too badly broken down to assess, the second molar is substituted. If the second molar is missing or cannot be used, the third molar is then substituted. If all three molars are missing or cannot be used, an M is placed on the recording chart.

If the designated central incisor is missing or cannot be used, the adjacent central incisor is substituted. If both central incisors are missing or cannot be used, again an M is placed on the chart.

To assess the debris on each surface, the examiner must mentally divide the tooth into five sections. The clinical crown is subdivided longitudinally into mesial, middle and distal thirds. The mesial and distal thirds make up the first two subdivisions; each area extends to the middle third of its adjacent proximal surface. The remaining middle third is then subdivided horizontally into the gingival, middle, and occlusal thirds (Fig. 7.1). Each of the subdivisions is examined for the presence of the pink-stained oral debris. If no debris is present, 0 is assigned to that section; if debris is present, 1 is assigned. The value of 1 is assigned only to those areas on which debris is definitely present. The lesser score of 0 is assigned to all questionable areas.

The debris score for each tooth is determined by adding the values of each of the five subdivisions.

PHP Index Value for the Individual

Total the scores for the individual teeth and divide by the number of teeth examined (Value 0–5).

PHP index Value for a Group

Total the individual scores and divide by the number of people examined.

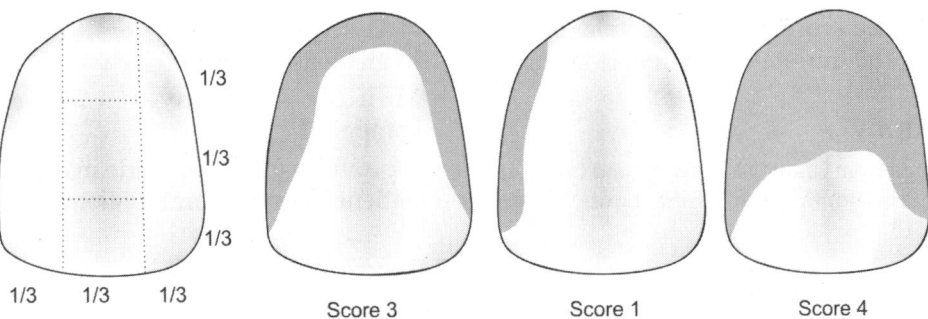

Fig. 7.1: Patient hygiene performance index

Bibliography

Podshadley AG, Haley JV. A method for evaluating oral hygiene performance. Public Health Reports 1968;83(3):259–64.

7.5 Modified Patient Hygiene Performance (PHP-M) Index

This was given by Leslie V and Lawrence H. Meskin in 1972. PHP-M is designed to be repeated following patient oral hygiene education. The areas of plaque are made known in this modification.

Method: Each of the six selected teeth is divided into five areas

- Gingival 3rd of middle area
- Middle 3rd of middle area
- Incisal 3rd of the middle area
- Distal area
- Mesial area.

An adequate representation of plaque accumulation in most mouths can be obtained by scoring the facial and lingual surfaces of the following teeth:

- The most posterior teeth in the upper right quadrant
- The upper right cuspid; if not present another anterior tooth.
- The upper left first molar or first bicuspid
- The most posterior tooth in lower left quadrant
- The lower left cuspid; if absent any other anterior tooth
- Lower left first molar or first bicuspid

The plaque is disclosed using any disclosing solution to assure the most objective evaluation. The patient is scored three times

1st—stained scored at the time of initial classification

2nd—patient is asked to brush as usual and then stained and scored

3rd—after receiving oral hygiene instructions at the end of 4 weeks.

The range of scores varies from 0 (best) to 60 (worst).

Bibliography

1. Martens LV, Meskin LH. A innovative technique for assessing oral hygiene. Journal of Dentistry for Children. 1972;39:12.

7.6 Plaque Free Score

It is a method for assessing the patients oral hygiene performance, was developed by Grant DA, Stern IB and Everett FG in 1958.

Method: To determine the location number and percent of plaque free surfaces for individual motivation and instruction. Interdental bleeding can also be recorded.

All erupted teeth are included. Missing teeth are recorded by a single horizontal line through the box in the chart form. Four surfaces are recorded for each tooth— facial, lingual, mesial and distal.

Apply disclosing agent and record each tooth for evidence of plaque using red when red disclosing agent is used. A light and mouth mirror can be used.

Plaque free score: Number of plaque free surfaces × 100/number of available surfaces

Bibliography

1. Adapted from Grant DA, Stern IB, and Listgarten MA. Periodontics, 6th ed. St. Louis, Mosby, 1988:613.

7.7 Hygiene Analysis Index

It was developed by William D Love, Juan M, Ramirez and R. Paul Fultz in 1975. It consists of identifying plaque or debris by using a suitable disclosing agent and then recording it. O'Leary, Drake and Naylor (1972) proposed such an index, but limited scoring only to that plaque in contact with the gingival margin.

Method: All teeth are included. Four surfaces are recorded for each tooth; facial, lingual, mesial, distal. A suitable disclosing agent is applied to all teeth and scored according to the following criteria.

0 — When there is no disclosed material on the tooth surface

1 — When there is disclosed material on the tooth surface

No attempt was made to determine if the material was plaque or some other material. Missing teeth are indicated by a horizontal line. To assume that all teeth are examined, it is advisable to place a circle in the middle of the box to indicate a clean tooth. Occlusal surfaces and third molars are excluded. After each examination, the number surfaces scoring "1" were totaled and the result divided by number of surfaces examined. The resulting percentage of surfaces with disclosed material constitutes the hygiene analysis index (HAI).

Advantages

- It is easy to perform
- It requires minimal time — no more than 2–3 minutes.
- Results are reproducible within acceptable limits.

- HAI scores reflect several levels of oral hygiene as performed by patients.
- Multiple scores over time are easily compared.
- It provides a helpful guide in educating the patient to proper oral hygiene procedures.

Bibliography

1. Love WD, Ramirez JM, Fultz RP. An oral hygiene measurement system for possible research and clinical use. J Public Health Dent 1975;35(4):227–30.

7.8 Clinical System for Scoring Patient's Oral Hygiene Performance

It was developed by John A Lenox, Raymond A, Kopezyk in 1970.

This system does not measure the severity of plaque; it only indicates the presence or absence of plaque. All teeth are included. Four surfaces are recorded for each tooth; facial, lingual, mesial, distal.

Method: The anatomical line angles are used as dividing points between the various tooth surfaces. A simple clinical technique is used after disclosing the plaque. The examiner calls "yes" when plaque is present and "no" when plaque is absent from the surface. If the examiner follows the sequence of surfaces then calling tooth number is not required. First, facial aspect of each quadrant is done and then lingual side is repeated the same way. Therefore, each proximal surface is evaluated twice (from facial and lingual aspects) but the examiner does not need to switch mirror positions from facial to lingual to view the entire proximal surface. Although each proximal surface is designated twice, it is charted in only one block.

Bleeding is evaluated with the tip of the probe placing it just into the opening of the gingival sulcus (1 mm or less) at the distal aspect of last molar. The probe is carried with a continuous motion along the entrance of the sulcus into the next interproximal area and this procedure is continued till midline. While the buccal mucosa is still retracted, the quadrant is observed (after 30 seconds) for bleeding. The presence or absence of bleeding is recorded the same way as plaque. Repeated evaluations at monthly intervals can be done to evaluate individual efficacy in maintaining oral hygiene.

Calculation: Bleeding points are calculated as a percent of the total tooth surfaces scored. The total number of surfaces with plaque or bleeding is divided by the total number of surfaces scored and then, multiplied by 100 to get the plaque retention or the percent of surfaces with bleeding. Scoring system permits correlation of plaque patterns with specific types of home care techniques. Facial and lingual scores are related to brushing efficiency and interproximal scores are related to flossing efficiency.

Bibliography

1. Lenox JA, Kopczyk RA. A clinical system for scoring a patients oral hygiene performance. J Am Dent Assoc 1973;86:849–52.

7.9 The University of Mississippi Oral Hygiene Index (UM-OHI)

UM-OHI was developed to provide a simple method for recording the presence of plaque in a patient's mouth. The index attempts to combine the best features of the patient hygiene performance index and the PSR. The UM-OHI utilizes the tooth demarcations of the PHP and the method and ease of recording, and the recording instrument of the PSR. Unlike the PSR, examiners record 6 observations from the buccal and the lingual aspect of each arch for a total of 12 observations. The resulting scores reveal the effectiveness of the patient's home care skills and provide adequate information for patient education.

Scoring Protocol

The oral cavity is divided into sextants, left and right posterior teeth and anterior teeth in each arch. Since home care skills vary for buccal and lingual surfaces, the UM-OHI is used on the buccal and the lingual sextants. Thus, there are 12 sections, or 2 sets of 6 observations. The scores reveal the effectiveness of the patient's current home care skills by area.

As with Podshadley and Haley's PHP index, each tooth is divided into 5 sections. The mesial and distal sections and the middle section, which is subdivided horizontally into the gingival, middle, and occlusal (or incisal) thirds. After staining, each of the 5 sections is scored for the presence or absence of plaque. If plaque definitely exists in the section it is scored a 1; if no plaque is present or the observation is questionable, the section receives a 0. Adding the scores of the 5 surface sections of the tooth with the most plaque in the sextant produces a score ranging from 0 to 5. In a manner similar to the PSR scoring, teeth are examined in each sextant until a maximum score is obtained or the sextant is completed. The highest score is recorded on the recording instrument and the examiner moves to the next sextant. In addition to the numerical score, if plaque is present on either of the proximal (P) sections or the gingival (G) section, the corresponding letter is appended to the numerical score entered in the box representing the sextant. The addition of the P and G helps in identifying specific areas of the tooth where there are brushing or flossing deficiencies.

Bibliography

1. Silberman SL, Le Jeune RC, Serio FG, Devidas M, Davidson L, Vernon K. A Method for Determining Patient Oral Care Skills: The University of Mississippi Oral Hygiene Index. J Periodontol 1998;69:1176–80.

8

Indices to Assess Calculus

Introduction

Early studies that were conducted to evaluate the effect of calculus inhibitory materials utilized, for the most part, clinical impressions obtained either from a direct visual examination or through use of intra-oral photographs. The direct visual examination was supplemented by the use of dental instruments, such as mouth mirrors, explorers, hoes, and periodontal probes. Supragingival calculus was quantitated on the basis dichotomized grading as "absence or presence" or on an ordinal scale "slight, moderate, severe". Very little effort was specifically directed toward the establishment of examiner standardization and reproducibility of these procedures.

During the decade from 1960 to 1970, a considerable clinical research effort was expended in an attempt to develop calculus quantitating procedures that were both as objective and quantitative as possible, and reproducible. Three major quantitating procedures for the direct in vivo measurement of calculus deposits were introduced. The three methods were the calculus surface index (and its companion calculus surface severity index), the Probe method of calculus assessment, and the marginal line calculus index.

Bibliography

Volpe AR. Indices for the measurement of hard deposits in clinical studies of oral hygiene and periodontal disease. J Periodontal Res 1974;9:S14:31–60.

8.1 Calculus Surface Index (CSI)

This was developed by Ennever, Sturzenberger and Radike in 1961. This method utilizes the four mandibular incisor teeth in the evaluation of calculus accumulation. The selection of these teeth was based upon the rate of calculus formation and the ease of observing the calculus on these teeth. In applying the scoring method, calculus was considered to be present if any amount, supragingival or subgingival, could be detected either visually or by touch. If the examiner was uncertain about the presence of calculus on a given surface, the surface was called calculus free. Each subject was examined through use of a number 23 dental explorer and a mouth mirror. Each of the mandibular incisors was considered on the basis of four surfaces: two proximals (scored from the lingual aspect), one labial and one lingual. At examination, a number of surfaces on which calculus had occurred were assigned to each tooth. The total number of surfaces (maximum of 16) on which calculus was detected was considered to be the subject's calculus score and is referred to as the CSI.

The CSI method has been shown to have excellent inter-examiner reproducibility and to be a relatively rapid and efficient scoring procedure for calculus deposits (either supragingival or subgingival). It is particularly advantageous in evaluating calculus deposits that have accumulated over a relatively short period of time (1–6 weeks). The CSI method was modified to include 6 lower anterior teeth and all of the natural teeth that are present.

Bibliography

1. Ennever J, Sturzenberger OP, Radike AW. The Calculus Surface Index method for scoring clinical calculus studies. J Periodont 1961;32:54.
2. Volpe AR. Indices for the measurement of hard deposits in clinical studies of oral hygiene and periodontal disease. J Periodontal Res 1974;9: Suppl 14:31–60.

8.2 The Calculus Surface Severity Index (CSSI)

It was developed by Ennever J et al in 1961 as a companion to their CSI. It is a measure of the quantity of calculus present on the facial, mesial, lingual and distal surfaces of the four mandibular incisors. Calculus is assessed on a severity scale from zero to three on each of the four surfaces of the mandibular incisors (maximum possible score of 48). The scoring scale is described in Table 8.1.

Table 8.1: The calculus surface severity index (CSSI)

Code	Criteria for CSSI
0	No calculus present
1	Calculus observable, but less than 0.5 mm in width and/or thickness
2	Calculus not exceeding 1.0 mm in width and/or thickness
3	Calculus exceeding 1.0 mm in width and/or thickness

Bibliography

1. Conroy CW, OP Sturzenberger. The rate of calculus formation in adults. J. Periodont. 1958;39;142.
2. Ennever J, Sturzenberger OP, Radike AW. The Calculus Surface Index method for scoring clinical calculus studies. J Periodont 1961;32:54.
3. Volpe AR. Indices for the measurement of hard deposits in clinical studies of oral hygiene and periodontal disease. J Periodontal Res. 1974;9:Suppl.14: 31–60.

8.3 Probe Method of Calculus Assessment

This was developed by Volpe and Manhold over a 7-year period (1960–1967). The first publication concerning this technique was a preliminary report which described a method of evaluating the effectiveness of potential calculus inhibitory agents. This report described the use of a periodontal probe, graduated in mm and tape-colored at the graduated end to facilitate obtaining accurate readings. Supragingival calculus accumulation was measured on the lingual surfaces of the six mandibular anterior teeth by bisecting the surfaces (in one vertical plane) with the periodontal probe and recording the calculus heights in mm.

This method was further developed and refined Volpe et al. (1965) over the next 3 years and more thoroughly described in a subsequent publication. This report provided a modification of the original technique which would allow for measurement of calculus in three constant planes, rather than the one vertical plane previously employed. It was indicated that these three readings for each lingual (and to a certain extent, interproximal) surface would incorporate the concept of calculus height and width (area), more accurately assess the amount (volume) of calculus present and provide a fixed reference point for subsequent re-examinations. The three measurement planes for the quantitation of calculus accumulations on the lingual surfaces of the mandibular six anterior teeth are described as follows:

The FIRST PLANE is for gingival measurements and is obtained by vertically positioning the probe so as to bisect the lingual (or facial) surface of the tooth (Fig. 8.1).

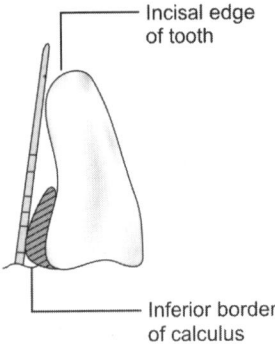

Incisal edge
of tooth

Inferior border
of calculus

Illustration of proper positioning of prope so that it contacts both the incisal edge of the tooth and calculus to be measured

Fig. 8.1: Probe method of calculus assessment

The SECOND PLANE is for distal measurements and is obtained by positioning the probe so as to bisect the mesio-incisal angle of the tooth and then placing the probe diagonally through the area of greatest calculus width on the distal aspect of the tooth. The THIRD PLANE is for mesial measurements and is obtained by positioning the probe so as to bisect the distoincisal angle of the tooth and then placing it diagonally through the area of greatest calculus width on the mesial aspect of the tooth.

Two recommendations have been presented in reference to the utilization of the Probe method of calculus assessment. In the first, it was recommended that the initial score of 0.5 units should be initially assigned to any calculus that is present, that is, even before it has reached 0.5 mm in height. In this manner, the Probe method would be based, for the earliest stages of calculus formation, on the "presence or absence" alternative, and later, on measurements of the increase in the extent or growth of calculus (Muhlemann, 1968). A relatively similar modification had independently been described in another publication (Volpe et al. 1967).

Calculation: Assuming a maximum height of 3mm of calculus, the total possible score for the six mandibular teeth with one measurement plane would be 18 units of calculus. With three

measurement planes, each tooth could then have 9 calculus units, for a total possible score of 54 units for the six teeth.

Bibliography

1. Volpe AR, Manhold JH. A method of evaluating the effectiveness of potential calculus inhibiting agents. NY State Dent J 1962;7:289.
2. Volpe AR, Manhold JH and Hazen SP. In vivo calculus assessment: Part I. A method and its examiner reproducibility. J Periodont 1965;36:294.
3. Volpe AR. Indices for the measurement of hard deposits in clinical studies of oral hygiene and periodontal disease. J Periodontal Res 1974;9: Suppl 14:31–60.

8.4 Glass's Criteria for Assessment of Calculus

Table 8.2: Glass index	
Code	Criteria
0	No calculus visible
1	Isolated calculus segments — not a continuous band – limited to the region of gingival crevice.
2	As above but a continuous band on a tooth surface (most calculus was observed was limited to the lingual of the lower anteriors)
3	Extends beyond the region of the gingival crevice, but less than the gingival third covered.
4	Gingival third or more of the tooth covered in part or whole by calculus.

Bibliography

1. Glass RL. A clinical study of hand and electric brushing. J Periodontol. 1965;36:322–7.

8.5 Marginal Line Calculus (MLC) Index

This was developed by Muhlemann and Villa in 1967. MLC was developed in order to provide an accurate measurement of supragingival calculus accumulation which is in the area of closest proximity to the gingiva. Thus, a greater precision is provided in correlating the rate of calculus formation with inflammatory gingival disease. Also, this procedure allows for the conduction of a calculus inhibitory clinical study in a relatively small number of subjects. The MLC index only scores supragingival calculus formed in the cervical area along the marginal gingivae on the lingual side of the four mandibular incisors. For more concise evaluation, this cervical band paralleling the free gingiva is divided into two parts by an axial plane which bisects the incisal edge of the incisors and which is directed towards the most apical position of the marginal free gingiva (Fig. 8.2). The resulting mesial and distal part of the band or line are scored separately by estimating the percentage of the distance covered by calculus deposits. In order to simplify the procedure only 0, 12½, 25, 50, 75, and 100 percentages are used. The smallest calculus score is given 12.5%. If the examiner is uncertain about the percentage to give, the higher percentage is assigned. The mesial and distal percentages per tooth are averaged. The means of the four teeth are averaged to give the subject's score, the maximum possible score being 100%. Since minute particles of calculus are not visible when wet, total dryness of the linguocervical area is essential for scoring. A warm stream of air is continuously blown on the lingual tooth surfaces until calculus is clearly visible in its full extent on the cervical band between two interdental papillae.

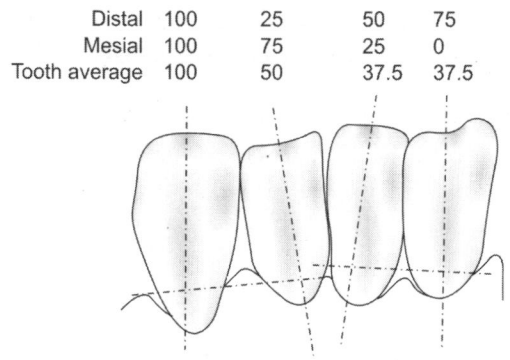

Distal	100	25	50	75
Mesial	100	75	25	0
Tooth average	100	50	37.5	37.5

Fig. 8.2: Marginal line calculus index

Bibliography

1. Muhlemann HR and Villa P. The marginal line calculus index. Helv Odont Acta. 1967;11:175.
2. Volpe AR. Indices for the measurement of hard deposits in clinical studies of oral hygiene and periodontal disease. J Periodontal Res 1974;9: Suppl 14: 31–60.

8.6 Calculus Along Wire Index (CalcWI)

Artun proposed a system for assessment of calculus accumulation along the retainer wire in subjects wearing bonded lingual retainer following orthodontic treatment. The criteria are shown in Table 8.3.

Table 8.3: CalcWI	
Score	Criteria
0	No calculus along wire
1	Moderate amount of calculus along wire
2	An abundance of calculus along wire

CalcWI was scored both incisally and gingivally along the retainer wire in areas corresponding to all interproximal surfaces from the mesial aspect of one canine to the mesial aspect of the other canine and in areas corresponding to all lingual surfaces from canine to canine.

Bibliography

1. Artun J. Caries and periodontal reactions associated with long-term use of different types of bonded lingual retainers. Am J Orthod. 1984;86(2):112–8.

8.7 Sign Grading System for Calculus

This system was proposed by Amit A Agarwal (2011). The oral cavity is divided into six sextants: 18–14, 13–23, 24–28, 38–34, 33–43 and 44–48. A typical examination usually starts with the maxillary right third molar and is continued, sextant wise, in a clockwise direction until all the teeth required to be assessed are through. All surfaces of the tooth should be examined for each grade and the surface with the highest grade should be allocated to that particular tooth based on the criteria described in Table 8.4. This will help

Table 8.4: Sign grading system

Grade	Criteria
–	Absence of supra or subgingival calculus
+	Isolated flakes or continuous band of calculus present supragingivally not covering more than one-third of the crown and without presence of subgingival calculus (or) supragingival/subgingival calculus present only on the proximal surface
++	Isolated flakes or continuous band of subgingival calculus present on labial/lingual surface of crown without presence of supragingival calculus (or) supragingival calculus in cervical one-third of labial or lingual surface of crown along with presence of subgingival calculus (or) supragingival calculus extending more than one-third but less than two-thirds of labial or lingual surface or crown, with or without the presence of subgingival calculus
++	Supragingival calculus extending more than two-thirds of the crown, with or without the presence of subgingival calculus

in simpler data management and assessment of overall condition of the patient, rather than mentioning different grades for each tooth surface. Similarly, grading of the sextants will depend on the highest grade of the tooth within that sextant. In all classification, "crown" means clinical crown and not anatomic crown.

Scoring requires adequate light and mouth mirror. If optimal conditions and chair-side assistance are provided and all teeth are to be examined, scoring according to this system requires approximately 4–5 minutes (Table 8.4).

For Field Study

The surface with highest grade is allocated to that particular tooth (t) and the tooth with highest grade is allocated to that sextant (X). Then consider signs – as 0; + as 1; ++ as 2 and +++ as 3.

For Clinical Research

As per the study requirement, either the sextant can be counted as above, or the grades allotted to each tooth are converted to numerical data (T). Then, sum all the numbers (sT) to be included in the study and divide by the total number of teeth examined (N).

The interpretation of the total average score is given in Table 8.5.

Table 8.5

Score	Interpretation
0–1	Mild (+)
1.1 – 2	Moderate (++)
2.1 – 3	Severe (+++)

Bibliography

1. Agrawal AA. A randomized clinical study to assess the reliability and reproducibility of "Sign Grading System". Indian J Dent Res 2011;22:285–90.

CALCULUS COMPONENT IN OTHER INDICES

8.8 Oral Hygiene Index (*refer* Section 7.1 in Chapter 7)

8.9 Simplified – Oral Hygiene Index (*refer* Section 7.2 in Chapter 7)

8.10 Calculus component of Periodontal Disease Index (*refer* Section 3A.2 in Chapter 3)

8.11 Calculus component of Irritant Index (refer Section 16.4)

9

Indices to Assess Tooth Mobility

INTRODUCTION

The special morphology of the periodontal structures anchoring the roots of teeth in the alveolar bone allows for physiological tooth mobility. It is somewhat more pronounced on erupting teeth than in the healthy adult dentition. It increases in the presence of apical abscesses and during orthodontic treatment. Clasped teeth often are more mobile than other teeth in the same dentition. Increased tooth mobility may be one of the cardinal symptoms of periodontal disease. The most primitive recommendation is to test the amount of tooth mobility (TM) by moving the crowns between two fingers.

Historically many devices were developed to standardize the assessment of tooth mobility. Elbrecht (1939) measured TM with a large dial indicator that was fixed on a tripod in front of the patient's mouth. The dial indicator registered the labiolingual crown excursions which were produced by digital pressure. The author points out the inaccuracy of the method, since movements of the head could interfere with the movements of the crowns. Only values over 0.75 mm in total labiolingual crown excursions could be determined.

Werner (1942) used an instrument called "oscillometer." It consisted of a rod with a scale attached and held on the front teeth. By moving the neighboring or proximal tooth labiolingually with a force of 700 grams, the resultant difference of tooth position could be read on the scale. Differences of tooth position smaller than 0.25 mm could not be evaluated.

Beyeler and Dreyfus (1947, 1949) approached the problem of TM differently. Their vibrometer does not measure labiolingual excursions of crowns but tries to determine the behavior of teeth when exposed to oscillatory vibrations of high frequency. These authors gave only preliminary laboratory results.

Mühlemann (1951) used intraorally attached dial indicators to determine the degree of crown excursions that were produced by known static forces which was called periodontometry.

Certain indices were developed to evaluate the tooth mobility to overcome the problems with devices. However, a degree of subjectivity could be observed when evaluating TM.

Bibliography

1. Mühlemann HR. The Measuring Method. Initial and Secondary Tooth Mobility 1954 Dec (22–29)

9.1 Tooth Mobility Index

The most subjective method used to assess tooth mobility was described by Miller SC in 1950.

Method: The tooth is held firmly between two instruments and moved back and forth. Mobility is scored from 0–3 as shown in Table 9.1.

Table 9.1	
Code	Criteria tooth mobility index
0	No detectable movement when force is applied
1	Barely distinguishable tooth movement
2	The crown of the tooth moves up to 1 mm in any direction
3	Movement more than 1 mm in any direction or the teeth can be depressed or rotated in their sockets

This method is useful for diagnosis and treatment planning for an individual practitioner.

Bibliography

1. Miller SC. Textbook of Periodontia, 3rd edition, The Blakiston Co., Philadelphia and Toronto, 1950.
2. Mühlemann HR. The Measuring Method. Initial and Secondary Tooth Mobility 1954, Dec (22–29).

9.2 Mobility Index by Ramfjord

Ramfjord has suggested a mobility using the following criteria (Table 9.2).

Table 9.2	
Code	Criteria for mobility index by Ramfjord
M0	Physiologically mobility; firm tooth
M1	Slightly increase mobility
M2	Definite to considerable increase in mobility but no impairement of function.
M3	Extreme mobility; a loose tooth that cannot be used for normal function.

Bibliography

1. Ramfjord SP. The Periodontal Disease Index. J Periodontol 1967;38:602–10.

9.3 Mobility Index by Laster et al

Mobility is assessed by the application of lateral horizontal forces based on the criteria given in Table 9.3.

Table 9.3	
Code	Criteria for mobility index by Laster et al
0	Normal
1	Movement greater than normal
2	Mobility of 1 mm in lateral direction
3	Mobility greater than 1 mm laterally plus rotation and/or axial depression.

Bibliography

1. Laster L, Laudenbach KW, Stoller NH. An evaluation of clinical tooth mobility measurements. J Periodontol 1975, 46(10):603–7.

9.4 Mobility Index by Grace and Smales

This index can be useful to track the amount of mobility in teeth over a period of time (Table 9.4).

Table 9.4	
Grade	Mobility index by Grace and Smales
0	No apparent mobility
1	Tooth mobility is perceptible, but less than 1 mm buccolingually.
2	Mobility is between 1 and 2 mm.
3	Mobility exceeds 2 mm buccolingually or vertically.

Tooth Mobility Index by Lindhe (Table 9.5)

Table 9.5: Tooth mobility by Lindhe	
Degree	Interpretation for tooth mobility by Lindhe
1	Movability of the crown of the tooth 0.2–1 mm in horizontal direction
2	Movability of the crown of the tooth exceeding 1 mm in horizontal direction
3	Movability of the crown of the tooth in vertical direction as well.

10 Indices to Assess Dental Fluorosis and Enamel Defects

INTRODUCTION

Over the past 50 years, various indices have been proposed for measuring enamel defects, including fluorosis. These indices may be conveniently divided into two main groups: specific fluorosis indices and descriptive indices encompassing all types of defects. The fluorosis indices are designed to measure defects of enamel due to excessive fluoride ingestion, usually described as enamel mottling or fluorosis.

Numerous attempts have been made in the past to arrive at a rational method of classifying and measuring levels of enamel defects, including fluorosis, in population groups. The acceptance of these fluorosis indices rests in large measure, on the ability of an examiner to distinguish fluoride induced changes in the enamel from those that are not fluoride-induced. Several investigators have suggested that some diffuse opacities similar in appearance to dental fluorosis are not caused by fluoride and have developed descriptive indices for classifying changes in the enamel which require no consideration of etiology (Al-Alousi et al., 1975; Jackson et al, 1975; Ainamo and Cutress, 1982; FDI, 1982; Clarkson and O'Mullane, 1989). This approach, alleviates the need for making the sometimes difficult differential diagnosis between fluoride and non-fluoride opacities.

Classifications/Indices

Conflicting views on fluoride and nonfluoride defects lead to the development of two different approaches to measure the level of enamel defects in populations exposed to fluoride.

1. Use various criteria to distinguish between fluoride and non-fluoride defects and then to record only the fluoride defects by use of a specific fluorosis index.

2. The difficulty in differentiating between fluoride and non-fluoride defects and the confusion in the classifications of mottling, fluorosis and enamel defects led, not surprisingly, to the development of the second group of indices covering all types of enamel defects. This second approach is to use a purely descriptive index to record all defects seen and not to assign any etiology to them. If any differences are found between fluoridated and non-fluoridated groups when these descriptive indices are used, then, all other factors being equal, the cause may be attributed to fluoride.

A. SPECIFIC FLUOROSIS INDICES

1. Dean's index (Dean et al, 1934; 1942).
2. Thylstrup and Fejerskov index (Thylstrup and Fejerskov, 1978)
3. The tooth surface index of fluorosis (TSIF) (Horowitz et al, 1984).

4. Fluorosis risk index (Pendrys, 1990)
5. Chronological Fluorosis Assessment (CFA) index
6. Simplified fluoride mottling index
7. Visual analog scale

B. DESCRIPTIVE INDICES FOR ENAMEL DEFECTS AND OPACITIES

1. The Index of Al-Alousi et al (1975).
2. Young's classification (1973)
3. Al-Alousi and Jackson's classification (1975)
4. Murray and Shaws's classification (1979)
5. The developmental defects of enamel index (FDI, 1982).
6. The modified developmental defects of enamel index (Clarkson and O'Mullane, 1989).
7. Mottling index
8. Enamel defects index

Some common terminologies that are used in describing the enamel defects are listed in Table 10.1.

10A Specific Fluorosis Indices

Introduction: Dental fluorosis is a hypoplasia or hypomineralization of tooth enamel or dentine produced by chronic ingestion of excessive amounts of fluoride during the period of tooth development.

Obtaining accurate measurements of fluorotic conditions in humans is a demanding and tedious process. The effect of moisture on the scoring of a tooth or surface could be a factor, and patient information regarding residence histories or other potential exposure to fluoride can aid or detract an examiner's ability to make correct clinical judgments.

Many different factors can result in changes in the normal appearance of the enamel (Small and Murray, 1978; Pindborg, 1982). The single most studied causal factor is fluoride, which can result in a range of clinical manifestations referred to collectively as dental fluorosis. This condition can be distinguished from other defects of the enamel based on enamel color, distribution of the condition on the affected tooth or within the mouth and the extent to which the enamel is left intact.

Bibliography

1. Rozier RG. Epidemiologic indices for measuring the Clinical manifestations of dental fluorosis: Overview and critique Adv Dent Res 1994;8:39–55.

10A.1 Dean's Index

Dean HT realized the importance of providing a standard classification system for the clinical conditions described by McKay. Dean's collaboration with McKay and his experiences in completing examinations on approximately 2000 subjects in endemic areas of six states resulted in the original classification scale for dental fluorosis, presented in Table 10.2.

Table 10.1: Terminology for enamel defects

Common terms	Alternative terms
Dental fluorosis	Enamel fluorosis, mottling, fluorosed opacities
Enamel opacities	Internal enamel hypoplasia, developmental opacities, idiopathic opacities, demarcated, diffuse, confluent opacities.
Enamel hypoplasia	Aplasia, internal and external hypoplasia, hypocalcification, pits, grooves, missing enamel.
Discolored enamel	Pigmentation, tetracycline staining.
Developmental defects of enamel	Enamel defects, dental fluorosis, enamel opacities, hypoplasia and discolored enamel.

Scoring Criteria

Classification	Score	Original criteria (Dean, 1934)
		Table 10.2: Criteria for Dean's index
Normal	0	The enamel presents the usual translucent semi vitriform type of structure. The surface is smooth and glossy and usually of a pale creamy white color.
Questionable	0.5	Slight aberrations in the translucency of normal enamel, ranging from a few white flecks to occasional white spots, 1 to 2 mm in diameter.
Very mild	1	Small, opaque, paper-white areas are scattered irregularly or streaked over the tooth surface. It is principally observed on the labial and buccal surfaces, and involves less than 25% of the tooth surfaces of the particular teeth affected. Small pitted white areas are frequently found on the summits of the cusps. No brown stain is present in the mottled enamel of this classification.
Mild	2	The white, opaque areas on the surfaces of the teeth involve at least half of the tooth surface. The surfaces of molars, bicuspids, and cuspids subject to attrition show thin white layers worn off and the bluish shades of underlying normal enamel. Faint brown stains are sometimes apparent, generally on the upper incisors.
Moderate	3	No change is observed in the form of the tooth, but generally all of the tooth surfaces are involved. Surfaces subject to attrition are definitely marked. Minute pitting is often present, generally on the labial and buccal surfaces. Brown stain is frequently a disfiguring complication. It must be remembered that the incidence of brown stain varies greatly in different endemic areas, and many cases of white opaque mottled enamel, without brown stain, are classified as "moderate" and listed in this category.
Moderately Severe		Macroscopically, a greater depth of enamel appears to be involved. A smoky white appearance is often noted. Pitting is more frequent and generally observed on all the tooth surfaces. Brown stain, if present, is generally deeper in hue and involves more of the affected tooth surfaces.
Severe	4	The hypoplasia is so marked that the form of the teeth is at times affected, the condition often being manifest in older children as a mild pathologic incisal-occlusal abrasion. The pits are deeper and often confluent. Stains are widespread and range from a chocolate brown to almost black in some cases.

Modified Dean's Index, 1942

The "moderately severe" and the "severe" categories were combined into a single "severe" category providing the six-point measurement scale currently in use (Dean *et al.* 1939; Dean, 1942). The criteria for these six classifications are given in Table 10.3.

Classification	Score	Modified criteria (Dean, 1942)
		Table 10.3: Criteria for modified Dean's index
Normal	0	The enamel presents the usual translucent semi- vitriform type of structure. The surface is smooth and glossy and usually of a pale creamy white color.
Questionable	0.5	The enamel discloses slight aberrations from the translucency of normal enamel, ranging from a few white flecks to occasional white spots. This classification is utilized in those instances where a definite diagnosis of the mildest form of fluorosis is not warranted and a classification of "normal" not justified.
Very mild	1	Small, opaque, paper-white areas scattered irregularly over the tooth but not involving as much as approximately 25% of the tooth surface. Frequently included in this classification are teeth showing no more than about 1–2 mm of white opacity at the tips of the summits of the cusps of the bicuspids or second molars.

Contd...

Table 10.3: Criteria for modified Dean's index (Contd.)		
Classification	*Score*	*Modified criteria (Dean, 1942)*
Mild	2	The white opaque areas in the enamel of the teeth are more extensive but do not involve as much as 50% of the tooth.
Moderate	3	All enamel surfaces of the teeth are affected, and surfaces subject to attrition show marked wear. Brown stain is frequently a disfiguring feature.
Severe	4	Includes teeth formerly classified as "moderately severe" and "severe". All enamel surfaces are affected, and hypoplasia is so marked that the general form of the tooth may be affected. The major diagnostic sign of this classification is the discrete or confluent pitting. Brown stains are widespread, and teeth often present a corroded-like appearance.

Scoring Per Person

- The worst two teeth are used as a basis for the person-level score.
- Where two teeth are not affected to the same degree, the convention used in recent years seems to have been to assign a person-level score based on the lowest of the two highest scores (Horowitz *et al*, 1984; NIDR, 1991)

Dean's index is still in common use today and is the one recommended by the World Health Organization for oral health surveys (WHO, 1987, 1997).

Advantages

1. Simplicity and utility
2. Clinical manifestations of the response of enamel to fluoride are predictable by the Dean's index

Demerits

1. Since the index is based on the two most severely affected teeth, it does not allow for the measurement of the extent of defects on the remaining teeth.
2. It gives no indication of the location of the teeth or the tooth surfaces affected.
3. The use of the term "questionable" is too vague.
4. The index appears to describe the milder forms of fluorosis accurately but is not sensitive enough to distinguish between degrees of fluorosis in high-fluoride areas.
5. The statistical basis for using the arithmetic mean to calculate the CFI is questionable on the grounds that the classification is based on an ordinal and not an interval scale.

10A.2 Community Fluorosis Index (Dean, 1942)

An index of fluorosis is needed for the community in order to compare its prevalence in communities with different levels of fluoride in water supplies and later to correlate these findings with the caries experience of these communities. The variation of fluorosis within individuals is of less importance than among communities.

Scoring: In a given population, the proportion in each category was multiplied by the weight given to derive a score for the community. $F_{CI} = (n \times w)/N$.

Where, F_{CI} is the community index of fluorosis, n is the number of individuals in each category, w is weighting for each category and N is the total population.

Public health significance of CFI scores as defined by Dean (from Dean, 1946) are listed in Table 10.4.

Table 10.4: Cutoff Level's for CFI	
Range of scores for CFI	Public health significance
0.0–0.4	Negative
0.4–0.6	Borderline
0.6–1.0	Slight
1.0–2.0	Medium
2.0–3.0	Marked
3.0–4.0	Very marked

Bibliography

1. Dean HT. Classification of mottled enamel diagnosis. J Am Dent Assoc 1934;21:1421–26.
2.. Rozier RG. Epidemiologic indices for measuring the clinical manifestations of dental fluorosis: Overview and critique. Adv Dent Res 1994;8(1): 39–55.

10A.3 Moller's Modification of Dean's index

Moller in 1965 attempted to develop a modification for Dean's index to make it more sensitive. The criteria for this index are listed in Table 10.5.

Table 10.5: Criteria for Moller's modification

Weighting	Diagnosis	Clinical criteria
0	Normal	The enamel shows the usual translucency. The surface is smooth, shiny and usually of a pale, creamy white to grey white colour. In this group are also opacities, which are not considered to be of fluorotic character.
0	Optimal	The enamel is on clinical inspection completely homogeneously mineralized without hypomineralization of any sort. The enamel is smooth and mirror-like, and has a shiny, 'varnished' look. The colour is creamy white to yellowish white.
¼	Questionable	In areas with relatively low fluoride content in drinking water, there are cases which even the most experienced researcher cannot classify as either normal or very mild. These cases show mainly labially in the upper front teeth as very narrow, opaque, paper-white, horizontal lines in the tooth's incisal third especially. In the back teeth are now and then seen small, opaque spots (about 0.5 mm in diameter) directly on the cusp tips, while the rest of the tooth is completely normally mineralized. The features of these opaque lines and spots are so fine that they are often confused with perichymata. This fine feature shows more clearly with drying the tooth, a procedure which should always be done while diagnosing
½–1	Very mild	Clearer opaque, paper-white, transversely oriented striations or spots found spread especially on the upper incisal and labial surfaces and most concentrated in the incisal third. In the back teeth are seen opaque regions (<1 mm in diameter) directly on the cusp tips. Opaque, paper-white, narrow, transversely running lines reach down over the cusp, while the rest of the tooth is normal. The opaque regions cover at most a fourth of the surface of the tooth. When viewed from a distance, the tooth seems to have a slightly mother-of-pearl sheen. The lower grades of very mild dental fluorosis are rated 1/2 and the worse 1.
1½ – 2	Mild	The mainly transversely running opaque lines and spots are clear and stretch further down over the tooth's surface towards the outer circumference. One can detect that the opaque lines begin to merge together into diffuse regions, so that the tooth seen at a distance (40–50 cm) seems whiter — more opaque than a normally mineralized tooth. Seen close to, these opaque areas take up, however, at most half of the tooth's surface. Changes in the front teeth's lingual surfaces are considerably less obvious than on the labial. As far as the back teeth are concerned, the changes in labial and lingual surfaces are of more or less the same degree. On the cusps of canines, premolars and molars there are cases where the cusp tips are worn, so that the wear facets peripherally are bordered by a narrow, opaque ring (an expression of the fluorotic surface layer) surrounded by the clearer underlying enamel. In pronounced cases the development of pigment can be seen, especially in the upper incisors. Lower grades of mild dental fluorosis are scored 1½ and the worse degrees 2.

Contd...

Table 10.5: Criteria for Moller's Modification (Contd.)

Weighting	Diagnosis	Clinical criteria
2½ – 3	Moderate	The opaque regions take up practically all the tooth's surface. Tooth shape is normal, but a weak 'pit' development can be found, especially on premolar buccal and palatal surfaces, as well as upper incisor labial surfaces. Pigment where present can vary in colour from yellow to brown. The lower grades of moderate dental fluorosis are rated 2½ and the worse 3.
3½ – 4	Severe	The shape of the tooth can be changed. The development of pits is pronounced. Merging of pits is often seen. Sometimes the outer layer of enamel is partially or completely missing, and the tooth has a corroded look. Pigmentation varies in colour from brown, to dark brown, to black. Lower degrees of severe dental fluorosis score 3½ and the worse degrees 4.

Bibliography

1. Cited in book: Fluorides in caries prevention. 3rd edition. Murray JJ, Rugg-Gunn, Jenkins GN. Vargese Publishing House, India. Page: 226–227.

10A.4 Thylstrup and Fejerskov Index (TFI)

This index was developed to "refine, modify, and extend the original concepts established by Dean" (Fejerskov et al, 1978). It was developed to be more sensitive classification system for recording enamel changes found in areas with fluoride in the drinking water at levels above than that studied by Dean.

Originally facial and occlusal surface were scored. In the modified version, only facial surface is scored. A 10-point ordinal scale is used to classify enamel changes associated with increasing fluoride exposure (Table 10.6). Teeth are to be cleaned and dried for 2 minutes before examination.

Table 10.6: Criteria for TEI

Score	Original criteria (Thylstrup and Fejerskov, 1978)	Modified criteria (Fejerskov et al., 1988)
0	Normal translucency of enamel remains after prolonged air-drying.	The normal translucency of the glossy, creamy-white enamel remains after wiping and drying of the surface.
1	Narrow white lines located corresponding to the perikymata.	Thin white opaque lines are seen running across the tooth surface. The lines correspond to the position of the perikymata. In some cases, a slight "snow capping" of cusps/incisal edges may also be seen.
2	Smooth surfaces: More pronounced lines of opacity which follow the perikymata. Occasionally confluence of adjacent lines. Occlusal surfaces: Scattered areas of opacity < 2 mm in diameter and pronounced opacity of cuspal ridges.	The opaque white lines are more pronounced and frequently merge to form small cloudy areas scattered over the whole surface. "Snow capping" of incisal edges and cusp tips is common.
3	Smooth surfaces: Merging and irregular cloudy areas of opacity. Accentuated drawing of perikymata often visible between opacities. Occlusal surfaces: Confluent areas of marked opacity. Worn areas appear almost normal but usually circumscribed by a rim of opaque enamel.	Merging of the white lines occurs, and cloudy areas of opacity occur spread over many parts of the surface. In between the cloudy areas, white lines can also be seen.
4	Smooth surfaces: The entire surface exhibits marked opacity or appears chalky white. Parts of surface exposed to attrition appear less affected. Occlusal surfaces: Entire surface exhibits marked opacity. Attrition is often pronounced shortly after eruption.	The entire surface exhibits a marked opacity or appears chalky white. Parts of the surface exposed to attrition or wear may appear to be less affected.

Contd...

Table 10.6: Criteria for TEI (Contd.)		
Score	Original criteria (Thylstrup and Fejerskov, 1978)	Modified criteria (Fejerskov et al. 1988)
5	Smooth and occlusal surfaces: Entire surface displays marked opacity with focal loss of outer-most enamel (pits) < 2 mm in diameter.	The entire surface is opaque, and there are round pits (focal loss of the outermost enamel) that are less than 2 mm in diameter.
6	Smooth surfaces: Pits are regularly arranged in horizontal bands < 2 mm in vertical extension. Occlusal surfaces: Confluent areas < 3 mm in diameter exhibit loss of enamel. Marked attrition.	The small pits may frequently be seen merging in the opaque enamel to form bands that are less than 2 mm in vertical height. In this class, these are also included surfaces where the cuspal rim of facial enamel has been chipped off, and the vertical dimension of the resulting damage is less than 2 mm.
7	Smooth surfaces: Loss of outermost enamel in irregular areas involving <½ of entire surface. Occlusal surfaces: Changes in the morphology caused by merging pits and marked attrition.	There is a loss of the outermost enamel in irregular areas, and less than half the surface is so involved. The remaining intact enamel is opaque.
8	Smooth and occlusal surfaces:Loss of outermost enamel involving > ½ of surface.	The loss of the outermost enamel involves more than half the enamel. The remaining intact enamel is opaque.
9	Smooth and occlusal surfaces: Loss of main part of enamel with change in anatomical appearance of surface. Cervical rim of almost unaffected enamel is often noted.	The loss of the major part of the outer enamel results in a change of the anatomical shape of the surface/tooth. A cervical rim of opaque enamel is often noted.

Merit

More sensitive than Dean's index.

Demerits

1. Teeth are examined after a two-minute period of air-drying, which creates an unnatural situation.
2. +thetic significance of changes in score 1 and 2 is questionable since it is the effect of drying that these areas appear clearly.

Bibliography

1. Thylstrup AC, Fejerskov O. Clinical appearance of dental fluorosis in permanent teeth in relation to histologic changes. Community Dent Oral Epidemiol 1978;6: 315–28.

10A.5 Simplified Thylstrup and Fejerskov Index

Ana Karoline A et al., proposed a simplified version of TFI and they evaluated the accuracy in diagnosing dental fluorosis in rural communities. In this simplified version, only six upper anterior teeth were recorded instead of all the teeth present based on the criteria of TFI (Table 10.6).

Bibliography

1. Ana Karoline Adelário, Lívia FVN, Lia SC, Andréa Maria DV, Efigênia FF, Mauro Henrique NGA. Accuracy of the Simplified Thylstrup and Fejerskov Index in Rural Communities with Endemic Fluorosis. Int J Environ Res Public Health 2010,7,927–37.

10A.6 Tooth Surface Index of Fluorosis (TSIF)

It was developed in the early 1980's by Horowitz et al 1984. The TSIF was developed in part to allow for the separate assessment of cosmetic fluorosis, i.e. fluorotic discoloration, staining, or pitting on surfaces visible to others. This index was originally designed with an aim to assess the prevalence and severity of dental fluorosis which were of public health significance.

Method of Examination

Tooth surfaces are not dried before the examination, the rationale being primarily an esthetic one. The rationale is that teeth should be assessed in their natural state and that those opacities that are visible only after drying should not be included in the definition of fluorosis. Surfaces scored for anterior teeth are facial and lingual surface and for posterior teeth are buccal, occlusal, and lingual surface. The criteria for fluorosis are listed in Table 10.7.

Merits

1. Provides a useful indication of severity of fluorosis.
2. Distinction between discrete pitting and more advanced confluent pitting is made, making the index more sensitive than Dean's to higher degrees of fluorosis.
3. Criteria for scoring in the TSIF are clearer, and consequently, subjectivity should be reduced in their application.
4. The scoring of surfaces rather than individual teeth makes it more sensitive.

Demerits

1. Examiner reliability may be of more concern than with Dean's Index or the modified TFI because of the larger number of assessments to be made (72 surfaces vs. the usual maximum of 28 teeth or buccal surfaces in children).
2. The added lingual surfaces are more difficult to visualize than buccal surfaces,

which also adds to the concern about examiner reliability.

Bibliography

1. Horowitz HS, Driscoll WS, Meyers RJ, Heifetz SB, Kingman A. A new method for assessing the prevalence of dental fluorosis—the Tooth Surface Index of Fluorosis. J Am Dent Assoc. 1984;109: 37–41.

10A.7 Fluorosis Risk Index (FRI)

This was developed by Pendrys in 1990. Fluorosis Risk Index was designed to respond to the current pattern of fluoride exposure, which can be highly variable during the period when teeth are at risk of fluorosis.

The unique feature of the FRI is that each tooth is divided into zones that correspond to the age at which they begin development, and can be related to narrow age-bands of fluoride exposure, such as a 12-month time period. Buccal surface and the incisal edge/occlusal table of each permanent tooth (excluding third molars) have been divided into four scoring zones:

a. The incisal edge/occlusal table, defined as the enamel surface within one millimeter of the incisal edge of the tooth.

Table 10.7: The criteria for fluorosis for TSIF

Score	Criteria
0	Enamel shows no evidence of fluorosis.
1	Enamel shows definite evidence of fluorosis, namely, areas with parchment-white color that totals less than one-third of the visible enamel surface. This category includes fluorosis confined only to incisal edges of anterior teeth and cusp tips of posterior teeth ("snow capping").
2	Parchment-white fluorosis totals at least one-third of the visible surface, but less than two-thirds.
3	Parchment-white fluorosis totals at least two-thirds of the visible surface.
4	Enamel shows staining in conjunction with any of the preceding levels of fluorosis. Staining is defined as an area of definite discoloration that may range from light to very dark brown.
5	Discrete pitting of the enamel exists, unaccompanied by evidence of staining of intact enamel. A pit is defined as a definite physical defect in the enamel surface with a rough floor that is surrounded by a wall of intact enamel. The pitted area is usually stained or differs in color from the surrounding enamel.
6	Both discrete pitting and staining of the intact enamel exit.
7	Confluent pitting of the enamel surface exists. Large areas of enamel may be missing, and the anatomy of the tooth may be altered. Dark-brown stain is usually present.

b. The incisal/occlusal third of the buccal surface.

c. The middle third of the buccal surface.

d. The cervical third of the buccal surface.

Classification System

The classification I enamel surface zones: Portions of the enamel that begin formation during the first year of life, referred to as classification I enamel surface zones.

The classification II enamel surface zones: that begins formation during the third through sixth years of life.

Roughly 112 zones are scored, with 10 belonging to classification I, 48 to classification II, and the remaining 54 to unassigned zones. Scoring criteria are listed in Table 10.8.

Scoring

Subjects are identified as cases or controls for each of the two surface zones based on the distribution of scores within each.

At least two surfaces of a particular zone must have scores of 2 or 3 in order to be considered a case.

Table 10.8: Criteria for FRI

Score	Classification	Criteria
0	Negative	A surface zone will receive a score of 0 when there is absolutely no indication of fluorosis being present. There must be a complete absence of any white spots or striations, and tooth surface coloration must appear normal.
1	Questionable	Any surface zone that is questionable as to 1 whether there is fluorosis present (i.e. white spots, striations, or fluorotic defects cover 50% or less of the surface zone).
2	Positive: Mild-to-moderate	A smooth surface zone will be diagnosed as mild-to- being positive for enamel fluorosis if greater than 50% of the zone displays parchment-2 white striations typical of enamel fluorosis. Incisal edges and occlusal tables will be scored as positive for enamel fluorosis if greater than 50% of that surface is marked by the snow capping typical of enamel fluorosis.
3	Positive severe	A surface zone will be diagnosed as positive for severe fluorosis if greater than 50% of the 3 zone displays pitting, staining, and deformity, indicative of severe fluorosis.
7	Non-fluoride opacity	Any surface zone that has an opacity that appears to be a non-fluoride opacity.
9	Excluded	A surface zone is categorized as excluded 9 (i.e. not adequately visible for a diagnosis to be made) when any of the following conditions exist incomplete eruption: **Rule 1:** If a tooth is in proximal contact but the occlusal surface is not parallel with existing occlusion, the occlusal two-thirds of the tooth is scored, but the cervical one-third is recorded as excluded. **Rule 2:** If a tooth is erupted, but not yet in contact, the incisal/occlusal edge is scored, but all other surfaces are recorded as excluded. Orthodontic appliances and bands: **Rule 1:** If there is an orthodontic band present on a tooth only the occlusal table or incisal edge should be scored. **Rule 2:** If greater than 50 percent of the surface zones are banded, the subject should be excluded from the examination. Surfaces crowned or restored: **Rule 3:** Surface zones that are replaced by either a crown or restoration covering greater than 50 percent of the surface zone should be recorded as excluded. **Rule 4:** Any subject with gross deposits of plaque or debris on greater than 50 percent of the surface zones should be excluded from examination.

Demerits

1. Not suited to provide prevalence data
2. The index is complex, both from a biological perspective and in its application.
3. Acceptable levels of examiner reliability may be difficult to establish due to this complexity.
4. Results cannot be compared with those of any of the established indices used in determining prevalence. Therefore, the index cannot serve the dual purpose of providing prevalence estimates as well as estimates of risk
5. Case definition will affect the identification of risk factors.

Bibliography

1. Pendrys DG. The fluorosis risk index: a method for investigating risk factors. J Public Health Dent 1990;50:291–8.

10A.8 Chronological Fluorosis Assessment (CFA) Index

Evans RW developed an index for assessing dental fluorosis on the labial surfaces of the maxillary central incisors, since these teeth are among the first permanent teeth to erupt and are also of esthetic concern.

The labial surface of the maxillary central incisor crown is divided into three parts. The cervical, middle, and incisal third divisions are each scored separately according to the following criteria are listed in Table 10.9.

A tooth should be excluded unless 3 mm of the crown has emerged; this constitutes the incisal third. The middle third should be excluded unless eruption of the incisor has reached the point where the length of the erupted crown is equal to the incisal width. All three thirds are scored when, in principle, the ratio of crown length to incisal width is 3:2.

Uses: This index lends itself for assessment of the chronological development of dental fluorosis in relation to a given event, (1) within-individual fluorosis distribution across tooth thirds, (2) fluorosis distribution between tooth thirds both within and between cohorts of individuals, and (3) fluorosis distribution across tooth thirds where they are grouped by common developmental periods, as a means for controlling time-related variation in, for example, fluoride exposure.

The analysis was linked to the developmental period of the enamel crowns of the maxillary central incisors which commences at birth or soon afterward and is completed during the fourth year of life (Nielsen and Ravn, 1976). It was presumed that the rate of development proceeds linearly. Hence by the end of the first 16, 32 and 48 months of life, the respective development of the maxillary central incisor crown will be, on average, one-third, two-thirds and finally completed.

Table 10.9: Criteria for CFA index

Score	Criteria
0	The enamel has a normal appearance.
1	Signs of dental fluorosis-that is, opaque paper white areas scattered irregularly over the tooth surface (Dean, 1942)-affect less than 10% of the area.
2	10–49% of the area is affected.
3	50–89% of the area is affected.
4	90–100% of the area is affected.
5	The presence of pitting of fluorotic origin, as detected by the probing method described by Horowitz et al. (1984).
X	The surface is excluded from assessment, due either to non-eruption or to the presence of a defect that precludes a proper assessment, such as, for example tetracycline staining or caries.

Bibliography

1. Evans RW. An Epidemiological Assessment of the Chronological Distribution of Dental Fluorosis in Human Maxillary Central Incisors. J Dent Res 1993;72(5):883–90.

10A.9 Simplified Fluoride Mottling Index

This index was introduced in 1984 by Rahamatulla M and Rajasekar A.

It is based on the enamel opacities/lesion present on facial surfaces of the six upper and lower anterior teeth which are examined because of esthetic importance. The criteria are listed in Table 10.10.

Table 10.10: Criteria for simplified fluoride mottling index

Scores	Criteria
0	No involvement of facial surface.
1	Less than 1/3rd of the facial surface show evidence of lesion
2	About 1/3rd but less than 2/3rd of the surface affected
3	Over 2/3rd of facial surface involved
4	Brownish, black discoloration of entire facial surface

Bibliography

1. Rahamatulla M, Rajasekar A. A simplified method for assessment of community fluorosis index. IADR Abstract 1308; P316;1984.

10A.10 Visual Analog Scale

Despite the numerous advantages, the TFI, as well as the other dental fluorosis indices, are not on a continuous scale. All current dental fluorosis indices use ordinal scales and, therefore, the scores should be considered only arbitrary points along a continuum of change. Grading severity of dental fluorosis on a continuous scale is extremely important when the correlation between two factors is studied, as well as when evaluating the cause-and-effect relationship between two variables. Thus, the importance of creating a continuous scale for assessing the severity of dental fluorosis is evident.

Reference photographs were taken of patients' anterior teeth in areas of endemic fluorosis. The set examiners were asked to grade the amount of discoloration and malformation in the photographs on a 100 mm VAS. The left end of the scale was marked "best you can imagine," and the right end of the scale was marked "worst you can imagine." The photographs were shown in random order to each examiner. VAS score for each photograph, as perceived by each examiner, using a 100 mm ruler underneath the VAS and measuring the distance between the left end of the scale and the mark made by the examiner.

The visual analog scale (VAS) is a 100 millimeter continuous scale.

Advantages of VAS
1. VAS is completed rapidly, produces ratio data (that is, a linear scale)
2. Has high sensitivity to change
3. Is easy to score
4. Has good construct validity

Disadvantages: Perception regarding the fluorosis might vary among populations due to which scale need to be validated among different population groups.

Bibliography

1. Vieira APGF, Lawrence HP, Limeback H, Sampio FC, Grynpas M. A visual analog scale for measuring dental fluorosis severity. J Am Dent Assoc 2005;136:895–901.

10B. Descriptive Classifications

Indices based upon the clinical appearance of defects were proposed by various investigators (Losee et al., 1961; Young, 1973; Al-Alousi et al., 1975; Jackson et al., 975; Suckling et al., 1976; Murray and Shaw, 1979; FDI, 1982; Smith, 1983).

Each descriptive index is based on the principle that the recording of any condition, once the criteria are defined, must depend upon this definition and not be based on any presumed etiology.

10B.1 The Developmental Defects of Enamel Index (DDE Index) (FDI, 1982)

This was developed by working group of the FDI Commission on Oral Health, Research and Epidemiology.

Need for the Index
1. Lack of a well-defined and accepted classification of enamel defects and therefore a lack of comparability among various studies of such defects
2. Classification based on etiological considerations is premature, since only a few defects can be assigned an etiology
3. Classification based on descriptive criteria is the preferred basis of an epidemiological index

4. Descriptive classification should have flexibility for recording data on a person, tooth, or tooth-surface basis

Classification of enamel defects

1. *Types of defect:*

Normal

Opacity   (white/cream)

Opacity   (yellow/brown)

Hypoplasia   (pits)

Hypoplasia   (grooves: horizontal)

Hypoplasia   (grooves: vertical)

Hypoplasia   (missing enamel)

Discolored enamel   (not associated with opacity)

Other defects

Combination of defects

2. *Number and demarcation of defects:*

Single

Multiple

Diffuse (fine white lines)

Diffuse (patchy)

3. *Location of defects:*

Gingival one-half

Incisal one-half

Occlusal

Cuspal

Definitions of Terms used in the Classification

1. Types of Defects:

Developmental defects of enamel may be defined as disturbances in hard tissue matrices and in their mineralization arising during odontogenesis. Disturbances may be clinically obvious, they may be localized affecting single teeth or multiple teeth, systemic affecting groups of teeth developing at the period of disturbance or genetic. Defects may affect all teeth, primary only or permanent only and may also involve dentine or cementum or both.

Hypoplasia is defined as a quantitative defect of enamel visually and morphologically identified as involving the surface of the enamel (an external defect) and associated with a reduced thickness of enamel. The defective enamel may occur as (a) shallow or deep pits or rows of pits arranged horizontally in a linear fashion across the tooth surface or, generally distributed over the whole or part of the enamel surface; (b) the defective enamel may occur as small or large, wide or narrow grooves; (c) in some instances there may be partial or complete absence of enamel over small or considerable areas of dentine.

Opacity is defined as a qualitative defect of enamel identified visually as an abnormality in the translucency of enamel. It is characterized by a white or, discolored (cream, brown, yellow) area but in all cases the enamel surface is smooth and the thickness of enamel is normal, except in some instances when associated with hypoplasia.

Discolored enamel is defined as an obvious abnormal appearance of the enamel, which because of its color and distribution cannot be considered within the normal range of variation in color and shade of tooth enamel. This category excludes colored opacities.

2. Number and Demarcation of Defects:

Single: A defect well demarcated from the adjacent normal enamel. Only one lesion is visible on the tooth surface.

Multiple: More than one defect with margins well demarcated from the adjacent normal enamel.

Diffuse: Fine white lines. Distinct lines of opacity which follow the pattern of the perikymata. Confluence of adjacent lines may be observed.

Diffuse: Patchy, irregular, cloudy areas of opacity lacking well-defined margins.

3. Location of defects

The lingual and buccal surfaces (meeting at the incisal edge) of the anterior teeth have been arbitrarily divided into two halves: one half adjacent to the gingival margin, one-half adjacent to the incisal tip. Posterior teeth (premolars and molars) have an additional surface, the occlusal. This is the anatomical occlusal surface commencing at the cusp. Cuspal refers specifically to the tip of a cusp. It should not be confused with incisal or occlusal, and should be used only when a defect is distinctly confined to the cusp.

Clinical Examination

Tooth surfaces should be inspected visually, and defective areas tactilely explored with a probe to determine abnormalities of surface contour. Natural or artificial light can be used depending on field conditions. When using artificial light, the intensity and incidence of the source should be altered to overcome 'burning out' of the defects. Ideally the teeth should receive a prophylaxis and be dried at the time of examination.

- Unerupted, missing, heavily restored, badly decayed, fractured teeth and teeth (or tooth) Recording and coding of data should be done as described in Table 10.11

- Unerupted, missing, heavily restored, badly decayed, fractured teeth and teeth (or tooth surfaces) which for any other reason cannot be classified for defects must be coded 'X'. This implies that it will be disregarded from statistical evaluation.

- If the defect does not resemble any of the listed specific defects then it is coded as 'Other defect'. A written description can then be attached.

- Where more than one type of defect occurs on the same surface, each type is coded. This will produce two codes which will require recoding

Table 10.11: Codes for DDE		
	Permanent	*Primary*
Type of defect		
Normal	0	A
Opacity (white/cream)	1	B
Opacity (yellow/brown)	2	C
Hypoplasia (pits)	3	D
Hypoplasia (grooves: horizontal)	4	E
Hypoplasia (grooves: vertical)	5	F
Hypoplasia (missing enamel)	6	G
Discolored enamel (not associated with opacity)	7	H
Other defects	8	J
Combination of defects		
Number and demarcation of defects		
Single	1	A
Multiple	2	B
Diffuse (fine white lines)	3	C
Diffuse (patchy)	4	D
Location of the defect		
No defect	0	
Gingival one-half	1	
Incisal one-half	2	
Gingival and incisal halves	3	
Occlusal	4	
Cuspal	5	
Whole surface	6	
Other combinations	7	

- Number and demarcation: When the type of the defect has been classified the number of defects is coded.

Location of the Defect

The location of the defect is coded as in the gingival or incisal one-half, occlusally or cuspal. Where a lesion very obviously involves more than one segment, codes are available to identify all possibilities. However, there does not appear to be much value in attempting to be very precise in locating the segment and area covered by a lesion. The areas designated are arbitrary: it is sufficient to identify the primary location.

Demerits

1. Because of the multiple coding system and the examination of each tooth surface, the DDE Index is time-consuming and complicated to use and analyze.
2. Reproducibility of data using the index could be questionable.
3. Type of defect section in the index refers primarily to white and yellow opacities and to hypoplasia. Differentiation between opacities, whether white or yellow, is less important than the distinction between whether they were demarcated or diffuse.
4. Another major deficiency with the Index is that it is unable to record the severity of defects (Clarkson, 1987).

10B.2 The Modified Developmental Defects of Enamel Index

This was developed by Clarkson and O' Mullane (1989) for use in general purpose epidemiological studies. The criteria are listed in Table 10.12.

For screening and surveys, the criteria for modified DDE index has been simplified further (Table 10.13).

The major differences between the modified and the original DDE Index are:
1. A single score (instead of two scores) applies to each defect recorded

Table 10.12: Codes for modified DDE

	Code	Criteria
	0	Normal
Demarcated opacities	1	white/cream
	2	yellow/brown
Diffuse opacities	3	Diffuse – lines
	4	Diffuse – patchy
	5	Diffuse – confluent
	6	Confluent/patchy + staining + loss of enamel
Hypoplasia	7	Pits
	8	Missing Enamel
	9	Any other defects
Extent of defect	0	Normal
	1	<1/3rd
	2	At least 1/3rd to 2/3rd
	3	At least 2/3rd

Table 10.13: Codes for modified DDE for screening

Code	Criteria
0	Normal
1	Demarcated opacity
2	Diffuse opacity
3	Hypoplasia
4	Other defects

2. The demarcation of an opacity (demarcated or diffuse) instead of its color is the main factor recorded
3. The diffuse opacity section is expanded to allow for the recording of more extensive types of these opacities seen, i.e. confluent (score 5) and confluent in combination with staining and loss of enamel (score 6)
4. The scores for hypoplasia have been reduced from four to two by omitting scores for Grooves
5. The score for discoloration has been excluded
6. The severity of defects is included by recording the extent of defects.
7. The extent of a defect is derived by visually condensing all areas affected by a defect and then relating the total area affected to that of the total visible tooth surface area.

Bibliography

1. Clarkson J, O'Mullane D. A Modified DDE Index for Use in Epidemiological Studies of Enamel Defects. J Dent Res 1989;68(3):445–50.

10B.3 Young's Classification to Quantify Enamel Opacities

Table 10.14: Young's classification

Class	Classification
1	White fleck areas of enamel not greater than 2 mm in any direction
2	Colored flecks same as white flecks but usually varying shades of yellow or brown
3	White patches — opaque white areas > 2 mm when measured in any direction, well demarcated from the surrounding enamel
4	Outline and form same as white patches, but also colored. Usually varying shades of yellow or brown
5	Spaced white lines, These are seen as fine opaque lines in the enamel, Ill–defined areas of chalky white appearance also seen occasionally
6	As for class 5, but associated with hypoplasia
7	A mixture of white lines, opaque and colored areas. Lines often difficult to distinguish from the diffuse illdefined areas.
8	As for class 7, but associated with hypoplasia

Demerits

1. The scores are not arranged in a well-ordered fashion.
2. The use of such criteria as "areas greater or less than 2 mm" does not take into account the total area of a tooth surface which may be affected.
3. The criteria do not cover the full range of defects and there is no attempt to differentiate between the demarcation of opacities.
4. The criteria of diagnosis are not clearly stated, e.g. if two defects occur on the same surface, no indication is given as to which should be recorded.

10B.4 Al-Alousi and Jackson Classification of Enamel Defects

The main principle of this index was that the recording of any condition once defined must be made on the basis of that definition and not on the basis of a presumed etiology.

Table 10.15: AL-Alousi and Jackson classification

Type	Classification
A	White areas less than 2 mm in diameter.
B	White areas of, or greater than, 2 mm in diameter.
C	Colored (brown) areas less than 2 mm in diameter, irrespective of there being white areas.
D	Colored (brown) areas of, or greater than, 2 mm in diameter, irrespective of there being any white areas.
E	Horizontal white lines. Irrespective of there being any white non-linear areas.
F	Colored (brown) or white areas or lines associated with pits or hypoplastic areas.

This classification is similar to that used by Young (1973).

Examination

The occlusal, buccal and lingual surface of each tooth was examined and scored separately for the presence of any enamel opacity.

All missing or traumatized teeth and those with areas classified as questionable early carious lesions to be excluded.

Merits

It is simple to use and is not based on etiological factors.

It permits the study of a large number of persons in a limited amount of time and at minimum cost.

It is sensitive enough to detect small changes.

Bibliography

1. Al-Alousi W, Jackson D, Crompton G, Jenkins OC. Enamel mottling in a fluoride and in a non-fluoride community — A Study. Br Dent J. 1975;138,9.

10B.5 Murray and Shaw Criteria for Diagnosing Opacities

The occlusal, buccal and lingual surfaces of each tooth were examined and scored separately for the presence of any enamel opacity according to the criteria described in Table 10.16.

Table 10.16: Murray and Shaw criteria	
Type	Criteria
1	White opaque spots (or flecks) less than 2 mm in diameter.
2	White opaque spots (or patches) greater than 2 mm when measured in any direction. Well demarcated from the surrounding area.
3	Colored spots, flecks or patches.
4	Horizontal white lines, irrespective of there being any white non-linear lines. Not associated with deficiency of enamel substance (hypoplasia).
5	Hypoplasia, in association with any of categories 1–4.
6	Possible early carious lesions.
7	Missing.

Bibliography

1. Murray JJ, Shaw L. Classification and prevalence of enamel opacities in the human deciduous and permanent dentition. Arch Oral Biol. 1979;24:7–13.

10B.6 Mottling Index

Enamel defects were divided into three categories; mottling, opacities, and pigmentation. Their absence, presence, and severity were assessed by use of a standardized classification and recorded for the maxillary permanent incisors and canines only. For mottling, a six-point scale was used, based upon a modification of Dean's classification as described by Hodge & Smith. By definition, mottling was determined as such when at least four of the six maxillary teeth were affected in a linear fashion with or without concomitant pitting of the enamel surface. The description of the six point classification is described in Table 10.17.

Table 10.17: Criteria for mottling index	
Score	Mottling
M0	Normal—The enamel presents the usual translucent semi-vitriform type of structure with a smooth, glossy surface.
M1	Questionable — Slight aberrations from the normal translucency of enamel present, ranging from a few white flecks to occasional white areas.
M2	Very mild—Small, opaque, white lines or areas scattered irregularly over the tooth, but not involving as much as approximately 25% of the tooth surface.
M3	Mild — More extensive white opaque lines or areas in the enamel not involving as much as 50% of the tooth.
M4	Moderate — All labial enamel surfaces affected with possible attrition and wear, and brown stain sometimes a disfiguring feature.
M5	Severe — All labial enamel surfaces affected and hypoplastic, so that the general form of the tooth may be affected. Discrete or confluent pitting with widespread brown stains giving a corroded-like appearance.
Opacities were determined as isolated white flecks, spots, or patches randomly placed. These spots were only considered as opacities when involving one or two of the labial surfaces of the six teeth examined.	
O1	White opaque flecks, spots or patches involving less than 25% of the labial surface enamel.
O2	White opaque flecks, spots or patches involving 25–50% of the labial surface enamel.
O3	White opaque flecks, spots or patches involving more than 50% of the labial surface enamel.
Pigmentations were defined as the presence of a yellow or brown area similarly distributed as the opacities.	
P1	Yellow or brown pigmented patches involving less than 25% of the labial surface enamel.
P2	Yellow or brown pigmented patches involving 25– 50% of the labial surface enamel
P3	Yellow or brown pigmented patches involving more than 50% of the labial surface enamel.

Bibliography

1. Hodge, Smith 1965 cited in Curzon MEJ and Spector PC. Enamel mottling in a high strontium area of the USA. Community Dent Oral Epidemiol. 1977;5:243–7.

10B.7 Enamel Defects Index

Enamel defects index (EDI) was created based on three innovative principles: (i) A basic level of the three major categories of defects; (ii) more detailed subcategories of each major category; and (iii) each category scored independently as present or absent, thus simplifying decision making. The basic-level categories are hypoplasia, opacity, and post-eruptive breakdown scored by clinical diagnosis, resulting in a three-digit score per tooth surface examined, ranging from 000 to 111. Of the 3-digit score, the first digit relates to hypoplasia, the second to opacities, and the third to post-eruptive breakdown (Table 10.18).

Category definitions of the basic version of the enamel defects index as shown in Table 10.18.

Bibliography

1. Elcock C, Lath DL, Luty JD, Gallagher MG, Abdellatif A, Backman B, Brook AH. The new Enamel Defects Index: testing and expansion. Eur J Oral Sci 2006; 114: 35–8.

Table 10.18: Enamel defects index	
Defect	*Definition*
Hypoplasia	A defect involving the surface of enamel and associated with a reduced thickness; this may be translucent or opaque
Opacity	A defect involving an alteration in the translucency of enamel, which can be variable in degree. The enamel is of normal thickness, with a smooth surface. The opacity may be white, yellow or brown in color, with a demarcated or diffuse border.
Post-eruptive breakdown	A defect including the loss of surface enamel, after tooth eruption

11

Indices to Assess Malocclusion

INTRODUCTION

Many indices have been used with some success for recording other dental disorders (caries and periodontal diseases). Malocclusion is unique in presenting as a group of often unrelated traits to which, in social psychological terms, there may be considerable variability of adjustment. Despite these problems, several malocclusion indices have been developed and have been used for diagnostic classification, epidemiological data collection, recording treatment need/priority and assessment of the success of treatment.

There are five types of index, each for a distinct purpose. Indeed it is the purpose rather than content or conventions of an index that distinguishes it.

Diagnostic Classification

Angle's classification is the best known of this type, its subclasses often being used to describe incisor and buccal segment relationships separately. These classifications serve their purpose reasonably well, allowing ease of communication between orthodontists.

Epidemiologic Indices

These indices record every trait in a malocclusion to allow estimation of the prevalence of malocclusion in a given population; for example, the epidemiologic registration of malocclusion described by Bjork, Krebs and Solow, the FDI method, or Summer's occlusal index. Other indices of this type score tooth alignment in a way that allows study of tooth irregularity and periodontal disease, or treatment stability.

Treatment Need (Treatment Priority) Indices

Many indices have been developed to allow categorization of malocclusion according to the level of treatment need. Examples of these are Draker's HLD index, Grainger's treatment priority index and Salzman's handicapping malocclusion assessment. Summer's occlusal index, primarily designed for epidemiologic purposes, has also been used to determine treatment priority. These indices yield a score for each trait or component that is then weighted to calculate an overall score.

Treatment Outcome Indices

Assessment of the outcome of treatment or the changes resulting from treatment is a further potential use of occlusal indices. Several indices have been developed to evaluate treatment success. Summer's index and PAR index has also been used to assess the outcome of treatment.

Treatment Complexity Index

At present only one index, i.e. Index of Complexity, Outcome and Need (ICON) has been described to measure treatment complexity.

Bibliography

1. Shaw WC, Richmond S, O'Brien KD. The use of occlusal indices: A European perspective American J Orthodontics 1995;1–10.

11.1 Index of Tooth Position by Massler and Frankel

Angle's variations were modified for the purpose of this study by combining some (a tooth could not be both buccal and lingual or mesial and distal at the same time, nor could it be both supracluded and infracluded), and adding the category of "missing" tooth. Therefore the following descriptive classification of malpositions was used.

- Buccal (labial) or lingual displacement
- Mesial or distal displacement
- Rotated
- Infracluded or supracluded

A given tooth can therefore be in only one to three positions within the arch: correct occlusion, malpositioned or missing. If malpositioned, the tooth can be displaced in as many as four different spatial relationships. Table 11.1 shows codes for various tooth positions.

In all cases, even minor deviations from the contact line and the ideal plane of occlusion as defined by Angle were noted. The occlusal and buccal examinations were recorded separately. The exact deviation of each tooth from its ideal position in the plane of occlusion could thus be readily recorded without the

Table 11.1: Codes for tooth positions

Codes	
BR	Labial displacement and rotated
B	Labial displacement
M	Mesial displacement
LR	Lingual displacement and rotated
LMR	Lingual and mesial displacement, rotated
X	Lost by extraction
DR	Distal displacement and rotated
D	Distal displacement
S	Supra-erupted
I	Infra-erupted

necessity of making time consuming models of the teeth and arches of each child.

Any tooth which was not in perfect occlusion from both the occlusal and buccal aspects was considered maloccluded. Third molars are not considered. Each maloccluded tooth was assessed a value of one without regard to the degree of its displacement. Thus a given tooth might have been recorded as having been malposed in four different ways, but was counted only once as one maloccluded tooth. The number of maloccluded teeth in each individual was then counted. The evaluation of the occlusion of a given individual resulted in a number from 0 to 28. Missing teeth were considered only as absent. The effects of missing teeth, particularly lower first molars were assessed and counted although the missing tooth was itself not counted as maloccluded tooth. Newly erupted teeth which had not yet reached their full occlusal position were not counted as infraerupted. Rather this classification was reserved for those teeth which were pathologically prevented from erupting.

The designation of malocclusion was reserved for those patients in whom the malpositioning of the teeth was sufficiently severe in degree to require orthodontic treatment and, or any case having more than 10 malpositioned teeth.

Bibliography

1. Massler M, Frankel JM. Prevalence of malocclusion in children aged 14 to 18 years. Am J Orthod 1951;37(10):751–68.

11.2 Handicapping Labio-lingual Deviation (HLD) Index

The intent of the HLD index is to measure the degree of handicap caused by the different components of malocclusion. The Medicaid statutes in the early 1960s recognized there was a need for a method to identify those with a medically handicapping malocclusion. Draker HL developed the handicapping labio-lingual deviation (HLD) index which was one of the first indices used in the United States to identify those with handicapping mal-occlusions. The HLD selects deviations from ideal and these are scored and weighted. The HLD index has been modified by some states to determine and prioritize eligibility for the state-funded orthodontic treatment. The original cut-off point of 13 selected for the HLD index.

The Maryland's version of HLD, the HLD (Md) index, modified the HLD's original scoring formula for overjet and overbite. The HLD (Md), changed the cut-off from 13 to 15 points and modified the Draker's scoring formula by subtracting 2 mm from overjet and 3 mm from overbite measurements.

The state of Washington HLD modification has five qualifying conditions and the cut-off point has changed to 30. The original form of the HLD index is not a reliable index to assess the orthodontic treatment need because it does not record missing, impacted teeth, spacing between teeth and transverse discrepancies such as midline deviations and crossbites.

The HLD index was modified in the state of California, the HLD (CalMod) index and used the cut-off point of 26 (Table 11.2). CalMod HLD index has been created because of the settlements originating from two lawsuits against the state of California claiming the state of California failed to comply with the orthodontic provisions of the Medicaid statutes (Brown V. Kizer, 1989; Duran V. Belshe, 1994). As a result of these lawsuits, two qualifying exceptions that cause tissue damage were added to the original HLD index, namely the deep impinging bites and crossbites of individual anterior teeth with tissue destruction (Parker, 1998). In addition, overjets greater than 9 mm and reverse overjets more than 3.5 mm were added as additional qualifying exceptions. The ectopic eruption and unilateral posterior crossbite were also added as weighted factors (Parker, 1998).

No	Condition	Score
	Table 11.2: The California modification of the HLD (CalMod) index	
1	Cleft palate deformity	
2	Cranio-facial anomaly	
3	Deep impinging overbite: When the lower incisors are destroying the soft tissue of the palate. Tissue laceration and/or clinical attachment loss must be present.	
4	Crossbite of individual anterior teeth: When clinical attachment loss and recession of the gingival margin are present.	
5	Severe traumatic deviations: Attach a description of condition, i.e. loss of a pre-maxilla by burn, trauma or pathology.	
6	Overjet greater than 9 mm: Reverse overjet greater than 3.5 mm	
7	Overjet (≤ 9 mm)	(mm)
8	Overbite including the reverse overbite	(mm)
9	Mandibular protrusion (reverse overjet ≤ 3.5 mm)	(mm) × 5
10	Open bite	(mm) × 4
11	Ectopic eruption: Count each tooth, excluding third molars	(count) × 3
12	Anterior crowding: Score one point for the maxilla, and/or one point for mandible; two points maximum for anterior crowding.	(0, 1, or 2) × 5
13	Labio-lingual spread: Arch length insufficiency must exceed 3.5 mm excluding mild rotations that may react favorably to stripping or mild expansion procedures.	(mm)
14	Posterior unilateral crossbite: Must involve 2 or more adjacent teeth, one of which must be a molar and not including the posterior bilateral crossbite	4
Total Score		

Conditions 1 to 6 are the qualifying conditions and if present further scoring is not needed. Otherwise, the sum of other conditions (7–14) must be 26 or above to be considered as a handicapping malocclusion. All measurements are recorded in the order given and rounded off to the nearest millimeter. If both anterior crowding and ectopic eruption are present in the anterior portion of the mouth, the most severe condition will be scored, not both conditions. Overjet is recorded with the patient's teeth in centric occlusion and measured from the labial portion of the lower incisors to the labial of the upper incisors. This index is recommended for use on individuals of 13 years of age and older.

Bibliography

1. Ali Borzabadi-Farahani (2011). An Overview of Selected Orthodontic Treatment Need Indices, Principles in Contemporary Orthodontics, Dr. Silvano Naretto (Ed.), ISBN: 978-953-307-687-4.
2. Parker WS. The HLD (CalMod) index and the index question. Am J Orthodontics and Dentofacial Orthopedics 1998;114:134–41.

11.3 Handicapping Malocclusion Assessment Record

The handicapping malocclusion assessment record form is not designed to ascertain the presence of occlusal deviations ordinarily included in epidemiologic surveys of malocclusion or for clinical orthodontic examinations. Etiology, diagnosis, planning and complexity of treatment, and prognosis are not factors in this assessment.

Assessments can be made from casts or directly in the mouth of the patient. An additional record form is provided for direct mouth assessment which permits recording and scoring of mandibular function, facial asymmetry, lower lip malposition in relation to the maxillary incisor teeth and desirability of treatment. In order to avoid being influenced by considerations of etiology, treatment planning, difficulty and duration of treatment, and other professional value judgments not pertinent to this assessment, the assessor should not spend undue time in examining the casts. Scoring should be based on the first impression.

The teeth in malocclusion are assessed according to the criteria and the weights or point values assigned to them. The relative point values are based on clinical orthodontic experience from the standpoint of the usual contributory effects of various types of malocclusion on dental health, function and esthetics. The assessor should score 2 points for each affected maxillary incisor and 1 point for each affected maxillary posterior tooth and for each affected mandibular anterior and posterior tooth.

The maxillary anterior segment includes the four incisors only. Two points should be scored for deviated maxillary incisor and 2 points for each visible crest of the interdental papilla of spaced maxillary teeth from canine to canine. The mandibular anterior segment also includes the four incisors, for which only 1 point is scored for each deviated incisor tooth and 1 point for each visible crest of the interdental papilla from canine to canine when incisors are spaced.

The posterior segments in the maxilla and in the mandible include the canines, first and second premolars, and first molars. One point only is scored for each posterior tooth deviation and for each spaced posterior tooth (not papilla) when both the crests of the mesial and distal interdental papillae are visible. When the maxillary anterior score under A (intra-arch deviation) plus the score of the anterior segment under B (inter-arch deviation) equals 6 points or more, 8 additional points are added to the grand total score to denote the presence of an esthetic handicap.

A. *Intra-arch Deviation*

Intra-arch deviation assessment is made by placing the casts, teeth upward, in direct view of the assessor. The number or teeth affected is recorded as indicated on the handicapping malocclusion assessment record form. When series of assessments are made, the score can be computed at a later time.

Missing anterior and posterior teeth are assessed by actual count.

An unerupted tooth, a severely carious non-functioning tooth, or a tooth with only the roots remaining is recorded as missing.

- Crowded anterior and posterior teeth.
- Rotated anterior teeth
- Rotated posterior teeth
- Open spacing of anterior teeth
- Closed spacing of anterior teeth
- Open spacing of posterior teeth
- Closed spacing of posterior teeth.

B. *Inter-arch Deviation*

The casts are approximated in terminal occlusion as indicated by a wax bite so as not to extend beyond the buccal and labial surfaces of the occluded teeth.

- Overjet
- Overbite
- Cross bite of incisors
- Cross bite of posterior teeth
- Open bite of incisors
- Open bite of posterior teeth
- Anteroposterior deviation of posterior teeth.

C. *Dentofacial Deviations: 8 Points are Scored for Each Dentofacial Deviation*

- Facial and oral clefts
- Lower lip palatal to maxillary incisor teeth
- Occlusal interference
- Functional jaw limitation
- Facial asymmetry
- Speech impairment.

Bibliography

1. Salzmann JA. Handicapping malocclusion assessment to establish treatment priority. American J Orthodontics 1968;54:749.

11.4 FDI System (A Method for Measuring Occlusal Traits)

This was developed by the FDI Commission on Classification and Statistics for Oral Conditions (COCSTOC).

The method proposed in this system is designed for application to subjects who, considering their age, should have full complements of permanent teeth, except for third molars. This method is not designed for use on subjects who are still in a mixed dentition stage of development because of the dynamic nature of the mixed dentition stage and because many problems of occlusion in that stage of development are self-correcting. Observations and measurements are designed to be made directly in the mouth.

Measurements are limited to certain assessments of the teeth themselves, to relations among teeth in the same arch and to inter-arch relations of teeth; no general assessments of soft tissues are indicated, e.g. soft tissue profiles, because such assessments are too subjective. The measurements made on each child are divided into three general categories: dental measurements, intra-arch measurements and inter-arch measurements. Under each of these categories the following specific variables are measured and recorded:

A. *Dental Measurements*

1. Anomalies of development
   a. Congenitally absent teeth
   b. Supernumerary teeth
   c. Malformed teeth
   d. Impacted teeth
2. Missing teeth due to extraction or trauma
3. Retained primary teeth

B. *intra-arch Measurements*

1. Crowding
2. Spacing
3. Anterior irregularities
4. Upper midline diastema

C. *Inter-arch measurements*

1. Lateral segments
   a. Anteroposterior — molar relation
   b. Vertical — posterior openbite
   c. Transverse — posterior crossbite
2. Incisal segments
   a. Anteroposterior — Overjet
   b. Vertical — overbite, anterior openbite
   c. Transverse — midline deviation
   d. Soft tissue management

Bibliography

1. Baume LJ et al. A method for measuring occlusal traits. Int Dent J 1970;20:563–656.

11.5 Occlusal Index (OI)

Nine characteristics are scored in the occlusal index: dental age, molar relation, overbite, overjet, posterior cross-bite, posterior open-bite, tooth displacement (actual and potential), midline relations, and missing permanent teeth.

Scoring of Nine Characteristics

Dental age: By classifying the occlusion in to a dental age, based on the stage of occlusal development, differences in chronologic age, sex, and sequence of tooth eruption are corrected:

1. Dental age 0 begins at birth and ends with the eruption (appearance of any portion of the clinical crown) of the first deciduous tooth. This dental age is characterized by having no erupted teeth.
2. Dental age I begins with the eruption of the first deciduous tooth and ends when all deciduous teeth are in occlusion. This dental age is characterized by the development of the deciduous dentition.
3. Dental age II begins when all deciduous teeth are in occlusion and ends with the eruption of the first permanent tooth. This dental age is characterized by the presence of the completed deciduous dentition.
4. Dental age III begins with the eruption of the first permanent tooth and ends when all permanent central and lateral incisors and first molars are in occlusion. This dental age is characterized by the first stage of the mixed dentition, sometimes referred to as the "early mixed dentition."
5. Dental age IV begins when all permanent central and lateral incisors and first molars are in occlusion and ends with the eruption of any permanent canine or premolar. This dental age, which is characterized by a "dormant" period during which no permanent teeth are erupting, is sometimes referred to as the "middle mixed dentition."
6. Dental age V begins with the eruption of any permanent canine or premolar and ends when all the permanent canines and premolars are in occlusion. This dental age is characterized by the last stage of the mixed dentition, sometimes referred to as the "late mixed dentition."
7. Dental age VI begins when all permanent canines and bicuspids are in occlusion. This dental age is characterized by the presence of the completed permanent dentition (second molars may or may not have erupted).

Second permanent molars are not considered in the assessment of dental age, in as much as canines and premolars usually erupt before second molars and fix the anteroposterior position of the first permanent molar. Subsequent eruption of the second molars, therefore, usually has no effect on molar relation. Several of the described dental ages either begin or end when groups of teeth have completely erupted into occlusion. Occlusal contact, however, does not occur in the child who has an open-bite or in whom one or more teeth, for a variety of reasons, have failed to erupt to the occlusal plane. When extenuating circumstances, such as sucking habits or tongue-thrusting, have produced the lack of occlusal contact, the mere presence in the mouth of the required teeth for a specific dental age is used in making the assessment.

Molar relation: The scoring of molar relation has the following properties:

1. Defined "cut-off" points, where one type of relation ends and another begins.
2. No classification into Angle Class I, II, or III; Angle's classification, however, may be derived from these measurements.
3. The relation of the deciduous second (E) and permanent first molars (6) is considered for each side.

Five relations each for the deciduous and permanent molars were used. This is best described by considering dental age II (for the relation of E) and dental age VI (for the relation of 6). The "cut-off" points are as follows: (Table 11.3):

A. Deciduous Teeth

1. Mesial: The mesiobuccal cusp of upper E occludes with the distobuccal cusp of lower E.
2. Distal: The mesiobuccal cusp of upper E occludes with the mesiobuccal cusp of lower E

B. Permanent Teeth

1. Mesial: The mesiobuccal cusp of upper 6 occludes with the distobuccal cusp of lower 6.
2. Distal: The mesiobuccal cusp of upper 6, occludes with the mesiobuccal cusp of upper 6. The flush terminal plane also occurs when these cusps are vertical; the flush terminal plane can be used to score

"cusp to cusp," distal of 6, because the plane is more easily visualized and its position is determined from a normal E relation.

Overbite: Positive overbite is scored as the distance the maxillary central incisor occludes past the mandibular central incisor, and this distance is scored in "thirds" of the length of the clinical crown of the mandibular central incisor. Negative overbite (open-bite) is scored as the vertical distance from the incisal edge of the maxillary central incisor to the incisal edge of the mandibular central incisor in millimeters.

Overjet: The scores may be positive, zero, or negative.

Posterior cross-bite (osseous type): Cross-bite may be dental, functional, or osseous. Therefore, in order for posterior cross-bite to be an indicator of the osseous relation, it must be differentiated from other types of cross-bite.

In dental cross-bite this tooth will not be in normal arch alignment and will be scored as a displaced tooth rather than a cross-bite. Functional cross-bite involves muscular adjustment to tooth interferences. The teeth seem to be in normal arch alignment, but the lower jaw will not close without shifting, thereby causing the functional cross-bite.

Osseous cross-bite may be unilateral or bilateral and is scored similarly to molar relation, in that posterior cross-bite has definite "cut-off". The buccal cusp of the

Molar	Code		Molar relation
1	E	0	>cusp to cusp distally
	6	5	
2	E	1	cusp to cusp distally; flush terminal plane
	6	6	
3	E	2	<cusp to cusp, either mesially or distally; normal relation
	6	7	
4	E	3	cusp to cusp, mesially
	6	8	
5	E	4	>cusp to cusp mesially
	6	9	

Table 11.3: Cut-off points for molar relationship

mandibular posterior tooth is used as the cusp which determines the posterior cross-bite cuspal relation. Posterior cross-bite is scored the same for the deciduous, mixed, or permanent dentitions, i.e. counting the number of teeth in the maxillary arch which are in each type of posterior cross-bite cuspal relation.

Posterior open-bite: Posterior open-bite may be defined as the lack of occlusal contact between any opposing posterior teeth (posterior teeth include the deciduous canines and molars, and the permanent canines, premolars, and molars) with the jaws in "centric occlusion." Posterior open-bite may be unilateral or bilateral and may accompany an anterior open-bite (negative overbite). Posterior open-bite is scored as either present or not present and if present, as either unilateral or bilateral. Generally, two or more adjacent posterior teeth will be in open-bite. Tooth displacement: The scoring procedures for tooth displacement will be discussed by dividing the dentitions into the non-mixed (deciduous and permanent) and mixed dentitions.

Non-mixed dentitions: The scoring of tooth displacement for the non-mixed dentition includes two degrees of displacement: (1) 1.5 to 2.0 mm deviation or 35 to 45 degrees of rotation from normal arch alignment (scored as 1 or single weight) and (2) > 2 mm deviation or > 45 degrees of rotation from normal arch alignment (scored as 2 or double weight).

Premolars and molars are not scored for rotation in the occlusal index. A tooth may be in normal arch alignment buccolingually, but, because of space deficiency, it may be blocked by the adjacent teeth and fail to erupt completely.

A tooth in this situation is sometimes referred to as being in infraversion and is scored as "1.5 to 2.0 mm deviation."

Mixed dentition: Tooth displacement in the mixed dentition can be divided into two types, depending on the cause.

1. Tooth displacement not associated with space deficiency. A displaced tooth not associated with space deficiency is any maxillary or mandibular incisor or canine which is displaced (either deviated 1.5 mm. or more or rotated 35 degrees or more) when, at the same time, there is sufficient space in the arch line for normal alignment. Causes of this type of displacement are usually habits or eruption disorders. These teeth are weighted (1 or 2) as in the displacement scoring procedures for the non-mixed dentitions.

2. Tooth displacement associated with space deficiency. During the mixed dentition, if the space necessary for proper adjustment of the completed permanent dentition is known, probable tooth displacement may be predicted. A method of assessing potential space deficiency is to measure the mesiodistal widths of the permanent teeth and subtract the length of the arch perimeter. If the width of the teeth exceeds the arch perimeter, tooth displacement will occur. The mesiodistal widths of some permanent teeth, however, are unknown during the mixed dentition.

The mixed dentition analysis (MDA), can predict the mesiodistal widths of the canines and premolars with certain degrees of probability from measurements of the mesiodistal widths of the mandibular permanent incisors. By subtracting the predicted widths of the canines and premolars from the available space, one can estimate the expected amount of tooth displacement. Preliminary studies indicate that n + 1 mm of space deficiency produce n displaced teeth. This information is factored into the weighting mechanism of the occlusal index to make the index valid over time. When an occlusion is scored during the mixed dentition and a space deficiency is noted, the weighted value for the space deficiency will be similar to the weighted value for tooth displacement which the occlusion will have when examined during the permanent dentition. The procedure for scoring tooth displacement associated with space deficiency is as follows (all measurements are in millimeters):

(a) Measure the greatest mesiodistal width of each of the four permanent mandibular incisors; divide the total of the sum of the widths by 2.

For each quadrant:

(b) Add 10 to the sum in (a), if measuring the maxillary quadrants, or add 9 to the sum in (a), if measuring the mandibular quadrants.

(c) Determine any mandibular incisor overlap in millimeters and add this value to the sum in (b); if there is no incisor overlap, measure any spacing between the mandibular incisors in millimeters and subtract this value from the sum in (b).

(d) Measure the arch length from the distal surface of the permanent lateral incisor to the mesial surface of the first permanent molar; subtract this from the score in (c).

(e) Repeat steps (b) through (d) for each quadrant.

(f) Add the positive scores in (d) from each quadrant. The final score is the total estimated amount of space deficiency, in millimeters. This score will be "weighted" in the computation of the OI score.

Midline Relations

Diastema: If the incisors are not in occlusion (dental age III), the observation is not recorded. When the diastema equals or exceeds 2 mm, it is given a weight in the OI. Jaw Deviation: If any central incisor is missing, the procedure is not recorded. Jaw deviations of 3 mm or more are given a weight in the OI. Missing permanent teeth: Only missing maxillary incisor teeth which have not been replaced by a prosthesis are scored. Normally, in a child with at least any four of the twelve permanent canines or premolars in occlusion

all incisors should be erupted. After this stage of dental development, measurement can be made. One simply records the number of missing maxillary incisors.

In keeping with the concept of validity during time, an index of occlusion should consider the stages of dental development. The OI incorporates separate weighting mechanisms for each stage:

1. Deciduous dentition stage-dental ages I and II.
2. Mixed-dentition stage-dental ages III, IV, and V.
3. Permanent dentition stage-dental age VI.

The calculating form to be used is determined by the dental age of the subject. After the dental age is ascertained, the appropriate form can be used. The sum of the weights in all columns is then determined. Based on the total score, the individual can be rated as shown in Table 11.4.

Table 11.4: Average score range of the individual

Class	Suggested range of OI scores for class
Good occlusions	0.0 to 2.5
No treatment	2.6 to 4.5
Minor treatment	4.6 to 7.0
Definite treatment	7.0 to 11.0
Worst occlusions	11.1 to 16.0

Bibliography

1. Summers CJ. The occlusal index: a system for identifying and scoring occlusal disorders. Am J Orthod 1971;59(6):552–67.

11.6 Dental Aesthetic Index (DAI)

The DAI is an orthodontic index based on socially defined aesthetic standards. The development of the DAI employed the public's ratings of the aesthetics of 200 occlusal conditions representing the wide range of occlusal conditions found in a population of half a million people. The ratings were linked by factor analysis and step-wise regression procedures to the occlusal trait measurements that were available for each of the 200 occlusal configurations. The resulting regression equation calls for ten measured components (intraoral measurements of occlusal traits) to be multiplied by their regression coefficients (weights) and the addition of the products plus a constant to give a DAI score (Table 11.5). After an individual's score has been calculated it can be placed on a continuum to determine the point at which the score falls between most and least aesthetic dental appearance. Based on the total score, the individual can also be categorized as shown in Table 11.6.

Limitations

- Lack of assessment of occlusal anomalies such as buccal crossbite, impacted teeth, centre-line discrepancy, and deep overbite

weakens the index (Otuyemi and Noar, 1996; Danyluk et al., 1999).
- Does not account for missing molars.
- No distinction between varying degrees of arch length discrepancy.

Bibliography

1. Jenny J, Cons NC, Kohout FJ, Jakobsen J. Predicting handicapping malocclusion using the Dental Aesthetic Index (DAI). Int Dent J 1993;43(2):128–32.
2. Ali Borzabadi-Farahani (2011). An Overview of Selected Orthodontic Treatment Need Indices, Principles in Contemporary Orthodontics, Dr. Silvano Naretto (Ed.), ISBN: 978–953–307–687–4

11.7 Malocclusion Severity Index (MSI)

MSI was developed by applying a series of weighting scores to the various occlusal anomalies recorded. The following features were assessed (Table 11.7).

1. Details of previous orthodontic care.
   a. Orthodontic extractions
   b. History of appliance wear
2. Occlusal anomalies. The dentition was assessed for the presence of the following nine occlusal anomalies, anyone of which was considered to be indicative of a state of malocclusion and orthodontic treatment need.

Based on the total score, the individual can be rated as shown in Table 11.8.

Bibliography

1. Hill PA. The prevalence and severity of malocclusion and the need for orthodontic treatment in 9, 12 and 15 year old Glasgow school children. Br J Orthodontics 1992;19:87–96.

Table 11.5: Coeficient for DAI	
Component	Weight
Constant	13
Missing incisor, canine and premolar teeth — number	6
Crowding in incisal, segments — number segments crowded	1
Spacing in incisal segments — number segments spaced	1
Diastema — in mm	3
Largest anterior irregularity, maxilla — in mm	1
Largest anterior irregularity, mandible — in mm	1
Anterior maxillary overjet — in mm	2
Anterior mandibular overjet — in mm	4
Vertical anterior openbite —in mm	4
Anteroposterior molar relation — Largest deviation from normal (½ cusp = 1, full cusp or more = 2)	3
Total score	

Table 11.6: Cut off level's for malocclusion severity using DAI		
DAI score	Malocclusion severity	Treatment need category
≤ 25	Normal/minor	No treatment need/slight need
26–30	Definite	Treatment elective
31–35	Severe	Treatment highly desirable
≥ 36	Very severe/handicapping	Treatment mandatory

Table 11.7: Criteria and weight's for MSI

Parameter	Criteria	Weight
Anterior openbite	> 3 mm is scored	10
Traumatic overbite	Tissue impingement or stripping involving palatal or labial mucosa	18
Anterior crossbite	1 tooth	14
	2 teeth	16
	3 teeth	18
	4 teeth	20
Posterior crossbite	One or more maxillary posterior teeth occlude lingually to the mandibular arch and there is an associated displacement of the mandible on closure into centric occlusion.	16
Upper anterior spacing	3 mm or more of spacing between the mesial aspect of the canine tooth on one side of the arch to that on the opposing side of the arch.	14
Incisal overjet spacing	1 mm or less	0
	2–5 mm	0
	6–9 mm	8
	10 mm	24
Upper incisor rotations	rotation of an upper incisor through 30° or more, about its long axis. A tooth scored as rotated was not also scored as being crowded.	
	1 tooth	10
	2 teeth	14
	3 teeth	16
	4 teeth	18
Upper and lower posterior crowding	Unilateral	8
	Bilateral	10
Upper and lower anterior crowding	Number of lower anterior	4
	Number of upper anterior	4

Table 11.8: Cut off level's for malocclusion severity using MSI

0–7	Ideal occlusion or minimal malocclusion	No treatment need
8–17	Moderate malocclusion	Treatment elective
18–32	Sever malocclusion	Treatment desirable
33 or more	Very severe malocclusion	Treatment essential

11.8 WHO Method for the Epidemiological Assessment of Malocclusion

Dental aesthetic index criteria are used as described above. It is recommended that this index be used for age groups in which there are no longer primary teeth, usually from 12 years. The CPI probe is used when measuring anterior irregularities, overjet and openbite. The following traits are assessed.

- Missing incisor, canine and premolar teeth — number
- Crowding in incisal segments — Number segments crowded
- Spacing in incisal segments — Number segments spaced
- Diastema — In millimetres
- Largest anterior irregularity, maxilla — In mm
- Largest anterior irregularity, mandible — In mm
- Anterior maxillary overjet — In mm
- Anterior mandibular overjet — In mm
- Vertical anterior openbite — In mm
- Anteroposterior molar relation
- Need for immediate care and referral

Bibliography

1. Oral Health Surveys 4th edition WHO 1997.

11.9 Index of Orthodontic Treatment Outcome/Peer Assessment Rating (PAR) Index

PAR index was developed to record the malocclusion at any stage of treatment. The index was formulated over a series of six meetings in 1987 with a group of 10 experienced orthodontists (British Orthodontic Standards Working Party).

The concept is to assign a score to various occlusal traits which make up a malocclusion. The individual scores are summed to obtain an overall total representing the degree a case deviates from normal alignment and occlusion. Normal occlusion and alignment is defined as all anatomical contact points being adjacent, with a good inter-cuspal mesh between upper and lower buccal teeth, non-excessive overjet and overbite. The score of zero would indicate good alignment and higher scores (rarely beyond 50) indicating increased levels of irregularity. The overall score is recorded on the pre- and post-treatment dental casts. The difference between these scores represents the degree of improvement as a result of orthodontic intervention and active treatment. There are 11 components of the PAR Index as shown in Table 11.9.

Buccal and anterior segments: The dental arch is divided into three recording segments, left buccal, right buccal and anterior. Scores are recorded for both upper and lower arches.

Buccal segments: The recording zone is from the mesial anatomical contact point of the first permanent molar to the distal anatomical contact point of the canine.

Anterior segment: The recording zone is from the mesial anatomical contact point of the canine on one side to the mesial anatomical contact point of the canine on the opposite side. The occlusal features recorded are crowding, spacing, and impacted teeth. Displacements are recorded as the shortest distance between contact points of adjacent teeth parallel to the occlusal plane. The greater the displacement the greater the PAR score. The displacements between first, second, and third molars are not recorded as these contacts are so broad and are extremely variable within the normal range. An impacted tooth is recorded when the space for this tooth is less than or equal to 4 mm. Impacted canines are recorded in the anterior segment.

Scores for the displacements and impactions are added to give an overall score for each recording zone (Table 11.10).

If there is potential crowding in the mixed dentition, average mesio-distal widths are used to calculate the space deficiency as given in Table 11.11.

Buccal occlusion: The buccal occlusion is recorded for both left and right sides. The fit of the teeth is scored with respect to the three planes of space. The recording zone is from the canine to the last molar, either first, second, or third. All discrepancies are recorded when

Table 11.9: Component's for PAR index
1. Upper right segment
2. Upper anterior segment
3. Upper left segment
4. Lower right segment
5. Lower anterior segment
6. Lower left segment
7. Right buccal occlusion
8. Overjet
9. Overbite
10. Centreline
11. Left buccal occlusion

Table 11.10: Score for each zone	
Score	*Discrepancy*
0	0 to 1 mm
1	1.1 to 2mm
2	2.1 to 4mm
3	4.1 to 8rnm
4	Greater than 8 mm
5	Impacted teeth

Table 11.11: Mixed dentition crowding assessment using average mesio-distal widths

Upper		
Canine	8 mm	Total = 22 mm (impaction ≤ 18 mm)
1st premolar	7 mm	
2nd premolar	7 mm	
Lower		
Canine	7 mm	Total = 21 mm (impaction ≤ 17 mm)
1st premolar	7 mm	
2nd premolar	7 mm	

the teeth are in occlusion. The antero-posterior, vertical and transverse irregularities are summed for each buccal occlusion based on the score given in Table 11.12.

Table 11.12: Buccal occlusion assessments. (Temporary developmental stages and submerging deciduous teeth are excluded.)

Score	Discrepancy
Antero posterior	
0	Good interdigitation Class I, II and III
1	Less than half unit discrepancy
2	Half a unit discrepancy(cusp to cusp)
Vertical	
0	No discrepancy in intercuspation
1	Lateral open bite on at least two teeth greater than 2 mm
Transverse	
0	No cross-bite
1	Cross-bite tendency
2	Single tooth in cross-bite
3	More than one tooth in cross-bite
4	More than one tooth in scissor bite

Overjet: Positive overjet as well as teeth in cross-bite are recorded as per the criteria given in Table 11.13. The recording zone is from the left to right lateral incisors. The most prominent aspect of any one incisor is recorded. When recording the overjet the ruler is held parallel to the occlusal plane and radial to the line of the arch. It is not uncommon to see two upper laterals in cross-bite as well as

an increased overjet on the central incisors. In this situation if the overjet were 4 mm, the score would be 3 for the cross-bite and 1 for the positive overjet (4 in total).

Table 11.13: Overjet and cross-bite criteria

Score	Discrepancy
Overjet	
0	0–3 mm
1	3.1–5 mm
2	5.1–7 mm
3	7.1–9 mm
4	greater than 9 mm
Anterior cross bites	
0	No discrepancy
1	One or more teeth edge to edge
2	One single tooth in cross–bite
3	Two teeth in cross-bite
4	More than two teeth in cross-bite

Overbite: Records the vertical overlap or open bite of the anterior teeth are recorded as per the scores given in Table 11.14. Overbite is recorded in relation to the coverage of the lower incisors or the degree of open bite. The recording zone includes the lateral incisors. The tooth with the greatest overlap is recorded.

Table 11.14: Open bite and over-bite criteria

Score	Discrepancy
Open bite	
0	No open bite
1	Open bite less than and equal to 1 mm
2	Open bite 1.1–2 mm
3	Open bite 2.1–3 mm
4	Open bite greater than or equal to 4 mm
Overbite	
0	Less than or equal to one third coverage of the lower incisor
1	Greater than one-third, but less than two-thirds coverage of the lower incisor
2	Greater than two-thirds coverage or the lower incisor
3	Greater than or equal to full tooth coverage

Centreline: The centreline discrepancy in relation to the lower central incisors is recorded as per the score given in Table 11.15. If a lower central incisor has been extracted the measurement is not recorded.

Table 11.15: Criteria for centerline discrepancy	
Score	*Discrepancy*
0	Coincident and up to one-quarter lower incisor width
1	One quarter to one-half lower incisor width
2	Greater than one half lower incisor width

The PAR Ruler

A ruler has been designed to make measurement easier. The information briefly summarizes the recording features of the index and facilitates quick assessments, and allows contact points to be viewed through the ruler.

Conventions

General

1. All scoring is accumulative.

2. There is no maximal cut-off level.

3. The occlusion should be scored disregarding functional displacement (this cannot be determined from dental casts alone).

4. The contact points between first, second, and third molars are not recorded. The contact points between molars are so variable, however, severe deviations will produce a cross-bite, and will be noted in the buccal occlusions.

5. If the contact point displacement is as a result of poor restorative work (restorations or crowns), the displacement is not recorded.

6. Contact points between deciduous teeth are not recorded.

7. Extraction spaces are not recorded if the patient is to receive a prosthetic replacement. However, if space closure is intended, the distance between adjacent teeth should be noted.

Canines

1. Where there are missing canines, displacements resulting from discrepancies between the mesial contact point to the first premolar and the distal of the lateral incisor should be recorded in the anterior segment.

2. Canine cross-bites should be recorded in the overjet section.

3. Contact points between the canines and premolars are scored as follows: the distal contact point of the canine to the midpoint on the mesial surface of the adjacent premolar. (These contact points are so variable. When untreated normal occlusions were assessed this relationship seemed to be the most acceptable.)

Impactions

1. If a tooth is unerupted and displaced from the line of the arch either buccally or palatally due to insufficient space, this is regarded as an impaction. However, if the tooth is erupted and displaced, the displacement score is recorded.

Incisors

1. If there is agenesis of the upper incisor or the tooth has been lost due to trauma or caries the procedure is as follows: (a) if the space is maintained (for a prosthesis), the distance between adjacent teeth is not recorded; (b) if the space is to be closed, the distance between adjacent teeth is recorded.

2. When recording an overjet, if the tooth falls on the line the lower grade is recorded.

3. If a lower incisor has been extracted or is missing, the centreline is not recorded.

Molars

1. Contact points between first and second molars are not recorded,

2. If the first molars have been extracted, the contact point of the second molar is recorded.

Bibliography

1. Richmond S, Shaw WC, O'Brien KD, Buchanan IB, Jones R, Stephens CD, Roberts CT, Andrews M. The development of the PAR Index (Peer Assessment Rating): reliability and validity. Eur J Orthod 1992 Apr;14(2):125–39.

11.10 The Swedish Medical Board Index (SMBI)

The original form of this Swedish index was developed having 4 categories of need (grade 1 to 4). Later on, Linder-Aronson et al., 1976 revised the index and with addition of fifth category, the grade zero for individuals with no need for treatment. The SMBI calls for the subjective views and patient's wishes to be considered when deciding on the treatment need (Table 11.16).

Bibliography

1. Cited in Ali Borzabadi-Farahani (2011). An Overview of Selected Orthodontic Treatment Need Indices, Principles in Contemporary Orthodontics, Dr. Silvano Naretto (Ed.), ISBN: 978-953–307–687–4.

11.11 Index of Orthodontic Treatment Need (IOTN)

Brook P and Shaw W developed this index and initially named it as the Index of Orthodontic Treatment Priority. Later, it was renamed to the Index of Orthodontic Treatment Need (IOTN). The IOTN is one of the most commonly used occlusal indices that assess the orthodontic treatment need among children and adults. The Index of Treatment Need consists of two independent components: the Dental Health Component (DHC), based on the Swedish index described below, and the Aesthetic Component (AC). The DHC of IOTN is similar to an index used by the Swedish Medical Health Board 'the Swedish Medical Board Index (SMBI).

The dental health component: This component has five categories ranging from 1 (no need (or treatment) to 5 (great need), which may be applied clinically or to patients study casts (Table 11.17). The most severe occlusal trait is identified for any particular patient. The scores for individual traits are not summed: thus, a series of multiple minor

Grade		
4	Very urgent need	Aesthetically and/or functionally handicapping anomalies, such as cleft lip and palate, extreme post-normal or pre-normal occlusion, retained upper incisors, extensive aplasia.
3	Urgent need	Pre-normal forced bite, deep bite with gingival irritation not only on incisive papilla, large overjet with lower lip behind upper centrals, extremely open bite, crossbite causing transverse forced bite, scissors bite interfering with articulation, severe frontal crowding or spacing, retained canines, aesthetically and/or functionally disturbing rotations.
2	Moderate need	Aesthetically and/or functionally disturbing proclined or retroclined incisors, deep bite with gingival contact but without gingival irritation, severe crowding or spacing, infra-occlusion of deciduous molars and permanent teeth, moderate frontal rotations.
1	Little need	Mild deviations from normal (ideal) occlusion, such as pre-normal occlusion with little negative overjet, post-normal occlusion without other anomalies, deep bite without gingival contact, open bite with little frontal opening, crossbite without a forced bite, mild crowding or spacing, mild rotations of only little aesthetic and/or functional significance.
0	No need	Normal (ideal) occlusion without deviations.

Table 11.16: The modified 5-grade index (ISMHB) for orthodontic treatment need

variations, each of which is unimportant with respect to dental health, cannot be added together to place an individual in a higher category. A ruler has been developed to aid diagnosis. The following characteristics are assessed for the dental health component: missing teeth; overjet; cross bites; contact point displacement; and overbite.

Table 11.17: Dental health components in IOTN

Grade 1 (none)

1	Extremely minor malocclusions, including displacements less than 1 mm

Grade 2 (little)

2a	Increased overjet greater than 3.5 mm but less than or equal to 6 mm with competent lips.
2b	Reverse overjet greater than 0 mm but less than or equal to 1 mm
2c	Anterior or posterior Crossbite with less than or equal to 1 mm discrepancy between, retruded contact position and intercuspal position.
2d	Displacement of teeth greater than 1 mm but less than or equal to 2 mm.
2e	Anterior or posterior open bite greater than 1 mm but less than or equal to 2 mm.
2f	Increased overbite greater than or equal to 3.5 mm without gingival contact
2g	Pre-normal or post-normal occlusions with no other anomalies. Includes up to half a unit discrepancy.

Grade 3 (moderate)

3a	Increased overjet greater than 3.5 mm but less than or equal to 6 mm with incompetent lips
3b	Reverse overjet greater than 1 mm but less than or equal to 3.5 mm.
3c	Anterior or posterior crossbites with greater than 1 mm but less than or equal to 2 mm discrepancy between retruded contact position and intercuspal position.
3e	Lateral or anterior open bite greater than 2 mm but less than or equal to 4 mm.
3f	Increased and complete overbite without gingival or palatal trauma.

Grade 4 (great)

4a	Increased overjet greater than 6 mm but less than or equal to 9 mm.
4b	Reverse overjet greater than 3.5 mm with no masticatory or speech difficulties.
4c	Anterior or posterior crossbites with greater than 2 mm discrepancy between retruded contact position and intercuspal position.
4d	Severe displacements of teeth greater than 4 mm.
4e	Extreme lateral or anterior open bites greater than 4 mm.
4f	Increased and complete overbite, with gingival or palatal trauma.
4h	Less extensive hypodontia requiring pre-restorative orthodontics or orthodontic space closure to obviate the need for a prosthesis.
4l	Posterior lingual crossbite with no functional occlusal contact in one or both buccal segments.
4m	Reverse overjet greater than 1 mm but less than 3.5 mm with recorded masticatory and speech difficulties.
4t	Partially erupted teeth tipped and impacted against adjacent teeth

Grade 5 (very great)

5a	Increased overjet greater than 9 mm.
5h	Extensive hypodontia with restorative implications (more than one tooth missing in any quadrant) requiring pre-restorative orthodontics.
5i	Impeded eruption of teeth (except for third molars) due to crowding, displacement, the presence of supernumerary teeth, retained deciduous teeth and any pathological cause.
5m	Reverse overjet greater than 3.5 mm with reported masticatory and speech difficulties.
5p	Defects of cleft lip and palate.
5s	Submerged deciduous teeth.

A grade is allocated according to the severity of the worst single occlusal trait and describes the priority for treatment. In recording the worst trait following hierarchical scale is used (in a descending order), Missing teeth, Overjet, Crossbites, Displacement of contact points, and Overbite (including open bite). To remember the hierarchical scale, the acronym of 'MOCDO' can be constructed and used. For instance, if two or more occlusal anomalies achieve the same DHC grade, the hierarchical scale is used to determine which dental anomaly should be recorded (i.e. dental anomaly with higher rank in the hierarchical scale is recorded). In recording the DHC, only the worst occlusal feature/anomaly is recorded.

The aesthetic component: This consists of a ten-point scale illustrated by a series of photographs which were rated for attractiveness by a lay panel and selected as being equidistantly spaced through the range of grades. A rating is allocated for overall dental attractiveness rather than specific morphological similarity to the photographs. The final value reflects treatment need on the grounds of aesthetic impairment, and by implication the sociopsychological need for orthodontic treatment. Both parents and children find this easy to apply, and there is a high level of agreement between the scores obtained by dentists, parents and children.

Bibliography

1. Brook PH Shaw WC. The development of an index of orthodontic treatment priority. Eur J Orthodontics 1989;20:309–20.
2. McGuinness NJ, Stephens CD. An introduction to indices of malocclusion. Dent Update 1994 May;21(4):140–4.
3. Ali Borzabadi-Farahani (2011). An Overview of Selected Orthodontic Treatment Need Indices, Principles in Contemporary Orthodontics, Dr. Silvano Naretto (Ed.), ISBN: 978–953–307–687–4.

11.12 The modified IOTN

The modified IOTN is a two-grade scale (need/no definite need), instead of 5 grade scale with 30 sub-categories. The modified IOTN is based on idea that the IOTN is not an index to measure the complexity; and therefore, there would be no benefit in recording the occlusal anomaly that placed the child in treatment need category. The modified IOTN simplifies identifying people in need of treatment and improves the reliability and validity of the index (Burden et al., 2001). By using the modified IOTN, every case with IOTN DHC ≥ 4 and/or IOTN AC ≥ 8 is classified as being in need of treatment. The criteria are listed in Table 11.18.

Table 11.18: The modified dental health component of IOTN
Definite need for orthodontic treatment: If any one of the occlusal anomalies below is present, there is a definite need for orthodontic treatment. (In brackets, for information and comparison, are given the sub-categories from the original dental health component of IOTN). The acronym "MOCDO" is used as an aide memoire: Missing teeth, overjet, crossbites, displacement of contact points (crowding), overbite.

M Hypodontia requiring pre-restorative orthodontics or orthodontic space closure to obviate the need for a prosthesis (4h, 5h).
   Impeded eruption of teeth (5i). Presence of supernumerary teeth (4x), and retained deciduous teeth (5s).
O Increased overjet greater than 6 mm. (4a, 5a) Reverse overjet greater than 3.5 mm with no masticatory or speech difficulties (5m, 4b).
   Reverse overjet greater than 1 mm but less than 3.5 mm with recorded masticatory and speech difficulties (4m).
C Anterior or posterior crossbites with greater than 2 mm discrepancy between retruded contact position and intercuspal position (4c).
D Contact point displacements greater than 4 mm (4d).
O Lateral or anterior open bites greater than 4 mm (4e).
   Deep overbite with gingival or palatal trauma (4f).

Bibliography

1. Burden DJ, Pine CM, Burnside G. Modified IOTN: an orthodontic treatment need index for use in oral health surveys. Community Dent Oral Epidemiol 2001;29:220–5.

11.13 Index of Complexity, Outcome and Need (ICON)

This was proposed by Daniels C and Richmond S (2000) to assess treatment need, complexity, treatment improvement, and outcome based on international professional opinion, intended for use in the context of specialist practice.

General Assumptions of the Index

- When the index is used to assess treatment outcomes, it is assumed that an appropriate level of co-operation was obtained from the patient.
- The index may require confirmation of the presence of teeth using radiography.
- Except for the aesthetic assessment, occlusal traits are not scored to deciduous teeth unless they are to be retained in the permanent dentition to obviate the need for a prosthetic replacement, for example, when the permanent tooth is absent.
- The index contains five components, all of which must be scored.

Dental Aesthetics: The dental aesthetic component of the IOTN (Shaw et al., 1991a) is used. The dentition is compared to the illustrated scale and a global attractiveness match is obtained without attempting to closely match the malocclusion to a particular picture on the scale. The scale works best in the permanent dentition. The scale is graded from 1 for the most attractive to 10 the least attractive dental arrangement. Once this score is obtained it is multiplied by the weighting of 7.

Crossbite: A normal transverse relationship in the buccal segments is observed when the palatal cusps of the upper molar and premolar teeth occlude, preferably into the occlusal fossa of the opposing tooth, or at least between the lingual and buccal cusp tips of the opposing tooth. Crossbite is deemed to be present if a transverse relation of cusp to cusp or worse exists in the buccal segment. This includes buccal and lingual crossbites consisting of one or more teeth, with or without mandibular displacement.

In the anterior segment, a tooth in crossbite is defined as an upper incisor or canine in edge-to-edge or lingual occlusion. Where a crossbite is present in the posterior or anterior segments or both, the raw score of 1 is given which is multiplied by the weighting of 5. When there is no crossbite the score for this trait is 0.

Anterior vertical relationship: This trait includes both open bite (excluding developmental conditions) and deep bite. If both traits are present only the highest scoring raw score is counted. Positive overbite is measured at the deepest part of the overbite on incisor teeth. The criteria are listed in Table 11.19.

Open bite may be measured with an ordinary mm ruler to the mid incisal edge of the most deviant upper tooth. The raw score obtained is multiplied by 4.

Upper arch crowding/spacing: This variable attempts to quantify the tooth to tissue discrepancy present in the upper arch or the presence of impacted teeth in both arches. The sum of the mesio-distal crown diameters is compared to the available arch circumference, mesial to the last standing tooth on either side. This may require the use of a mm ruler for accuracy, but with practice can be estimated by eye.

No estimation is made to account for the curve of Spee or the degree of incisor inclination. Once the crowding/spacing discrepancy has been worked out in mm, it is reduced on to the ordinal scale (0–5).

Note that an impacted tooth in either the upper or lower arch, immediately scores the

Table 11.19: Protocol for occlusal trait scoring

Score	0	1	2	3	4	5	Weights
Aesthetic	1–10 As judged using IOTN AC						7
Upper arch crowding	Score only the highest trait either spacing or crowding	Less than 2 mm	2.1 to 5 mm	5.1 to 9 mm impacted teeth	9.1 to 13 mm	13.1 to 17 mm	> 17 mm 5
Upper spacing	Up to 2 mm	2.1–5 mm	5.1–9 mm	>9 mm			5
Crossbite	Transverse relationship of cusp to cusp or worse	No crossbite	Crossbite present				5
Incisor open bite	Score only the highest trait either open bite or overbite	Complete bite	Less than 1 mm	1.1–2 mm	2.1–4 mm	> 4 mm	4
Incisor overbite	Lower incisor coverage	Up to 1/3 tooth	1/3 – 2/3 coverage	2/3 up to full covered	Fully covered		4
Buccal segment antero-posterior	Left and right added together	Cusp to embrasure relationship only, Class I, II or III to cusp	Any cusp relation up to but not including cusp	Cusp to cusp relation-ship			3

maximum for crowding. A tooth must be unerupted to be defined as impacted.

An unerupted tooth is defined as impacted under the following conditions:

- If it is ectopically placed or impacted against an adjacent tooth (excluding third molars but including supernumerary teeth);
- When less than 4 mm of space is available between the contact points of the adjacent permanent teeth.

Retained deciduous teeth (i.e. without a permanent successor) and erupted super-numerary teeth should be scored as space unless they are to be retained to obviate the need for prosthesis. In transitional stages average canine and premolar widths can be used to estimate the potential crowding. Suggested averages are 7 mm for premolar and lower canine and 8 mm for upper canine. The presence of erupted antimeric teeth allows more accurate estimation for this purpose. Spacing due to teeth lost to trauma and exodontia is also counted.

Post-treatment spaces created to allow prosthetic replacements should match the antimeric tooth width. Discrepancy between such spaces and the antimeric tooth can be counted as excess spacing or crowding, whichever is appropriate. The use of the index to assess spacing in relation to retained deciduous teeth demands that the fate of the deciduous teeth is known before the index can be applied.

Once the raw score has been obtained it is multiplied by the weighting 5.

Buccal Segment Antero-posterior Relationship: The scoring zone includes the canine premolar and molar teeth. The antero-posterior cuspal relationship is scored for each side in turn. The raw scores for both sides are added together and then multiplied by the weighting 3.

Derivation of the Final Score

Once all of the raw scores have been obtained and multiplied by their respective weights, they are added together to yield a single weighted summary score for a particular cast. The interpretation of the summary scores are described in Table 11.20.

Table 11.20: Interpretation for ICON score	
ICON complexity grade	*Score range*
Easy	< 29
Mild	29 to 50
Moderate	51 to 63
Difficult	64 to 77
Very difficult	> 77

The ICON uses the following formula to assess the orthodontic treatment outcome.

Improvement grade = Pre-treatment score – 4 × Post-treatment score. Based on the score derived from this orthodontic treatment outcome formula, subjects can be categorized as listed in Table 11.21.

Limitations

The index is heavily weighted for aesthetics (weighting of seven), which relies on subjective opinion of clinician.

Table 11.21: Improvement grades	
Improvement grade	*Score range*
Greatly improved	> –1
Substantially improved	–25 to –1
Moderately improved	–53 to –26
Minimally improved	–85 to –54
Not improved or worse	< –85

Overall, ICON is simple to use, measures relatively few traits, does not need hierarchy and can be used on patients or study casts without protocol modification.

Bibliography

1. Daniels C, Richmond S. The development of the index of complexity, outcome and need (ICON). J Orthod. 2000;27(2):149–62.

2. Ali Borzabadi-Farahani (2011). An Overview of Selected Orthodontic Treatment Need Indices, Principles in Contemporary Orthodontics, Dr. Silvano Naretto (Ed.), ISBN: 978–953–307–687–4.

11.14 Norwegian Index of Orthodontic Treatment Need

In Norway, a new orthodontic treatment need index was introduced in 1990 for allocation of refunds of treatment costs by the National health insurance system. As national subsidies for orthodontic care are limited, the treatment costs are reimbursed by the government in accordance with the severity of malocclusion. The index defines four groups or grades, denoting very great need, great need, obvious need and little/no need (100, 75, 40 and 0% reimbursement respectively).

The various dentofacial conditions and morphologic trails that constitute the four groups of the treatment need index are given below. Selection of traits and definitions of cut-off points are based on present scientific evidence and empirical orthodontic norms about the risks for detrimental effects of dentofacial anomalies on dental health, function and psychosocial well-being.

Group A: Very great need

1. Cleft lip–jaw-palate
2. Inherited or acquired craniofacial anomalies
3. Severe anomalies requiring a combination of orthodontics and orthognathic surgery
4. Anomalies of comparable severity

Group B: Great need

1. Overjet 9 mm or more

2. Unilateral buccal or lingual crossbite on three or more pairs of opposing teeth with forced bite and/or asymmetry
3. Anterior open bite with occlusal contacts on molars only
4. Impacted incisors and canines where appliance therapy is necessary
5. Anterior crossbite on all incisors
6. Anterior teeth missing due to agenesia or tooth loss
7. Increased overbite (deep bite) with labial or palatal impingement of the soft tissue with two or more teeth
8. Bilateral buccal crossbite (scissors bite) on two or more pairs of opposing teeth
9. Agenesis of two or more teeth in the same quadrant (3rd molars excepted)
10. Anomalies of comparable severity.

Group C: Obvious need
1. Overjet 6–9 mm
2. Open bite on three or more pairs of opposing teeth
3. Inversion of anterior teeth
4. Increased overbite (deep bite) without contact on anterior teeth, or with contact on the gingival ¼ of the palatal surface of the maxillary anterior teeth
5. Agenesis of single teeth in the lateral segments
6. Median diastema of 3 mm or more, or pronounced general spacing of anterior segment
7. Pronounced crowding of anterior teeth

8. Occlusal disorder combined with strong subjective dysfunction symptoms
9. Anomalies of comparable severity

Group D: Little/no need
1. Overjet less than 6 mm
2. Bilateral crossbite
3. Anterior and lateral open bite on fewer than three pairs of opposing teeth
4. Increased overbite (deep bite) with occlusal contact incisal to the gingival ¼ of the palatal surface of the maxillary anterior teeth
5. Local cross, and scissors bite without asymmetry or forced bite
6. Moderate crowding in anterior and lateral segments
7. Median diastema less than 3 mm
8. Moderate spacing in anterior and lateral segments

Based on the clinical examination, occlusal measurements on the study casts, and X-rays, each child was classified into one of the four groups defined by the index. All the traits defined by the index were recorded. The classification allocated to the child was determined by presence of the most severe trait.

Bibliography

1. Espeland LV, Ivarsson K, Stenvik A. A new Norwegian index of orthodontic treatment need related to orthodontic concern among 11-year-olds and their parents. Community Dent Oral Epidemiol 1992;20:274 9.

12

Indices to Measure Extrinsic Stains

INTRODUCTION

Snyder (1964) describes a Diversified Dental Index (Pigmentation) and Horowitz and Chamberlin developed a Dental Pigmentation Index for recording staining that occurred in clinical trials of stannous fluoride agents on children. Stain was assessed by tooth surface but quantitative estimates of the area covered were not made. An attempt at an accurate and detailed evaluation of extrinsic stain diagnosed clinically in adults was made by Lobene (1968). This index, with minor modifications, has also been used by Abbe et al (1971). However, according to Lobene (1968) a major disadvantage of the method is that moderately to highly stained teeth are necessary to permit statistical verification of results. Davis and Rees (1975) describe a method of evaluating stain by estimating the percentage area of labial incisor surfaces covered by stain and checking this estimate against planimeter measurements from photographs. Limited information is available on the reproducibility and sensitivity of this method.

12.1 Glass's Criteria for Stain Evaluation

The criteria for scoring extrinsic stains using glass index are given in Table 12.1.

Bibliography

1. Glass RL. A clinical study of hand and electric brushing. J Periodontol 1965;36:322-327.

12.2 Lobene's Stain Index

The labial surfaces of the eight incisor teeth were selected as surfaces to be evaluated. The labial surfaces of each incisors was divided into 2 regions: gingiva and the body region. The gingival region was crescent shaped band of the labial surface about 3 mm wide, adjacent to the free margin of the gingival and extending to the crest of the interdental papilla of the adjacent teeth. The remainder of the

Code	Criteria
0	No stain visible clinically
1	Slightest amount visible – limited to the gingival margin – discontinuous to be gray rather than black – less than 1mm in gingivo-occlusal height
2	As in no. 1 above, but continuous to form definite, dark band at gingival margin or more than 1 mm in height but no more than gingival third of the tooth involved
3	More than the gingival third involved
4	The entire tooth surface is generally stained

Table 12.1: Criteria for glass index

labial surface was designated as body region. The gingival and body region were scored separately for yellow stains by use of following criteria for stain intensity or severity: 0 – no stain, 1 – light stain, 2 – moderate stain and 3 – heavy stain.

The extent to which these yellow stains covered the gingival and body regions was scored according to the following criteria: 0 – no stain detected; only tooth color, 1 – stain over a third of the region, 2 – stain over two thirds of the region, and 3 – stain over more than two-thirds of the region. Subjects with missing or banded anterior teeth are excluded. The scores for the severity or extent for gingival and body region ranged from 0 – 24.

Bibliography

1. Lobene RR. Effect of dentifrices on tooth stains with controlled brushing. Journal of the American Dental Association 1968;77:849–55.

12.3 Dental Pigmentation Index

This was developed by Horowitz and Chamberlin to facilitate recording of pigmentation of teeth occurring in association with fillings or with non-carious tooth structure. For the purpose of evaluation, the definition of dental surfaces followed the criteria established in Snyder's Diversified Dental Index. The tooth was visualized as composed of two parts, a buccal and a lingual portion, separated by an imaginary plane running in the long axis of the tooth so that it bisected the mesial and distal surfaces. The width of the buccal surface encompassed, the distance from the midline of the mesial surface to the midline of distal surface and, in height, the distance from incisal or occlusal edge to gingival margin. For molars and premolars, the occlusal surface of the tooth was evaluated separately.

Evaluation: Stained filling material or marginal staining of dental structure bordering a filling was recorded as pigmentation associated with filling. The status of

pigmentation was recorded for each tooth as S – non-pigmented tooth; P – pigmented tooth; and F – pigmented restoration or pigmentation bordering a restoration. For those teeth with pigmentation recorded as P or F, the surfaces affected by pigmentation were recorded as follows: O – occlusal (for posterior teeth); B – buccal; and L – lingual.

Bibliography

1. Horowitz HS, Chamberlin SR. Pigmentation of teeth following topical applications of stannous fluoride in a non-fluoridated area. J Pub Health Dent1971:31:32–7.

12.4 Extrinsic Stain Index

This was proposed by Linda Shaw and Murray JJ in 1977. Accurate scale drawings from an atlas of tooth form were reproduced. Outlines of the labial and lingual surfaces of all eight incisor teeth were enlarged to scale (magnification × 4). Each tooth face was divided into 4 mm squares. There were total of 412 squares on the labial surfaces and 422 squares on the lingual surfaces (Fig. 12.1). The subjects were assessed for staining with a dental light and plane mouth mirror; the teeth were dried by compressed air before examination and any gross accumulation of plaque or debris was removed with a gauze

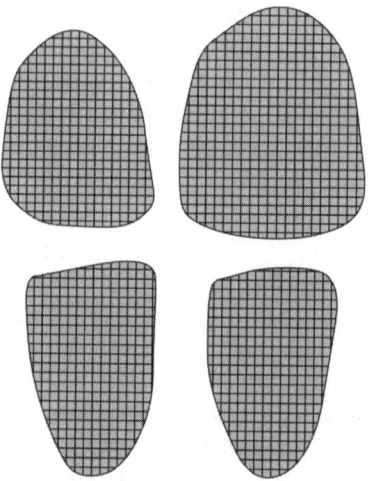

Fig. 12.1: Extrinsic stain index

dental napkin. All areas of extrinsic discoloration on the incisor teeth were drawn by the examiner on to the grid system and shaded in. The number of squares covered by stain was totaled separately for labial and lingual surfaces. If a square was not entirely covered by stain, only those where the shaded portion exceeded half the area were counted.

Advantages

The extrinsic stain index is simple to use and requires no specialized equipment. It is reproducible, sensitive to small changes and amenable to all types of statistical analysis.

Bibliography

1. Linda Shaw, JJ Murray. A new index for measuring extrinsic stain in clinical trials. Community Dent Oral Epidemiol 1977:5;116–20.

12.5 Eriksen Harald M and Gjermo P Criteria for Stain Evaluation

The discoloration of all the tooth surfaces present was recorded for each participant using the following clinical index system: 0 - no discoloration; 1 — small stained areas on a few teeth; 2 — teeth and front fillings moderately stained; 3 — heavy staining of large areas of the tooth surfaces and front fillings.

Bibliography

1. Eriksen Harald M, Gjermo Per. Incidence of stained tooth surfaces in students using chlorhexidine-containing dentifrices. Scandinavian Journal of Dental Research 1973;81:533–7.

12.6 Eriksen et al. Criteria for Stain Evaluation

A clinical evaluation of the extension and intensity of labial discolorations on the upper and lower front teeth was proposed by Eriksen and his associates in 1979. The following criteria were applied evaluating each tooth surface separately: Score 0: no staining, 1: staining located along the gingival 1/3rd of the surface, 2: half the surface stained and 3: staining covering more than half the surface.

An additional index system ranking the discolorations from 0–3 for increasing intensity was also used: Score 0: no stain visible, 1: slight staining, 2: distinct zones of stain and 3: heavy staining.

Scores 2 and 3 were regarded as cosmetically unacceptable.

Bibliography

1. Eriksen, HM, Jemtland B, Finckenhagen HJ and Gjermo P. Evaluation of extrinsic tooth discoloration. Acta Odontol Scand. 1979;37:371–5.

12.7 Discoloration Index System

This was advocated by Lang NP and Raber K in 1981. The score and criteria were described in Table 12.2.

Bibliography

1. Lang NP, Raber K. Use of oral irrigators as vehicle for the application of antimicrobial agents in chemical plaque control. Journal of Clinical Periodontology 1981;8, 177–88.

Table 12.2: Criteria for the discoloration index system (DIS)

Score	Criteria
0	No discoloration, clean and polished tooth surface, natural appearance in color
1	Slight yellowish discoloration, yellowish film over the entire extent of the clinical crown, slight brownish discoloration along the gingival margin
2	Moderate brownish discoloration on the interproximal surfaces and in the apical third of the clinical crown
3	Heavy brown and black discoloration over the entire extent of the tooth surface, black discoloration predominantly on the interproximal surfaces

12.8 Modification of the Lobene Stain Scoring Index

This was proposed by Macpherson et al in 2000. This involved visual stain assessment of the buccal/labial and lingual/palatal aspects of the index teeth. The modification consisted of dividing each aspect into 4 separate sites instead of only 2 (Fig. 12.2).

- **Gingival (G):** 2 mm wide strip running parallel to the gingival margin. The limit towards the incisal edge given by the end of the interdental papilla.
- **Body of tooth (B):** Central area of buccal/lingual aspect, between gingival and distal/mesial sites, extending to incisal edge.
- **Mesial (M):** Visible area between line angle and adjacent tooth, ending at the interdental papilla (i.e. start of gingival site).
- **Distal (D):** As for mesial (M) site.

Stain was recorded using 2 separate characteristics, namely intensity and area (extent) as suggested by Lobene (1968). The criteria for these 2 parameters were also slightly modified to provide better discrimination at the lower end of the scale and to take account of anatomical differences between the different sites. The criteria and codes for

intensity and extent are described in Table 12.3.

The area (extent) of the stain was recorded only if an intensity score of 2 or 3 was given. The area criteria and codes for the body of the tooth are shown in Table 12.4 and differed between the buccal/labial and lingual/palatal surfaces due to the normal difference in surface distribution of stain between these sites.

Procedure

Before scoring, the index teeth should be cleaned with a soft toothbrush and water to remove any plaque and food debris. The index teeth were then dried using a chair-side air syringe, and kept dry throughout the examination. Stain assessment was made without the aid of a magnifying glass. Only stain on natural tooth surfaces was recorded and staining in or adjacent to restoration margins was ignored. The index teeth selected

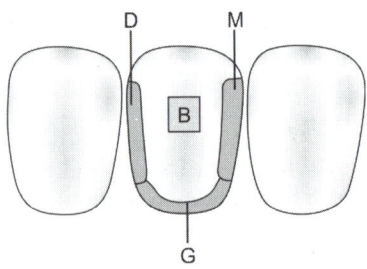

Fig. 12.2: Modification of the Lobene stain scoring index

Table 12.3: Modification of the Lobene stain scoring index

	Codes	Criteria
Intensity	0	No stain present, natural tooth colouration
	1	Faint stain
	2	Clearly visible stain, orange to brown
	3	Dark stain, deep brown to black
Extent (area code for approximal and gingival sites)	1	Thin line, can be continuous
	2	Thick line or band
	3	Covering total area

Table 12.4

Code	Buccal/labial surfaces	Lingual/palatal surfaces
1	Stain limited to pits/grooves	Up to 1/3 of area affected
2	Stain outside pits/grooves, up to 10% of area affected	Between 1/3 and 2/3 of area affected
3	Stain outside pits/grooves, more than 10% of area affected	More than 2/3 of area affected

were 11, 12, 21, 22, 31, 32, 41 and 42. If an incisor was missing, the nearest canine was substituted.

Bibliography

1. Macpherson LMD, Stephen KW, Joiner A, Schafer F, Huntington E: Comparison of a conventional and modified tooth stain index. J Clin Periodontol 2000; 27: 854–9.

12.9 Modification of the Lobene (1968) Stain Index (Gingival Modification of Stain Index)

The objective of this modification was to clearly define zones which separated the approximal, gingival and incisal surfaces where stain develops (Fig. 12.3). Therefore, each tooth was divided into 4 zones as has been suggested by Koertge and Gunsolley (1993). Intensity in each zone was scored by the criteria described by Lobene (1968), where 0 = no stain, 1 = light stain, 2 = moderate stain and 3 = heavy stain.

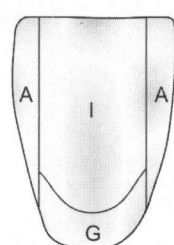

Fig. 12.3: Gingival modification of stain index

Bibliography

1. Grundemann LJMM, Timmerman MF, Ijserman Y, van der Velden U, van der Weijden GA. Stain, plaque and gingivitis reduction by combining chlorhexidine and peroxyborate. J Clin Periodontol 2000;27:9–15.
2. Koertge TE, Gunsolley JC. Comparison of two dentifrices in the control of chlorhexidine-induced stain. Journal of Clinical Dentistry 1993;4, 1–5.

12.10 Sign Grading System for Stains

This system was proposed by Amit A Agarwal (2011). The oral cavity is divided into six sextants: 18–14, 13–23, 24–28, 38–34, 33–43 and 44–48. A typical examination usually starts with the maxillary right third molar and is continued, sextants wise, in a clockwise direction until all the teeth required to be assessed are through. All surfaces of the tooth should be examined for each grade and the surface with the highest grade should be allocated to that particular tooth. This will help in simpler data management and assessment of overall condition of the patient, rather than mentioning different grades for each tooth surface. Similarly, grading of the sextants will depend on the highest grade of the tooth within that sextant. In all classification, "crown" means clinical crown and not anatomic crown. Grading of the stain were listed in Table 12.5.

Scoring requires adequate light and mouth mirror. If optimal conditions and chairside

Table 12.5: Sign grading system for stains

Grade	Criteria
–	Stains absent
+	Continuous line or isolated spots of stains along the gingival margin of clinical crown on labial or lingual surface, with or without involvement of proximal surface (or) Stains involving only proximal surface without involving labial or lingual surfaces (or) Isolated spots of stains limited to anatomic defects, restoration margins and/or orthodontic brackets
++	Stains covering up to half of the labial or lingual crown surface, with or without involvement of proximal surface
++	Stains covering more than half of labial or lingual crown surface, with or without involvement of proximal surface

assistance are provided and all teeth are to be examined, scoring according to this system requires approximately 4–5 minutes. Although this index, for stains, does not differentiate between extrinsic or intrinsic stains, it is recommended that it should be used preferably for extrinsic stains.

For field study: The surface with highest grade is allocated to that particular tooth (t) and the tooth with highest grade is allocated to that sextant (X). Then consider signs – as 0; + as 1; ++ as 2 and +++ as 3.

For clinical research: As per the study requirement, either the sextant can be counted as above, or the grades allotted to each tooth are converted to numerical data (T). Then, sum all the numbers (sT) to be included in the study and divide by the total number of teeth examined (N).

The average scores of the individual can be graded as mild, moderate and severe based on the cut-off scores listed in Table 12.6.

Table 12.6: Average score	
0–1	Mild (+)
1.1 – 2	Moderate (++)
2.1 – 3	Severe (+++)

Bibliography

1. Agrawal AA. A randomized clinical study to assess the reliability and reproducibility of Sign Grading System. Indian J Dent Res 2011;22:285–90.

13

Indices to Assess Tongue Coating

INTRODUCTION

Several methods have been described to measure the extent of tongue coating. Yaegaki and Sanada (1992) suggested a method to measure the tongue coating, in which tongue coating was carefully removed with a tongue scraper of the small spoon type, from the terminal sulcus to the apex of the tongue, then the tongue dorsal surface was cleaned with cotton pellets immersed in physiological saline. After removal of the tongue coating, the wet weight of the tongue coating was estimated (mg). Gross et al (1975) used an index to evaluate tongue coating. The scores were as follows: 0 = no coating; 1 = slight coating; 2 = moderate coating; 3 = heavy coating. Clinical description nor photographs were not given to visualise such an index. Bosy et al. (1994) estimated the amount of coating on the tongue's dorsal surface by visual examination as heavy, medium, light or none. Miyazaki et al. assessed the tongue-coating status according to the distribution area: score 0, none visible; 1, less than one-third of tongue dorsum surface covered; 2, less than two-thirds; and 3, more than two-thirds. Chen classified the tongue coating by colour (white, yellow, grey and black) and by quality of the tongue (dry, slippery, dry and rough, prickly, partially furred, completely furred).

Bibliography

1. Danser MM, Mantilla Gomez S, van der Weijden GA. Tongue coating and tongue brushing: a literature. Int J Dent Hygiene 1, 2003; 151–8.
2. Arthur Gross, George P, Barnes, Thayer C, Lyon. Effects of Tongue Brushing on Tongue Coating and Dental Plaque Scores. J Dent Res 1975;54:1236.

13.1 Addy et al. Criteria for Assessment of Area and Intensity of Staining of Tongue

A subjective determination of staining of the dorsum of the tongue was made both with regard to area and severity. The area of tongue stained was expressed as a percentage of the total area of the dorsum of tongue and scored according to the criteria as shown in Table 13.1.

Bibliography

1. Addy M, Moran J, Davies RM, Beak A, Lewis A. The effect of single morning and evening rinses of chlorhexidine on the development of tooth staining and plaque accumulation. A blind cross-over trial. J Clin Periodontol 1982 Mar;9(2):134–40.

Table 13.1: Scoring criteria (Addy et al)

Score	Criteria (area)	Score	Criteria (severity)
0	No staining	0	No staining
1	1–25% coverage	1	Slight staining
2	26–50% coverage	2	Moderate staining
3	51–75% coverage	3	Severe staining
4	76–100% coverage	4	Very severe staining

13.2 Modified Miyazaki Method for Evaluating Tongue Coating and Discoloration

Assessment of discoloration and coating: The procedure to assess coating was a modification of the method as described by Miyazaki et al. (1995). The tongue was divided in 9 parts. From the vallate papillae to the tip, i.e. back third, middle third and front third (according to Miyazaki et al., 1995). In addition from the left to the right, i.e. left third, middle third and right third. For each of the 9 sections discoloration and coating was visually assessed. The discoloration was scored on a scale from 0 to 4 and coating according to thickness on a scale from 0 to 2. Light-thin coating was scored when the pink color underneath was still visible through the coating. Heavy-thick coating was scored if no pink color could be observed under the coating. Each section of the tongue should be covered for more than 1/3 to obtain a score different than 0. Furthermore the presence or absence of fissures on the tongue was also recorded (Table 13.2).

Table 13.2: Scoring criteria for modified Miyazaki method

Score	Discoloration	Score	Coating
0	Pink	0	no coating
1	White	1	light-thin coating
2	Yellow/light brown	2	heavy-thick coating
3	Brown		
4	Black		

Bibliography

1. Gomez SM, Danser MM, Sipos PM, Rowshani B, Van der Velden U, Van der Weijden GA: Tongue coating and salivary bacterial counts in healthy/gingivitis subjects and periodontitis patients. J Clin Periodontol 2001; 28: 970–8.

13.3 Winkel Tongue Coating Index (WTCI)

The dorsum of the tongue was notionally divided into six areas, i.e. three in the posterior and three in the anterior part of the tongue.

Table 13.3: WTCI

0	No coating
1	Slight coating
2	Severe coating

The tongue coating in each sextant was scored as shown in Table 13.3.

The tongue coating value was obtained by the addition of all six scores, range 0–12.

Winkel tongue discoloration index (WTDI): In the six areas of the tongue, each sextant was scored as shown in Table 13.4.

The tongue discoloration value was obtained by the addition of all six scores, range 0–12 (WTDI).

Table 13.4: WTDI

0	No discoloration
1	Light discoloration
2	Severe discoloration

Bibliography

1. Winkel EG, Roldan S, Van Winkelhoff AJ, Herrera D, Sanz M. Clinical effects of a new mouthrinse containing chlorhexidine, cetylpyridinium chloride and zinc-lactate on oral halitosis. J Clin Periodontol 2003;30:300–6.

13.4 Tsai et al. (2008) Criteria Based on Miyazaki et al. (1995)

Tongue coating was assessed on a scale of 0–3 by inspecting the areas of the tongue (the tongue was divided into four areas by the sulcus terminalis and the linea mediana: anterior right, anterior left, posterior right and posterior left) and scoring the coating (0, no coating apparent; 1, less than one-third of the area of the tongue dorsum coated; 2, between one-third and two-thirds of the surface covered; and 3, more than two-thirds of the surface coated). The tongue coating score of a tongue could therefore range from 0 to 12.

Bibliography

1. Tsai CC, Chou HH, Wu TL, Yang YH, Ho KY, Wu YM, Ho YP. The levels of volatile sulfur compounds in mouth air from patients with chronic periodontitis. J Periodont Res 2008.

14

Indices to Assess Tooth Wear

INTRODUCTION

There exists both clinical and scientific ways to measure tooth wear and the literature prevails with many methods which can be broadly divided into quantitative and qualitative in nature. Quantitative methods rely on objective physical measurements, viz. depth of groove, area of facet or height of crown while qualitative methods rely on clinical descriptions. In a clinical intraoral examination, there will be an inclination towards descriptive assessment measures, such as mild, moderate or severe, rather than quantitative measurement, which is easier to perform reliably on a model or in the laboratory. Such methods tend to be more sensitive but do not lend themselves readily to clinical use—especially in epidemiology, where fieldwork data collection is often carried out in an environment lacking sophisticated equipment.

Many tooth wear indices have been developed for clinical and laboratory use. Unfortunately, the presence of so many indices does not allow for ready comparison of results between different studies, and this is especially important in epidemiology when trying to define the prevalence of a condition. Confusion is further generated in the literature as the majority of researchers, in their attempts to quantify the amount of tooth tissue loss due to tooth wear, have historically concentrated

on etiology only, and these indices tend to be surface limited. Often, the wear patterns described do not appear to reflect the etiology suggested and this relates to lack of uniformity with tooth wear terminology and translation errors. Many diagnostic indices do not properly reflect the morphological defects, and there is little international standardisation.

The literature identifies separate indices for use in clinical and laboratory situations and specific indices for attrition, abrasion, erosion and multifactorial tooth wear. There are common features to all of the indices, such as descriptive diagnostic criteria and criteria for quantifying the amount of hard tissue loss. These generally consider the size of the affected area—as a proportion of a sound surface and/or the depth of tissue loss—expressed as a degree of dentine exposure.

14.1 Tooth Wear Index (TWI)

Smith and Knight introduced the more general concept of measuring tooth wear per se, irrespective of the cause, and since then more recent indices have been developed or modified from Smith and Knight that do not rely on a prior diagnosis and are more clinically relevant. Most of these stress the importance of user training sessions and calibration exercises.

Smith and Knight in 1984 took Eccles ideas a stage further, producing the tooth wear index (TWI), a comprehensive system whereby all four visible surfaces (buccal, cervical, lingual and occlusal–incisal) of all teeth present are scored for wear, irrespective of how it occurred. This avoids the confusion associated with terminology and translation or differences in opinion for diagnosis of etiology based on clinical findings. Guidelines for using the criteria (Table 14.1) were produced in a booklet by the authors to aid training and standardization with other investigators; in cases of doubt, the lowest score is given.

Complete enamel loss (score 4) may, however, be misleading, as there is almost always a rim of enamel at the worn surface margins—the colloquial "enamel halo." This index was the first one designed to measure and monitor multifactorial tooth wear; a further pioneering feature was the ability to distinguish acceptable and pathological levels of wear, by comparison with threshold normal values for the age groups studied.

Tooth wear was defined as pathological if the teeth became so worn that they do not function effectively or seriously mar the appearance before they are lost through other causes or the patient dies. The index appears simple to use clinically intraorally or from models and photographs.

1. Each tooth surface susceptible to tooth wear is assessed by visual examination
2. Separate records are made of the cervical surface the remainder of the buccal or labial surface, the lingual or palatal surface, and the occlusal or incisal surface. The effect of tooth wear on occlusal or incisal surface. The effect of tooth wear on occlusal and incisal surface is not the same, so different criteria are used. The buccal and cervical surfaces are recorded separately because of the occurrence of cervical notch defects in some patients which may not be associated with wear of the entire buccal surface and which probably have a different etiology. The approximal surfaces are not recorded.
3. The total number of surfaces examined 128 surfaces.
4. Heavily restored surfaces and missing tooth are not recorded.
5. Despite the large number of surfaces, the assessment of each is straight forwards, and a complete record is usually made in under 5 minutes, including the time sometimes needed to clean the teeth sufficiently to make the visual assessments.
6. Index can be recorded either clinically or from photographs.

Table 14.1: Tooth wear index

Score	Surface	Criteria
0	B/L/O/I	No loss of enamel surface characteristics
	C	No loss of contour
1	B/L/O/I	Loss of enamel surface characteristics
	C	Minimal loss of contour
2	B/L/O	Loss of enamel exposing dentine for less than one-third of surface
	I	Loss of enamel just exposing dentine
	C	Defect less than 1 mm deep
3	B/L/O	Loss of enamel exposing dentine for more than one-third of surface
	I	Loss of enamel and substantial loss of dentine
	C	Defect less than 1–2 mm deep
4	B/L/O	Complete enamel loss–pulp exposure– secondary dentine exposure
	I	Pulp exposure or exposure of secondary dentine
	C	Defect more than 2 mm deep–pulp exposure – secondary dentine exposure

Limitations

The time necessary to apply to a whole dentition, amount of data generated and the comparisons with threshold levels for each age group.

The thresholds proposed were high, erring towards understatement rather than exaggerations of pathological wear.

Full use of the index as a research tool is not feasible without computer assistance.

Donachie and Walls (1996) outlined various flaws in the tooth wear index as an epidemiological tool in the ageing population and suggested a need to increase the sensitivity of TWI at extremes of tooth wear, to take account of the capacity of the elderly to have adequate function in cases of significant wear. They suggested altering threshold values, amplifying scoring criteria and creating a sixth point to distinguish between exposure of secondary dentine and frank pulp exposure.

Bibliography

1. Smith BG, Knight JK. An index for measuring the wear of teeth. Br Dent J 1984;156:435–8.
2. Donachie MA, Walls AW. The tooth wear index: a flawed epidemiological tool in an ageing population group. Community Dent Oral Epidemiol 1996;24(2):152–8.

14.2 Simplified TWI

Bardsley et al. (2004) pioneered a new, simplified version of TWI. Tooth wear scoring was essentially dichotomized into the presence or absence of dentine, with even cupping of dentine scoring one. A partial recording system was used, collecting data from 40 surfaces including occlusal surfaces of the four first molar teeth and the labial, incisal and lingual–palatal surfaces of the six upper and lower anterior teeth.

However, despite calibration and training, difficulties were experienced diagnosing dentine exposure in the epidemiological field and there is some debate as to the significance of dentinal cupping when exposed dentine does not relate to significant amounts of tissue loss.

Score	Criteria
	Table 14.2
0	No wear into dentine
1	Dentine just visible (including cupping) or dentine exposed for less than 1/3 of surface
2	Dentine exposure greater than 1/3 of surface
3	Exposure of pulp or secondary dentine

Bibliography

1. Bardsley PF, Taylor S, Milosevic A. Epidemiological studies of tooth wear and dental erosion in 14-year old children in North West England 1. The relationship with water fluoridation and social deprivation. Br Dent J 2004;197:413–6.

14.3 A System for Assessing Occlusal Tooth Wear

This was proposed by A Johansson, T Haraldson, R Omar, S Kiliaridis and GE Carlsson in 1993.

Method: A set of maxillary and mandibular study casts was obtained for each individual using standard alginate impressions and poured in stone. Only casts which permitted accurate scoring of wear were accepted. Third molars and heavily restored teeth were excluded from all evaluations.

Evaluations of the severity and the progression of wear were performed on the study casts on a tooth-by-tooth basis using ordinal scales (Tables 14.3 and 14.4). Intraoral photographs were used to determine grade 4 wear, which corresponded to 'wear into secondary dentine (Table 14.3). In the scale used for the evaluation of progression of wear, measurements of height reduction (grades 2 and 3, Table 14.3) were accomplished using the CEJ as the reference point. All assessments were performed in near standardized lighting conditions.

Table 14.3: Ordinal scale used for grading severity of occlusal wear	
Score	Criteria
0	No visible facets in the enamel. Occlusal/incisal morphology intact
1	Marked wear facets in the enamel. Occlusal/incisal morphology altered
2	Wear into the dentine. The dentine exposed occlusally/incisally or adjacent tooth surface Occlusal/incisal morphology changed in shape with height reduction of the crown
3	Extensive wear into the dentine. Larger dentine area (> 2mm^2) exposed occlusally/incisally or adjacent tooth surface. Occlusal/incisal morphology totally lost locally or generally. Substantial loss of crown height
4	Wear into secondary dentine (verified by photographs)

Table 14.4: Scale used for scoring progression of occlusal wear	
Score	Criteria
0	No definite change in previously recorded area(s)
1	Visible change, such as an increase of the facet area(s), without any measurable reduction of crown length; occlusal/incisal morphology changed in shape compared to the first examination
2	Measurable reduction of crown length, < 1 mm
3	Marked reduction of crown length, > 1 mm

Advantages

1. May be of value in determining the severity of occlusal wear and the rate of deterioration of the dentition.

2. From a clinical standpoint, the need for treatment, either immediate or at some future time, may in this way be more reliably assessed.

3. The reliability of the scales and its relative simplicity of use, are further advantages in the application suggested.

Bibliography

1. A Johansson, T Haraldson, R Omar, S Kiliaridis, GE Carlsson. A system for assessing the severity and progression of occlusal tooth wear. Journal of Oral Rehabilitation, 1993, Vol 20;125–131.

14.4 Occlusal Wear Criteria Given by Gunnar E Carlsson, Anders Johansson and Sture Lundqvist in 1985 (Tables 14.5 and 14.6)

The following scale of original attrition was applied.

The assessment was performed on casts, and, when available, intraoral photographs

Table 14.5	
Score	Criteria
0	No or little wear of enamel only
1	Marked wear facets of enamel
2	Wear into dentin
3	Extensive wear into dentin (>2 mm^2)
4	Wear into secondary dentin (verified by photographs)

taken at the first examination. An index of original wear was calculated by adding the highest value for each group of teeth (molars, premolars, canines, and incisors) in each jaw. The theoretical maximal value was thus 32.

Table 14.6: Continuation of occlusal wear was judged in accordance with the following scale by comparing and measuring casts and photographs from the first and the follow-up examination	
Score	Criteria
0	No certain change
1	Visible change, such as increase of facet areas, without measurable reduction of tooth length
2	Measurable reduction of tooth length <1 mm
3	Marked reduction of tooth length ≥ 1 mm

An index of continuing wear was calculated by adding the highest value for each group of teeth as described above for the original wear. The maximal value for this index was 24.

Bibliography

1. Carlsson GE, Johansson A, Lundqvist S. Occlusal wear. A follow-up study of 18 subjects with extensively worn dentitions. Acta Odontol Scand 1985;43:83–90.

14.5 Bjorn et al. Index of Dental Wear

This index was given by Oilo G, Dahl BL, Hatle G Gad AL in 1987. It consists of three categories of satisfactory degree of wear: Romeo (R), Sierra (S) and Mike (M) and two categories of not acceptable degree of wear: Tango (T) and Victor (V) (Table 14.7).

Table 14.7

Score	Criteria
R	No visible wear or change in anatomic form;
S	Limited (normal) wear; limited change in anatomic form
M	Considerable wear with obvious change in anatomic form but without need for treatment
T	Considerable wear with marked change in anatomic form; further damage to tooth and/or surrounding tissues is likely to occur;
V	Excessive wear; extreme change in anatomic form, esthetics, and function; pain on chewing; damage to tooth and/or surrounding tissues is occurring

All categories except Romeo contain subcategories (Table 14.8). To overcome the problem of grading the wear of restorations two extra subcategories of group M were introduced—that is, large wear facets in restorative material (MWR) and perforation of crown with hard, non-sensitive dentin exposed (MED-P).

Bibliography

1. Dahl BL, Oilo G, Andersen A, Bruaset O. The suitability of a new index for the evaluation of dental wear. Acta Odontol Scand 1989;47:205–10.

Table 14.8

Subcategories	Criteria
R	No visible wear
SOF	Wear facets in enamel
SDF	Small areas of exposed dentin
MLR	Obvious length reduction of tooth
MED	Large areas of exposed, hard dentin
MWR	Large wear facets in restorative material
MED-P	Perforation of crown with hard, non-sensitive dentin exposed
TLR	Considerable length reduction of tooth
TED	Large areas of exposed, soft dentin
VLR	Marked length reduction of tooth
VCA	Pain on chewing.

2. Oilo G, Dahl BL, Hatle G Gad AL. An index for evaluating wear of teeth. Acta Odontol Scand. 1987;45:361–5.

14.6 Hugoson Tooth Wear Diagnostic Criteria

It was given by Hugoson A, Bergendal T, Ekfeldt A, Helkimo M (1988). The degree of incisal or occlusal wear was evaluated for each single tooth in accordance with the following criteria (Table 14.9).

Table 14.9

Score	Criteria
0	No wear or negligible wear of enamel
1	Obvious wear of enamel or wear through the enamel to the dentin in single spots; score
2	Wear of the dentin up to one-third of the crown height
3	Wear of the dentin more than one-third of the crown height; excessive wear of tooth restorative material or dental materials on crown and bridgework, more than one-third of the crown height

Bibliography

1. Hugoson A, Bergendal T, Ekfeldt A, Helkimo M. Prevalence and severity of incisal and occlusal tooth wear in an adult Swedish population. Acta Odontol Scand 1988;46:255–65.

14.7 Individual Tooth Wear Index

This was proposed by Anders Ekfeldt, Anders Hugoson, Tom Bergendal and Martti Helkimo in 1990. The extent of incisal or occlusal wear was evaluated for each single tooth in accordance with the following criteria (Table 14.10).

Table 14.10	
Score	Criteria
0	No wear or negligible wear of enamel
1	Obvious wear of enamel or wear through the enamel to the dentin in single spots
2	Wear of the dentin up to one-third of the crown height
3	Wear of the dentin up to more than one-third of the crown height; excessive wear of tooth restorative material or dental materials in crown and bridgework, more than one-third of the crown height.

An individual incisal and occlusal tooth wear index (I_A) was created, on the basis of the scores of incisal or occlusal wear for each tooth of the individual.

$$I_A = \frac{10 \ G_1 + 30 \times G_2 + 100 \times G_3}{G_0 + G_1 + G_2 + G_3}$$

The index is the ratio between the weighted sum of all teeth with some degree of wear and the total number of existing teeth for that individual. The purpose was to obtain one single value for the degree of incisal and occlusal tooth wear. G_0, G_1, G_2 and G_3 = the number of teeth with score 0, 1, 2 and 3, respectively. The constants 10, 30 and 100 were chosen to reflect the differences in incisal and occlusal breakdown between teeth with scores 1, 2, and 3 respectively.

The index was proposed to study incisal and occlusal wear in adults from an epidemiologic point of view. The individual tooth wear index states the ratio between the weighted sum of all teeth with some degree of tooth wear and the total number of existing teeth for that individual. This relation will give a comparative measurement of the tooth wear in that individual. The values of the constants G_1, G_2, and G_3 were chosen to strengthen the difference in wear between teeth with scores 1, 2 and 3, respectively, in order to increase the discriminating power of this index. To emphasize the clinical and therapeutic importance of advanced wear, the difference between score 2 and 3 was deliberately made greater than the arithmetic difference between scores 0, 1 and 2.

Limitations

The index used describes well excessive wear of dentin and restorative material but has the limitation of not discriminating incisal and occlusal wear of restorative materials of degrees 0, 1 and 2. This limits the possibility of ranking slight to moderate tooth wear in individuals with occlusal restorations.

Bibliography

1. Ekfeldt A, Hugoson A, Bergendal T, Helkimo M. An individual tooth wear index and an analysis of factors correlated to incisal and occlusal wear in an adult Swedish population. Acta Odontol Scand 1990;48:343–9.

14.8 Tooth Wear Index Used in 1998 the UK Adult Dental Health Survey

The index used in this study confined the clinical examination to the palatal, labial and incisal surfaces of the six maxillary anterior teeth (Table 14.11) and the worst affected surface of the mandibular anterior teeth.

Bibliography

1. RN Rafeek, S Marchan, A Eder, WAJ Smith. Tooth surface loss in adult subjects attending a university dental clinic in Trinidad. International Dental Journal (2006) 56:181–6.

14.9 Smooth Wear Assessment

This was proposed by van Rijkom HM, Truin GJ, Frencken JE, König KG, van 't Hof MA, Bronkhorst EM, Roeters FJ (2002). Smooth wear is described as loss of tooth tissue with

Table 14.11

Score	Surface	Criteria
0	All	Sound; any TSL is restricted to enamel and does not extend into dentine
1	All	Loss of enamel, just exposing dentine: equivalent to mild TSL
2	B,L	Loss of enamel > 1/3 of surface area: equivalent to moderate TSL
	Incisal	Exposed dentine > 2 mm from widest point: equivalent to moderate TSL
3	B,L	Complete loss of enamel on a surface with pulp exposure or secondary dentine: equivalent to severe TSL
	Incisal	Pulp exposure/exposure of secondary dentine
8	All	Fractured tooth
9	All	Unscorable: Crown/bridge/no visible incisal edge/tip

the exception of caries and pure attrition, is independent of the etiology of wear. The criteria for the assessment of smooth wear were derived from the diagnostic criteria for oral and occlusal erosion developed by Lussi (1996). In order to differentiate between slight and deep enamel wear, the grade for enamel loss was split into 2 categories, extending the original index by one grade, since in the present index, etiology was not determined in advance, in contrast to the Lussi index which is focused on erosion, the indices for occlusal, oral and facial surfaces were combined. After this modification the applied ordinal classification for severity of smooth wear included (Table 14.12).

In case of doubt between two grades, the less advance grade was chosen. When it was questionable if dentine was involved,

Table 14.12

Grade	Criteria
0	No visible smooth wear
1	Slight smooth enamel wear with silky-shining, 'melted' appearance
2	Deep smooth enamel wear, more pronounced signs than grade 1, dentine is shining through (light yellow)
3	Smooth wear into dentine on lingual/palatal/occlusal surface or less than one-half of buccal/labial surfaces
4	Smooth wear into dentine on more than one half of the buccal/labial surfaces

sensitivity to cold air as well as careful probing was included.

Bibliography

1. van Rijkom HM, Truin GJ, Frencken JE, König KG, van 't Hof MA, Bronkhorst EM, Roeters FJ. Prevalence, distribution and background variables of smooth-bordered tooth wear in teenagers in Hague, the Netherlands. Caries Res. 2002 Mar-Apr;36(2):147–54.

14.10 The Exact Tooth Wear Index

This was proposed in 2009 by J Fares, S Shirodaria, K Chiu, N. Ahmad, M. Sherriff and D Bartlett. This index was developed according to the basic principles of the Smith and Knight Index. It uses an air syringe, a disposable mirror and WHO periodontal probe. All subjects were examined in the supine position under good lighting and with an assistant present. Before scoring each tooth, it was wiped with a cotton roll and then air syringed to dry its surface.

The wear on teeth was graded separately for enamel and dentine using 5- and 6-point scales, respectively (Table 14.13). Any surface change resulting from wear, irrespective of the etiology, was scored on the cervical, buccal, occlusal /incisal and palatal/lingual surfaces of the upper first molar to the contralateral first molar in both arches. In cases of doubt the lower score was recorded. Changes to the enamel surface texture or anatomy were graded according to the criteria listed as below:

Table 14.13

Score	Criteria
Exact tooth wear index for Enamel	
0	No tooth wear: no loss of enamel characteristics or change in contour
1	Loss of enamel affecting less than 10% of the scored surface
2	Enamel loss affecting between 10% and one-third of the scored surface
3	Enamel loss affecting at least one-third but less than two-thirds of the scored surface
4	Enamel loss affecting two-thirds or more of the scored surface
Exact tooth wear index for dentine	
0	No dentinal tooth wear: no loss of dentine
1	Loss of dentine affecting less than 10% of the scored surface
2	Dentine loss affecting between 10% and one-third of the scored surface
3	Dentine loss affecting at least one third but less than two-thirds of the scored surface
4	Dentine loss affecting two thirds or more of the scored surface, no pulpal exposure
5	Exposure of secondary dentine formation or pulpal exposure
Depth on cervical buccal surfaces (measured with a standard W and H periodontal probe)	
0	No tooth wear: no loss of tooth contour
1	< 1mm loss of tooth surface depth
2	Tooth surface loss in depth measuring $\geq$ 1 mm but < 2 mm
3	Tooth surface loss in depth measuring $\geq$ 2 mm

A separate score was given to the area around the cervical margin and to the buccal/facial surface following the protocols defined by Smith and Knight (1984). In brief, the area around the enamel/cemental junction or the zone just above the gingival margin, if this was not visible, was considered as the cervical area. Any part of the tooth coronal to this area was considered to be on the facial/buccal surface. Restorations covering more than 25% of any tooth surface (cervical, buccal, occlusal/incisal and palatal/lingual surfaces) and missing teeth were recorded separately.

Criteria

- Illuminate the teeth using a halogen light source
- Teeth dried prior to examination
- Mirrors front reflecting and un-scratched
- State the location of the examination
- Score all permanent teeth except third permanent molars
- The surfaces scored are: buccal/facial, occlusal/incisal, lingual/palatal and buccal–cervical in that order

- Once some part of the tooth is present in the mouth it is scored, all unerupted surfaces are scored 0
- Enamel is scored first and then dentine.

Conventions

- When in doubt with regard to a score the lower score should be applied.
- A tooth surface with a restoration covering more than 25% of a surface is scored R (excluded).
- Orthodontically banded surfaces are scored R.
- When tooth wear has occurred so that clinical crown height is lost, the buccal/facial and palatal/lingual surfaces are scored.
- For loss of tooth wear as well as the incisal/occlusal surface, otherwise no indication of future wear can be incorporated.

Bibliography

1. J Fares, S Shirodaria, K Chiu, N Ahmad, M Sherriff and D Bartlett. A New Index of Tooth Wear Reproducibility and Application to a

Sample of 18- to 30-year-old University Students. Caries Res 2009;43:119–125.

2. D Bartlett, M Harding, M Sherriff, S Shirodaria and H Whelton. A new index to measure tooth wear – methodology and practical Advice. Community Dental Health (2011) 28, 182–7.

14A. Indices to Assess Dental Erosion

14A.1 Malcolm and Paul Criteria

Malcolm and Paul (1961) observed that any estimation of the degree of erosion must be subjective, since the original dimensions of the teeth are not known. Nevertheless they divided the degrees of erosion into etching of the enamel surface and three groups of erosion, based on an estimate of tooth loss deduced from an assumed size of tooth crown. In their group 1, this loss did not exceed one fifth (2 mm) of the incisal enamel; in group 2 there was loss of one-fifth to one-half of the tooth crown; and in group 3 there was loss of more than half of the tooth crown.

Limitations: It is difficult to estimate loss by subtracting the remaining tooth substance from assumed dimensions for the original crown. The transition from group 1 to group 2 could not easily be defined.

Bibliography

1. Cited in: Ten Bruggen Cate HJ. Dental erosion in Industry. Brit J Industrial Medicine 1968;25:249–66.

14A.2 Ten Bruggen Cate Classification

Considering the difficulties with past criteria, Ten Bruggen Cate classified dental erosion in industrial workers into 5 grades as summarized below (Fig. 14.1):

Etching (Et): This consisted of a dull, ground-glass appearance of the enamel surface without loss of contour

- **Grade 1 erosion (G 1):** Loss of enamel only
- **Grade 2 erosion (G 2):** Loss of enamel with involvement of dentine
- **Grade 3 erosion (G 3):** Loss of enamel and dentine with exposure of secondary dentine
- **Grade 4 erosion (G 4):** Loss of enamel and dentine resulting in pulpal exposure

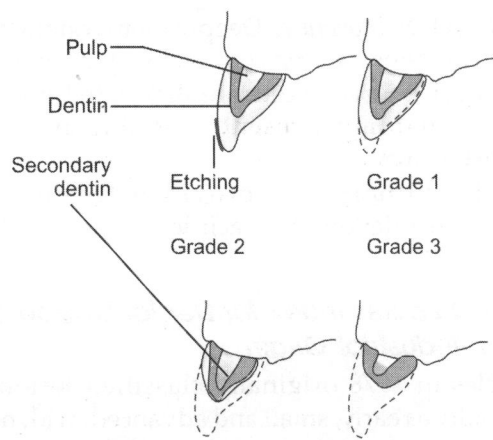

Fig. 14.1: Ten Bruggen Cate classification

Bibliography

1. Ten Bruggen Cate HJ. Dental erosion in Industry. Brit J Industrial Medicine 1968;25:249–66.

14A.3 The Keels–Coffield Clinical Severity Scale of Dental Erosion

Keels and Coffield proposed a clinical severity scale to assess dental erosion among individuals with gastroesophageal reflux disease (GERD). The severity of erosion was on scale of 0–3 (Fig. 14.2). The criteria are as follows:

- **Level 0:** No erosion
- **Level 1:** *Mild:* Only the cusp tips are affected; Shallow "moon craters" are present.

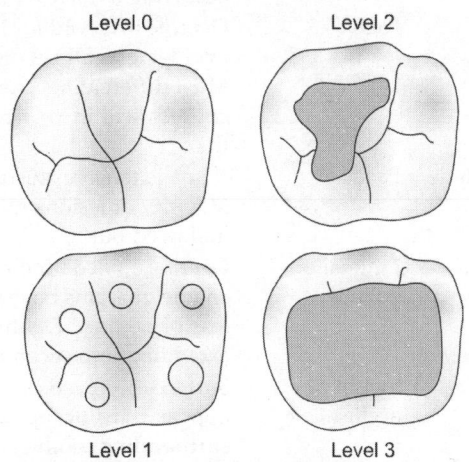

Fig. 14.2: Keels–Coffield clinical severity scale of dental erosion

- **Level 2:** *Moderate:* Deep moon craters or depressions are present and may coalesce
- **Level 3:** *Severe:* Teeth are slick with little or no anatomy present; possible pulpal exposures

The authors also provided treatment recommendations for each level specifically for GERD.

14A.4 Eccles Index for Dental Erosion of Non-industrial Origin

Eccles in 1978 originally classified lesions broadly as early, small and advanced, with no strict criteria definitions, thus allowing wide interpretation. Later, the index was refined and expanded in 1979, with greater emphasis on the descriptive criteria. It was presented as a comprehensive qualitative index, grading both severity and site of erosion due to non-industrial causes, and is considered as one of the cardinal indices from which others have evolved. In essence, it breaks down into three classes of erosion, denoting the type of lesion, assigned to four surfaces, representing the surface where erosion was detected. The criteria are discussed in Table 14.14.

Bibliography

1. Eccles JD. Dental erosion of nonindustrial origin. A clinical survey and classification. J Prosthet Dent 1979;42:649–53.
2. Wiktorsson AM, Zimmerman M Angar-Mansson B. Erosive tooth wear: Prevalence and severity in Swedish winetasters. Eur J Oral Sciences 1997;105:544–50.

14A.5 Erosion Criteria from the Modified Scoring System of Linkosalo and Markkanen (1985)

Vestibular/oral surfaces: Concavities located coronally from the enamel-cementum junction, the breadth of which greatly exceeds their depth, thus distinguishing them from wedge-shaped defects, Grade 0: no visible erosion, Grade 1: shallow concavities less than one-third of the surface, Grade 2: deep concavities or shallower concavities both more than one-third of the surface.

Occlusal surfaces: Grade 0: no visible erosion, Grade 1: small pits and slightly rounded cusps, fissures flattened, moderate cupping, occlusal surface morphology preserved, Grade 2: depression of the cusps

Class	Surface	Criteria
I		Early stages of erosion, absence of developmental ridges, smooth, glazed surface occurring mainly on labial surfaces of maxillary incisors and canines
II	Facial	Dentine involved for less than one-third surface; two types Type 1 (commonest): ovoid–crescentic in outline, concave in cross section at cervical region of surface. Must differentiate from wedge shaped abrasion lesions Type 2: irregular lesion entirely within crown. Punched out appearance, where enamel is absent from floor
IIIa	Facial	More extensive destruction of dentine, affecting anterior teeth particularly. Majority of lesions affect a large part of the surface, but some are localised and hollowed out
IIIb	Lingual or palatal	Dentine eroded for more than one-third of the surface area. Gingival and proximal enamel margins have white, etched appearance. Incisal edges translucent due to loss of dentine. Dentine is smooth and anteriorly is flat or hollowed out, often extending into secondary dentine
IIIc	Incisal or occlusal	Surfaces involved into dentine, appearing flattened or with cupping. Incisal edges appear translucent due to undermined enamel; restorations are raised above surrounding tooth surface
IIId	All	Severely affected teeth, where both labial and lingual surfaces are extensively involved. Proximal surfaces may be affected; teeth are shortened

Table 14.14: Criteria for dental erosion (non-industrial origin)

with severe cupping and grooving, restoration margins raised above the surrounding tooth level, occlusal surface morphology flattened.

Facets (attrition) defined as flat areas with clear cut borders and with corresponding wear of the antagonists were excluded.

In addition, an "erosion index" (EI) was determined for the permanent dentition of each subject:

$$EI = \frac{\Sigma \text{ of number of surfaces with an erosive lesion}}{\Sigma \text{ of the total number of surface at risk}} \times 100$$

Bibliography

1. Linkosalo E, Markkanen H. Dental erosions in relation to lactovegetarian diet. Scand J Dent Res 1985;93:436–41.
2. Ganss C, Klimek J, Giese K. Dental erosion in children and adolescents – a cross-sectional and longitudinal investigation using study models. Community Dent Oral Epidemiol 2001; 29: 264–71.

14A.6 Erosion Index

It was proposed by Lussi in 1991 (Table 14.15).

Bibliography

1. Lussi A, Schaffner M, Hotz P, Suter P. Dental erosion in a population of Swiss adults. Community Dent Oral Epidemiol 1991;19 (5):286–90.

14A.7 Aine Index for Erosion

Aine et al developed a grading system for dental erosions in children with gastro-esophageal reflux disease using 4 grades (Table 14.16). This can be used for both primary and permanent teeth.

Table 14.16: Aine index

Changes in teeth	Grade
Normal (no erosions)	0
Mild opacities, white spots, etched appearance	1
Punched-out holes along occlusal surfaces, incisal edges thinned, cusps flattened	2
Dentin exposed at the bottom of the punched-out holes along the occlusal surfaces; dentin exposed on other surfaces	3

Bibliography

Aine L, Baer M, Mai M. Dental erosions caused by gastroesophageal reflux disease in children. J Dentistry for Children. 1993; 60 (May-June): 210–4.

14A.8 Eccles and Jenkins Criteria

The codes used to measure tooth surface loss were graded as follows:
- Grade 0 indicated no clinical evidence of tooth surface loss;
- Grade 1 represented loss of enamel surface, giving a smooth glazed surface with no dentine involvement;

Table 14.15: Erosion index

Surface	Score	Criteria
Facial	0	No erosion. Surface with a smooth, silky glazed appearance, possible absence of developmental ridges
	1	Loss of surface enamel. Intact enamel cervical to the erosive lesion; concavity on enamel where breadth clearly exceeds depth, thus distinguishing it from toothbrush abrasion. Undulating borders of the lesion are possible and dentine is not involved
	2	Involvement of dentine for less than half of tooth surface
	3	Involvement of dentine for more than half of tooth surface
Occlusal/ lingual	0	No erosion. Surface with a smooth, silky glazed appearance, possible absence of developmental ridges
	1	Slight erosion, rounded cusps, edges of restorations rising above the level of adjacent tooth surface, grooves on occlusal aspects. Loss of surface enamel. Dentine is not involved
	2	Severe erosions, more pronounced signs than in grade 1. Dentine is involved

- Grade 2 showed involvement of the dentine for less than one-third of the area of the tooth surface
- Grade 3 indicated involvement of the dentine for more than one-third of the area of the tooth surface.

The calculations of the number of tooth that had a tooth surface loss score of 1, 2 or 3, were adjusted for missing tooth surfaces (i.e. teeth coded 8 and 9 were eliminated from the calculations).

The number of surfaces on which any Tooth Surface Loss (Tsl) of Grade 1, 2 or 3 occurred were added together to provide an unweighted composite score and referred to as the "Sum Surface 123". When only the severe scores, namely Grades 2 and 3 were added together, this unweighted composite score is referred to as the "Sum Surface 23". Another method used was to weight the Grades according to the severity and then add it together. The more severe instances of tooth surface loss were weighted by means of ordinal constants, e.g. a score of 2 was multiplied by 2 and a score of 3 was multiplied by 3. This weighted composite score is referred to as the "Weighted Sum Surface".

Bibliography

1. Eccles JD, Jenkins WG. Dental Erosion and Diet. Journal of Dentistry 1974;2:153–9.

14A.9 Modified version of Eccles and Jenkins

This was proposed by Johansson AK et al in 1996 on an ordinal scale for grading severity of dental erosion on buccal and lingual surfaces of maxillary anterior teeth. The criteria are as follows:

- **0:** No visible changes; developmental structures remain and macro-morphology intact;
- **1:** Smoothened enamel; developmental structures have totally or partially vanished; enamel surface is shiny, matt, irregular, 'melted', rounded or flat and macro-morphology generally intact.
- **2:** Enamel surface as described in grade 1; macro-morphology clearly changed; Facetting or concavity formation within the enamel and no dentinal exposure.
- **3:** Enamel surface as described in grades 1 and 2 macro-morphology greatly changed (close to dentinal exposure of large surfaces) or dentin surface exposed ≤ 1/3rd .
- **4:** Enamel surface as described in grades 1, 2 and 3; dentin surface exposed > 1/3rd ; pulp visible through the dentin.

Note: Approximal erosion and presence of 'shoulder' should be recorded.

Bibliography

1. Johansson AK, Johansson A, Birkhed D, Omar R, Baghdadi S, Carlsson GE. Dental erosion, soft-drink intake, and oral health in young Saudi men, and the development of a system for assessing erosive anterior tooth wear. Acta Odontol Scand 1996;54:369–78.

14A.10 Kunzel Criteria for Dental Erosion

Kunzel W, Cruz MS, Fischer T (2000) proposed the following criteria as some indices are based on the clinical severity of the erosion, focusing on accessible teeth and others based their measurements on the severity of the erosive process which were inadequate individuals with V-shaped erosion was typically located on upper central and lateral incisors. Hence following metric grades of progression were therefore employed (Table 14.17).

Bibliography

1. Kunzel W, Cruz MS, Fischer T. Dental erosion in Cuban children associated with excessive consumption of oranges. Eur J Oral Sci 2000;108: 104–9.

14A.11 A Clinical Index for Evaluating and Monitoring Dental Erosion

Larsen et al. (2000) proposed clinical index which is based on a clinical examination as well as photographs and casts of the teeth. The registration includes the following procedures:
1. Because teeth should be free from plaque to allow examination and scoring of the

Table 14.17: Kunzel criteria

Grade	Criteria
0.5	Objectionable: First sign of enamel wear on 11 and 21; mesial edges are rounded and smooth. It is difficult to distinguish these definitively from the effects of natural attrition. Different examiners may make different diagnoses (reliability)
1	The crown is markedly shortened at the mesial edge (> 1 mm) producing a linear slope in the tooth's profile, intersecting the tooth's axis at the incisal edge. Dentin is not affected. The eroded enamel is rounded towards the vestibular and oral surface. The tooth crown seems to be smaller in its medial-dorsal dimension
2	The incisal destruction has progressed mesiodistally to involve the distal edges of both central incisors. The mesial loss of enamel is more extensive (2 to 3 mm) and the dentin could be involved. At this stage the coronal defect has become unaesthetic
3	Further loss of incisal hard tissue, now involving the mesial edges of the lateral incisors. These are, at this stage, directly exposed to acid attack. The marked V-shaped gap now involves both adjacent teeth

surfaces, supragingival scaling and polishing must be performed, if needed, before air-drying. The teeth are then examined and photographed before impressions are taken.

2. Recording of teeth present, caries, mineralization disturbances, restorations, crowns and bridges, presence of erosion of the tooth surfaces, gingival shoulders, cervical abrasion lesions, and incisal as well as occlusal wear.

3. Intraoral color photographs are taken at frontal, right and left lateral as well as occlusal views.

4. Impressions in a silicone material for preparing casts in epoxy resin.

5. In the classification procedure the color photographs and data from the clinical records serve primarily as supplementary information for the identification of defects in the tooth surfaces, restorations, crowns and bridges. The final classification of tooth substance loss is thus based on visual inspection of the casts at 10X magnification of the facial surfaces, the oral surfaces, the incisal and occlusal surfaces and the cervical root surfaces separately. For each tooth every single surface is given a score value as per the criteria. Fractured teeth and teeth with restorations covering more than three fourths of the surface or crowns are excluded from evaluation of tooth substance

loss, as well as tooth surfaces that are insufficiently reproduced in the casts.

Grading of erosions

The presence of erosion is assessed by separate evaluation of single surfaces of the teeth, including the facial (buccal or labial), the oral (lingual or palatal) and the incisal or occlusal surfaces, as well as the cervical root surface in case of gingival recession. The severity of erosion on each tooth surface is scored in accordance with a classification system modified from that of Smith and Knight, comprising six grades of severity (Tables 14.18 and 14.19). In case of doubt between two scores when grading the surfaces, the lower score is chosen. Class V restorations in a surface with erosion are registered as covering less than half of the surface or covering between half and three-fourths of the surface. Teeth with crowns, bridges or multiple restorations leaving less than one-fourth of the tooth substance of a surface to be evaluated are disregarded. The raw scores from each patient are recorded on a registration form.

An additional finding characteristic of erosion on the facial and oral surfaces is the cervical shoulder. This is the result of loss of enamel and appears as a shoulder preparation parallel to the gingival margin. It is recorded as present or absent on facial or oral surfaces.

Table 14.18: Criteria for facial and oral crown surfaces	
Score	Criteria
0	Original developmental structures, perichymata, are present on part of or on the entire surface.
1	Signs of erosion indicated by absence of developmental ridges extending over the entire enamel surface resulting in a smooth, glazed enamel, but without distinct loss of the original morphology of the tooth.
2	Signs of erosion and loss of enamel with a change of the original morphology of the tooth surface resulting in a flattening of the surface or a concavity in enamel, the width of which clearly exceeds its depth. Dentin is not involved.
3	Signs of erosion and loss of enamel with exposure of dentin in less than one-third of the tooth surface.
4	Signs of erosion and loss of enamel with exposure of dentin in more than one-third of the tooth surface.
5	Signs of erosion and loss of tooth substance, changes of the original morphology of the facial or the oral surface as well as of one or both approximal surfaces

Table 14.19: Criteria for incisal and occlusal surfaces	
Score	Criteria
0	Original developmental structures are present on the entire surface
1	Loss of enamel resulting in a smooth, glazed appearance either locally or extending over the entire enamel surface. Areas worn into flat-faceted shapes or rounded cusps are possible. Dentin is not involved
2	Loss of enamel with exposure of dentin in minor areas
3	Loss of enamel with exposure of dentin on the entire incisal surface or in larger areas of one or more cusps
4	Considerable loss of enamel and dentin with lack of one- to two-thirds of the original height of the tooth crown
5	Excessive loss of enamel and dentin with lack of more than two-thirds of the original height of the tooth crown

Exposure of dentin on eroded incisal and occlusal surfaces may result in cupping, which appears as grooving of the incisal edges of the anterior teeth and depression of the cusps of the posterior teeth.

Criteria for Cervical Root Surfaces

The maximum depth and extension in the gingivo-occlusal direction of cervical abrasion lesions, characterized by a rounded or V-shaped groove in the area of the cemento-enamel junction on the facial root surface, is measured with a periodontal probe. Both the depth and the extension in the gingivo-occlusal direction is registered according to the scores as shown in Table 14.20.

Table 14.20: Criteria for cervical root surfaces	
Score	Criteria
0	No change of contour on the cervical surface
½	Cervical defect 0.5 mm
1	≥ 0.5 mm and <1.5 mm
2	≥ 1.5 mm and <2.5 mm
3	≥ 2.5 mm and <3.5 mm
4	≥ 3.5 mm

Mean indices are calculated on the basis of score values for the tooth surfaces. However, the presence of a Class V restoration in a surface with erosion increases the erosion score, as it is assumed that the need for restoration treatment is caused by the erosion. When a Class V restoration covers less than half of a surface, the value 3 is added to the erosion score for the surface. When a Class V restoration covers between half and three-fourths of a surface, the value 4 is added to the erosion score, which in such a case obtains a maximum value of 1. Likewise, the presence of erosion and a cervical shoulder on the same surface increases the erosion score by the value 1. The size of a cervical lesion in a tooth is expressed by multiplying the score value of the depth by the score value of the extension.

Calculation of Index Values

Index values for each individual are calculated for facial surfaces, oral surfaces, incisal/occlusal surfaces and cervical root surfaces by adding the ascribed values for a group of tooth surfaces and dividing by the number of surfaces. The groups of tooth surfaces used are the anterior teeth (incisors and canines) and the posterior teeth (premolars and molars), recorded in the maxilla and in the mandible separately.

Bibliography

1. Larsen IB, Westergaard J, Stoltze K, Larsen AI, Gyntelberg F, Holmstrup P. A clinical index for evaluating and monitoring dental erosion. Community Dent Oral Epidemiol 2000;28:211–7.

14A.12 Index of Erosion for Children

This index was proposed by O'Sullivan EA in 2000. It was designed to include site of erosion, severity and area of tooth surface affected. Every tooth was examined and given a score for surface affected, worst depth of erosion on the tooth and area of tooth surface affected with this worst depth. This way a three "digit" score for each tooth will be obtained. Several criteria's were used as guided to diagnose erosion which were absence of developmental ridges, concavities, the breadth of which exceeded the depth (in comparison with an abrasion cavity), edges of restorations proud of tooth surface or depression of cusps of posterior teeth (cupping) (Table 14.21).

Table 14.21: Site of erosion of each tooth	
Code	Criteria
A	Labial or buccal only
B	Lingual or palatal only
C	Occlusal or incisal only
D	Labial and occlusal or incisal
E	Lingual and occlusal or incisal
F	Multi-surface
Grade of severity (worst score for an individual)	
0	Normal enamel
1	Matt appearance of the enamel surface with no loss of contour
2	Loss of enamel only (loss of surface contour)
3	Loss of enamel with exposure of dentine (ADJ visible)
4	Loss of enamel and dentine with exposure beyond ADJ
5	Loss of enamel and dentine with exposure of the pulp
9	Unable to assess (crown or large restoration)
Area of surface affected by erosion	
–	Less than half of the surface affected
+	More than half of the surface affected

Bibliography

1. O'Sullivan EA. A new index for measurement of erosion in children. European Journal of Paediatric Dentistry 2000;2:69–74.

14A.13 Basic Erosive Wear Examination (BEWE)

This was described by D. Bartlett and C. Ganss and A. Lussi in 2008. The BEWE has been designed to provide a simple scoring system that can be used with the diagnostic criteria of all existing indices aiming to transfer their results into one unit which is the BEWE score sum. The aim of the BEWE is to be a simple, reproducible and transferable scoring system for recording clinical findings and for assisting in the decision-making process for the management of erosive tooth wear. The BEWE is a partial scoring system records the most severely affected surface in a sextant (Table 14.22).

Table 14.22: BEWE

Score	Criteria
0	No surface loss
1	Initial loss of enamel surface texture
2	Distinct defect, hard tissue loss (dentine) less than 50% of the surface area
3	Hard tissue loss more than 50% of the surface area

The differentiation between lesions restricted to enamel and dentine can be difficult particularly in the cervical area. Buccal/facial, occlusal, and lingual/palatal surfaces are examined with the highest score recorded. The examination is repeated for all teeth in a sextant but only the surface with the highest score is recorded for each sextant. The score are added for all the sextants and score sum is obtained.

Bibliography

1. Bartlett D, Ganss C, Lussi A. Basic Erosive Wear Examination (BEWE): a new scoring system for scientific and clinical needs. Clin Oral Invest (2008) 12 (Suppl 1):S65–S68.

15

Indices to Assess Treatment Need

INTRODUCTION

Dental epidemiology encompasses the quantitative study of oral diseases in order that the frequency and severity of these conditions in a population can be determined. If dental health programs are to be initiated, the needs of a population for treatment must be known with a reasonable degree of accuracy whenever manpower and budgetary requirements are to be determined. Evaluation also must be made periodically after programs are in operation, so that their effectiveness can be determined.

The use of the DMF to assess caries-experience was anticipated by Munblatt in 1933 and subsequently was developed by Klein, Palmer, and Knutson in 1938. The method for classification of orthodontic conditions was established by Angle in 1899, and modified by Broadbent in 1937. Indexes to indicate the severity of periodontal disease were developed by Massler and Shour in 1949 and Russell in 1956.

Modifications of the DMF index to approximate unmet treatment needs as well as attempts to create oral status indices and a multidimensional index of dental need are reviewed by Cohen and Jago. Most attempts to predict treatment needs involved some use of the DMF index (D component and/or the unmet dental treatment need evaluated as the proportion of D/DMF). Heloe used the DMF index, the GI index and the OHI index in an effort to determine realistic estimates of treatment needs. Conchie et al., reported treatment time by use of the "Simplified descriptive survey method suggested by WHO (1967). However, this simplified method does not count carious lesions. It is important to consider that the DMFT/S indices reflecting the summative caries experience are neither identical nor specific enough to describe treatment need. They neither adequately indicate treatment need pertinent to manpower and financial considerations nor are sufficient to evaluate the severity and potential complications of dental caries.

15A Simplified Quantitative Indices

The simplified approaches included both subjective (i.e. selfperceived) and objective (i.e. professionally assessed dental treatment need). These approaches usually robustly differentiated among the diverse treatment needs. For example, the need for the dental care was discriminated either among the need for emergency-oriented care, dental check-ups, and any other type of dental care, or between the two levels. For the self-perceived oral treatment need in children, an even more simplified approach was used, i.e. asking the question "Do you feel you need any dental treatment now?" (answer: yes/no).

Another simplified approach was to estimate the percent of people in need for the specific treatment, e.g. the percentage of people in need of an extraction or a conservative treatment. The problem with this approach is that people do not consider the extent of treatment needed, e.g. the need for one extraction is equally considered as the need for more extractions.

Dental treatment needs assessment according to the WHO criteria: The standard WHO methodology and criteria for the normative dental treatment needs assessment were developed and have been used. However, there has been inconsistency in how these criteria have been applied in the previous studies. Some examples were as follows:

- The need assessment included six types of basic needs: those relating to dental caries, traumatic dental injuries, enamel defects, periodontal, orthodontic, and prosthodontic problems.

- The need for prevention and the need for restorative treatments.

- Number of individuals needed a one-surface filling, a two-surfaces filling, or dental extraction

- no treatment needed, preventive treatment, fissure sealants, initial conservative restorations, advanced conservative restorations, and radical treatments

- Preventive (diet modification, prophylaxis, oral hygiene instructions, and sealants), restorative (restorations, pulp care, and crowns), and rehabilitative (tooth removal) treatments where a person or a tooth could be assigned to a maximum of two treatment categories

- Low (no visible disease or incipient disease), moderate (cavitated, asymptomatic decay, or moderate gingivitis), and high-urgency need (infection, tooth or jaw fracture, pulpitis, or severe periodontal condition with bleeding)

The problem with this discrimination is that different treatments were summed under one score.

15B Complex, Quantitative, Summative Indices

15B.1 Oral Health Status Index

- The Oral Health Status Index (OHSI) developed by Marcus M, Koch AL, Gershen J A in 1980 integrated the assessments of the teeth and periodontium into one numerical composite score which was an improvement over the multiple health profiles of earlier instruments.

- DMFT and 15 other variables such as TMJ dysfunction, degree of periodontal disease and tumors.

- Prior planning is needed to develop an examination protocol.

Marcus M, Koch AL, Gershen JA later modified in 1983 and 1985 by using weights for bone loss, missing/free ends, decayed/fractured and replaced teeth.

Later the index is validated in 2000 by Spolsky et al which is as follows:

- The sequence of the dental examination was: tooth status, gingival inflammation, calculus, gingival recession, probe depth, and bleeding on periodontal probing.

- The Oral Health Status Index (OHSI) is an outcome measure that integrates the status of the teeth and the periodontium into one numerical score ranging from −54 to 100. A completely edentulous person without replacement prostheses would be a zero.

Criteria used in Dental Caries Assessment

Coronal caries

Frank lesions detected as gross cavitation

Incipient lesions divided into: Pits and fissures on occlusal, buccal, and lingual surfaces.

The explorer catches after insertion with moderate to firm pressure accompanied by one or more of the following:

- Softness exists at the base;
- Opacity is adjacent to the area;
- Softened enamel adjacent to the area may be scraped away with the explorer.

Smooth areas on buccal (labial) or lingual surfaces. The area is carious if decalcified or if a white spot is present, as evidence of subsurface demineralization, and the presence of softening as determined by penetration or scraping away of the enamel by the explorer.

Proximal Surfaces

- If exposed to direct visual and tactile examination, the same as smooth areas (noted above).
- If not exposed to direct visual-tactile examination, the criteria are as follows:
- There is a discontinuity of the enamel in which the explorer will catch
- In anterior teeth, there is a characteristic shadow or loss of translucency upon transillumination.

Root Caries

Appears on the cementum when gingival recession exposes the root surface and excludes abrasion and erosion.

Detection is based on

- Softness of the root surface, i.e. softer than surrounding cementum
- Discoloration.

Missing Teeth

Missing teeth were classified into three categories:

- M = Tooth was lost as a result of caries or periodontal destruction; including clinically missing third molars
- ME = Tooth was lost with space closed so that contact exists with adjacent teeth (probably lost for orthodontic reasons)
- MT = Tooth was lost due to trauma (verified by questioning of the subject)

Filled Teeth: Defined as a tooth with a sound filling, permanent or temporary. Types of restorations and their acceptability were classified as follows:

- F = Sound filling, including inlay/onlay
- CF = Crown filling
- PF = Pontic restoration
- DF = Defective fillings were defined according to the "Victor" criteria of Ryge and Snyder (1973), which included assessment of the surface and color (anterior teeth), anatomic form, and marginal integrity. "Victor" is defined as clinical quality so unacceptable that it must be "replaced and/or immediately treated because damage is now occurring or because serious inadequacies exist" (California Dental Association, 1995).

Sound Teeth

Defined as a permanent tooth that included: those with sound coronal surfaces and roots; teeth with intact pit and fissure sealants; non-vital teeth with a sealed filling.

Gingival Assessment (Marginal Bleeding, MBI)

After gentle drying of the gingival tissues, the NIDCR probe was inserted not more than 2 mm into the gingival sulcus at the mid-buccal and swept along the buccal and mesial sites (one-half arch at a time) of all teeth according to the following criteria:

- 0 = No bleeding.
- 1 = Bleeding is present.
- 9 = Not scorable.
- X = Missing tooth.

Calculus Assessment (CI)

After gentle drying of the teeth, the NIDCR probe was used to determine supragingival and/or subgingival calculus at one site per tooth (even though both sites per tooth were examined by tactile exploring) according to the following criteria:

- 0 = No calculus is present.
- 1 = Supragingival calculus* but no subgingival calculus is present.

- 2 = Supragingival and subgingival calculus or subgingival calculus only is present.
- 9 = Not scorable.
- X = Missing tooth.

* Includes supragingival calculus located on the exposed crown and root of the tooth and extends to 1 mm below the free gingival margin.

Periodontal Destruction Assessment

All periodontal assessments were made at the mid-buccal and mesial sites of all scorable teeth by means of the NIDCR probe and were recorded in mm to the lowest whole mm. The criteria are as follows:

- Pocket depth (PD) = Distance in mm from the free gingival margin (FGM) to the base of the sulcus/pocket.
- Gingival recession (GR) = Distance in mm from the free gingival margin (FGM) to the cementoenamel junction (CEJ). Recorded as positive value if CEJ is exposed.
- Attachment loss (AL) = Distance in mm from the CEJ to the base of the sulcus/ pocket. Calculated as difference between PD and GR.

Bleeding on Probing Assessment (BOP)

The presence or absence of bleeding on probing was noted after 30 sec for each site examined (after completion of one-half of an arch) following the probe depth examination. The following criteria were used:

- 0 = No bleeding is present.
- 1 = Bleeding occurred after apical probing.
- 9 = Not scorable.
- X = Tooth is missing.

Bibliography

1. Spolsky VW, Marcus M, Coulter ID, Der-Martirosian C and Atchison KA. An Empirical Test of the Validity of the Oral Health Status Index (OHSI) on a Minority Population. J Dent Res 2000 79: 1983.
2. Spolsky VW, Marcus M, Coulter ID, Der-Martirosian C, and Atchison KA. An Empirical Test of the Validity of the Oral Health Status Index (OHSI) on a Minority Population. J Dent Res 79(12) 2000.

15B.2 Oral Health Status Index for Children

The oral health status index for children measures four parameters: decayed teeth, missing teeth, occlusion, and tooth position. For both the decay and missing variables, the index distinguishes between the primary anterior teeth and all other teeth (the primary posterior plus the permanent teeth) to reflect the consequences of these conditions as children mature. The coefficients for the primary anterior teeth are exactly half the weights for the primary molars and the permanent teeth. Because developmental patterns are ambiguous for many orthodontic characteristics, coefficients holding the same values represent occlusion and position for both types of dentition.

The children's index holds intuitive appeal in the quantitative sense. For example, the coefficient for a decayed tooth is half as large as that for a missing tooth. After decay has been restored, the index increases by the amount of the decay coefficient. As with the adult index, however the children's index does not numerically distinguish between a filled tooth and one that is intact.

Many orthodontic considerations are elucidated by the children's index. The occlusion and position parameters take into account characteristics of the child's face and dentition. Each tooth is evaluated along with each segment of the mouth.

Five components of the occlusal variables that are included are crossbite, overbite, overjet, profile and lips. The relevant occlusion variables affected in a child are checked in the recording form. Abnormal position by segment is assessed according to three factors: space loss, crowding in primary dentition and crowding in permanent dentition. Abnormal position is also evaluated for each tooth is evaluated when one or more of the following circumstances exist: displacement of at least 2 mm, rotation of at least 45°, tipping of at least 15°, ankylosis and ectopic eruption. Similar to the occlusion, number of units which are in abnormal position are counted and checked in the recording form.

In addition to abnormal position, other characteristics of the dentition are examined on a tooth-by-tooth basis. The primary teeth are numbered A to T using standard nomenclature. The secondary teeth are labeled, but the third molars have been excluded. The examiner determines whether each tooth is missing (M), decayed (D), or sound (S) and circles one for each tooth number or letter on form. A tooth is classified as missing if space occurs for any reason other than normal exfoliation for primary teeth when the succedaneous tooth has not erupted into the mouth. A tooth is classified as decayed if there is definite involvement of the dentin (for example, obvious decay). Next, the letter or number of each tooth present in the mouth is circled on the examination form. For each erupted tooth, "M" is circled and slashed. The results of the foregoing assessments are entered in the tally box at lower right of the form and the value each variable is multiplied by its negative coefficient (Table 15.1). Any value entered other than zero will reduce the index from 100.

Bibliography

1. Koch LA, Gershen JA, Marcus M. children oral health status index based on dentists judgment. J Am Dent Assoc 1985;110:36–42.

15B.3 Index of Restorative Dental Treatment Need

This was developed Falcon HC, Richardson P, Shaw MJ, et al. An outline framework for the index was developed and comprised three main components:

- Patient identified need for treatment
- Complexity of treatment (assessed by clinician)
- Priority for treatment (assessed by clinician).

Steps in Assessment

The assessment process involves examining the patient and applying a complexity code (range 1–3) for each component of the examination that relates to restorative dentistry. The complexity codes are divided into four main components, involving a periodontal treatment assessment, a root canal treatment assessment, and separate assessments in fixed and removable prosthodontics (Fig. 15.1). Each component of the assessment should be considered separately and may be the only relevant component for the complexity assessment for that patient. Each complexity component has a series of clinical descriptors that are ranked as low (code 1), moderate (code 2) or high complexity (code 3) (Table 15.2). To these complexity components, a modifying factor may apply. The modifying factors are similar for each component of the index although there are small variations. They are predominantly related to patient management issues. Modifying factors only increase

Variable	Coefficient	
	Primary anterior	*Primary posterior and permanent all teeth*
Decayed teeth	– 1.12	– 2.24
Occlusion	– 4.38	– 4.38
Position	– 1.73	– 1.73
Missing teeth	– 2.27	– 4.55

Table 15.1: Oral health status index for children

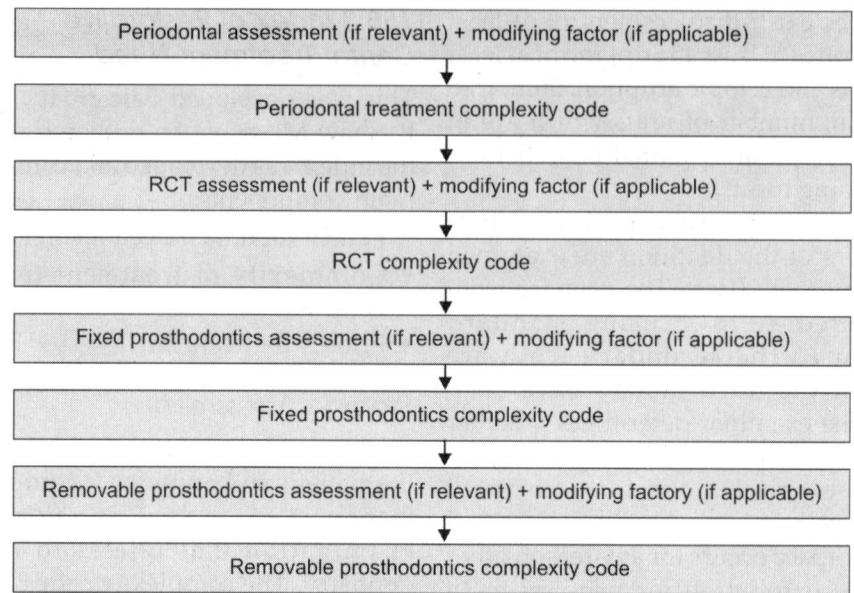

Fig. 15.1: Process flow (Index of restorative dental treatment need)

complexity by one code increment; they are not cumulative (Table 15.3). The highest complexity is code 3.

Step 1

Following a clinical examination and assessment of the patient's oral status, appropriate codes are selected which most closely describes the patient's condition or treatment requirement.

Step 2

The highest code achieved in any of the individual components is the overall restorative dentistry complexity score.

Step 3

The complexity codes are then recorded on a data collection sheet, together with an indication of whether modifying factors apply. Application of a modifying factor increases the score by one increment, unless the maximum score has already been achieved. This is the final restorative dentistry complexity score.

Complexity code 1 Able to be performed by any dental graduate

Complexity code 2 Able to be performed by any experienced dentist

Complexity code 3 Able to be performed by any dentist with skills developed following specialist training

Table 15.2: Complexity scores for the components of index of restorative dental treatment need

Component 1: periodontal treatment assessment

Complexity	Criteria
1	BPE score 1 – 3 in any sextant
2	BPE score of 4 in any sextant
	Surgery involving the periodontal tissues
	Surgical procedures associated with osseointegrated implants
3	Surgical procedures involving periodontal tissue augmentation and/or bone removal (e.g. crown lengthening surgery).

Contd.

Table 15.2: Complexity scores for the components of index of restorative dental treatment need (*Contd.*)

BPE score of 4 in any sextant and including one or more of the following factors:

Patients under the age of 35

Smoking 10+ cigarettes daily

A concurrent medical factor that is directly affecting the periodontal tissues

Root morphology that adversely affects prognosis

Rapid periodontal breakdown > 2 mm attachment loss in any one year

Component 2: Root canal treatment assessment (permanent teeth)Conventional root canal treatment or retreatment is the clinical procedure of choice. Surgical treatment should only be considered when conventional treatment is inappropriate.

Complexity	Criteria
1	Single/multiple root canals with curvature < 15° to root axis that are considered negotiable from radiographic or clinical evidence through their entire length. No root canal obstruction or damaged access Surgical treatment – Single root canals – Radiolucency < 6 mm diameter
2	Single/multiple root canals with curvature > 15° but < 40° to root axis that are considered negotiable from radiographic or clinical evidence through their entire length. Surgical treatment – Single root canals – No evidence of radiolucency – Hemisection of mandibular molars Teeth with incomplete root development
3	Single/multiple root canals with curvature > 40° Single/multiple root canals that are *not* considered negotiable from radiographic or clinical evidence through their entire length Surgical treatment – Multi rooted teeth – Single root canals – Radiolucency > 6 mm diameter Teeth with iatrogenic damage or pathological resorption Teeth with difficult root morphology

Component 3: Fixed prosthodontics treatment assessment: This basic assessment assumes that the proposed restorative dental treatment will conform to the existing occlusion. The principles apply to conventional and adhesive units fixed prosthodontic restorations include: Intracoronal restorations, veneer restorations, extracoronal restorations including pontic units

Complexity	Criteria
1	Restorations not involved in anterior guidance, where there are adequate sound or restored teeth to predictably maintain the existing occlusion
2	Restorations that contribute to anterior guidance where there are insufficient sound or restored teeth to predictably maintain the current guidance Extra coronal restoration of any one posterior sextant (all teeth), not involved in anterior guidance where a terminal unit is involved
3	Extra coronal restoration of the complete anterior guidance including pontic units. Extra coronal restoration of opposing sextants (all teeth). Restorations that are supported by osseointegrated implants

Contd.

Table 15.2: Complexity scores for the components of index of restorative dental treatment need (*Contd.*)

Component 4: Removable prosthodontics treatment assessment: Basic assessment assumes that the proposed treatment will conform to the existing occlusion

Complexity	Criteria
1	Prostheses with bounded saddles replacing posterior teeth
	All mucosal born prostheses
	Prostheses replacing anterior teeth where there are adequate sound or restored teeth to provide anterior guidance
2	Free end saddle prostheses which are dependent upon differential support
	Prostheses with problems involving the path of insertion and/or available undercuts where some tooth modification is involved
	Prostheses which contribute to anterior guidance
3	Prostheses where abutment teeth require extracoronal restoration to improve stability and retention
	The use of sectional prostheses
	Prostheses involving osseointegrated implant support
	Presence of orofacial defects requiring obturation/restoration

Table 15.3: Modifying factors that are relevant to each complexity assessment

A modifying factor can only increase complexity by one increment. Multiple factors are not cumulative.

- Co-ordinated medical and/or dental multi-disciplinary care
- Medical history that significantly affects clinical management
- Special needs for the acceptance or provision of dental treatment
- Mandibular dysfunction
- Atypical facial pain
- Undiagnosed facial pain
- Presence of a retching tendency
- Limited operating access

Modifying factors that are relevant to specific components of the complexity assessment:

Relevant to component 1: Periodontal treatment assessment

- Concurrent mucogingival disease

Relevant to component 2: Root canal treatment

- Root canal treatment
- Surgery in the proximity of important anatomical structures
- Surgery when periodontal attachment loss exeeds 3.5 mm

Relevant to component 3 and 4: Prosthodontic assessments

- Concurrent mucogingival disease
- Skeletal base discrepancy that affects the occlusion
- Evidence of significant parafunction
- Reorganization of the occlusion required
- Radiographic evidence of 50% reduction in bone support

Medical history that significantly affects clinical management

- Patients requiring IM or IV medication as a component of clinical management
- Patients with a history of head/neck radiotherapy
- Patients who are significantly immunocompromised or immunosuppressed
- Patients with a significant bleeding dyscrasia/disorder
- Patients with a potential drug interaction

Bibliography

1. Falcon HC, Richardson P, Shaw MJ, Bulman JS, Smith BG. Developing an index of restorative dental treatment need. Br Dent J. 2001;190(9):479-86.

15B.4 Quantitative Summative Dental Treatment Needs Index

In this assessment, the normative dental treatment need is recorded according to the WHO criteria. Subsequently, a QSDTNI is calculated for each subject. The calculation is based on the relative differences in monetary costs of diverse dental treatment services. To this end, the fee guide for dental treatment services, published annually by the British Columbia dental association (Canada, 2007), was used. The cost for a sealant is arbitrarily chosen as the basis for all calculations and is equaled to unity. Then, the relative ratio for each specific treatment is obtained by dividing the cost of a specific dental treatment by the cost of the sealant (Table 15.4). For example, the relative ratio for a one-surface filling (rrRF1) is calculated in the following way: rrRF1 = cost of one surface filling/cost of a sealant. The QSDTNI for each individual is calculated by summing relative ratios of all necessary specific treatment needs according to the following formula (n denotes the number of teeth requiring the specific treatment modality):

OSDTNI = n(rrPS) + n(rrRF1) + n(rrRF2) + n(rrRF3) + n(rrRE1) + n(rrRE2) + n(rrRE3) + n(rrPC) + n(rrPDmax) + n(rrPDman) + n(rrCDmax) + n(rrCDman) + n(rrSE)

One of the advantages of the QSDTNI is that it is a comprehensive and not a simplified assessment of dental treatment need. Additionally, this index is based on the WHO guidelines that are already widely applied, and subsequent calculations can be performed in a standardized way. It is important to emphasize that this index was not developed for clinical use. Another important consi-

Table 15.4: Relative ratios for the basic dental treatment needs*

Treatment modalities	Relative ratios for the specific treatments**
Preventive Sealant (PS)	RrPS = 1
Restorative filling***	
One surface (RF1)	rrRF1 = 3.93
Two surfaces (RF2)	rrRF2 = 4.97
Three surfaces (RF3)	rrRF3 = 5.86
Restorative endo	
Single-rooted (RE1)	rrRE1 = 16.90
Two-rooted (RE2)	rrRE2 = 22.02
Multi-rooted (RE3)	rrRE3 = 31.23
Restorative prosthetic	
Crown (PC)	rrPC = 26.71
Partial denture-cast frame	
Maxillary (PD max)	rrPDmax = 35.22
Mandibular (PD man)	rrPDman = 38.39
Complete dentures	
Maxillary (CD max)	rrCDmax = 27.80
Mandibular (CD man)	rrCDman = 30.94
Surgery	
Extraction (SE)	rrSE = 4.58

   * If a tooth needs several treatments, all treatments included, e.g. endodontic + restoration + crown.
  ** The relative ratio is the price of a specific dental treatment divided by the cost of a sealant.
 *** Filling due to a primary, secondary caries or trauma.

deration is that the suggested index includes assessments only of basic treatment needs.

Bibliography

1. Aleksejuniene J, Brukiene V. An assessment of dental treatment need: an overview of available methods and suggestions for a new, comparative summative index. J Public Health Dent. 2009;69:24–8.

15C. Specific Indices for Assessment of Disease Severity and Treatment Need

Some indices deal with disease component and with simultaneous assessment of treatment need of a specific disease. Indices like CPITN, PTNS deal with periodontal pockets, plaque and calculus with a provision to code the required treatment need. Similarly, indices like DMFT in conjunction with PUFA, modified DMFT index, Specific Caries Index, CAST index, etc. can assess the required treatment need for dental caries. Draker's HLD index, Grainger's treatment priority index and Salzman's handicapping malocclusion assessment, dental aesthetic Index, ICON can assess the treatment need for varying degrees of malocclusion.

15C.1 Dentition Status and Treatment Needs (1987)

A numerical coding system is used for recording the status of permanent teeth and an alphabetical coding system for primary teeth: Note that boxes pertaining to premolars or primary molars, cuspids and incisors are used for both primary and permanent teeth (Table 15.5). A distinction is made solely by the use of alphabetical or numerical codings. An entry must be made in every box on the chart. Codes for the dental caries status of primary and permanent teeth are as follows:

Criteria for diagnosis and coding (primary tooth codes within parentheses) are:

0 (A) Sound tooth: A tooth is recorded as sound if it shows no evidence of treated or untreated clinical caries. The stages of caries that precede cavitation, as well as other conditions similar to the early stages of caries,

Table 15.5: Dentition status codes		
Permanent Code		*Primary Code*
0	Sound	A
1	Decayed	B
2	Filled, with decay	C
3	Filled, no decay	D
4	Missing, as a result of caries	E
5	Missing, any other reason	–
6	Sealant, varnish	F
7	Bridge abutment or special crown	G
8	Unerupted tooth	–
9	Excluded tooth	–

are excluded because they cannot be reliably diagnosed. Thus, teeth with the following defects, in the absence of other positive criteria, should be coded as sound: white or chalky spots; discolored or rough spots; stained pits or fissures in the enamel that catch the explorer but do not have a detectably softened floor, undermined enamel, or softening of the walls; dark, shiny, hard, pitted areas of enamel in a tooth showing signs of moderate to severe fluorosis. All questionable lesions should be coded as sound.

1 (B) Decayed tooth: Caries is recorded as present when a lesion in a pit or fissure, or on a smooth tooth surface, has a detectably softened floor, undermined enamel or softened wall. A tooth with a temporary filling should also be included in this category. On approximal surfaces, the examiner must be certain that the explorer has entered a lesion. Where any doubt exists, caries should not be recorded as present.

2 (C) Filled tooth with decay: A tooth is scored as filled with decay when it contains one or more permanent restorations and one or more areas that are decayed. No distinction is made between primary and secondary caries (i.e. whether or not the carious lesions are in physical association with the restoration(s).

3 (D) Filled tooth with no decay: Teeth are considered filled without decay when one or more permanent restorations are present and there is no secondary (recurrent) caries or other area of the tooth with primary caries. A tooth with a crown placed because of previous decay is recorded in this category. A tooth that has been crowned for reasons other than decay, e.g. trauma or as a bridge abutment, is recorded as "bridge abutment or special crown" and coded 7 (G).

4 (E) Tooth missing due to caries: This score is used for permanent or primary teeth that have been extracted because of caries. For missing primary teeth, this score should be used only if the subject is at an age when normal exfoliation would not be a sufficient explanation for absence. In some age groups, it may be difficult to distinguish between unerupted teeth (code 8) and extracted teeth. Basic knowledge of tooth eruption patterns, the status of the corresponding contralateral tooth, the appearance of the alveolar ridge in the area of the tooth space in question, and the caries status of other teeth in the mouth may provide helpful clues in making a differential diagnosis between unerupted and extracted teeth. It is emphasized that code 4 should not be used for teeth judged to be missing for any reason other than caries.

5 Permanent tooth missing for any other reason: This code is used for permanent teeth judged to be absent congenitally, or extracted for orthodontic reasons or because of trauma, etc. This score is also used for permanent teeth that are judged to have been extracted because of periodontal disease. As for code 4, two entries of code 5 can be linked by a line in cases of fully edentulous arches.

6 (F) Sealant: This code is used for teeth in which a fissure sealant has been placed on the occlusal surface; or for teeth in which the occlusal fissure has been enlarged with a rounded or "flame-shaped" bur, and a composite material placed. If a tooth with a sealant has decay, it should be coded as 1 (decayed).

7 (G) Bridge abutment or special crown: This code is used to indicate that a tooth forms part of a fixed bridge, i.e. is a bridge abutment. This code can also be used for crowns placed for reasons other than caries. Note: Missing teeth replaced by a bridge are coded 4 or 5, as for other missing teeth.

8 Unerupted tooth: This classification is restricted to permanent teeth and used only for a tooth space with an unerupted permanent tooth but without a primary tooth. Teeth scored as unerupted are, of course, excluded from all calculations concerning dental caries. For differential diagnosis between extracted and unerupted teeth, see code 4.

9 Excluded tooth: This code is used for any tooth that cannot be examined.

Decayed, Missing and Filled Teeth (DMFT): Index The D-component includes all teeth with codes 1 or 2. The M-component comprises teeth with code 4 in subjects under 30 years of age, and teeth coded 4 and 5 for subjects 30 years and older, i.e. missing due to caries or for any other reason. Note: Previously only teeth missing due to caries were included in the DMFT index and in its M-component. The F-component includes only teeth with code 3. The basis for DMFT calculations is 32, i.e. all permanent teeth including wisdom teeth. Teeth with code 6 (sealant) or code 7 (crown, bridge abutment or element) are not included in the DMFT.

Treatment Needs of Individual Teeth

The codes and criteria for treatment needs were:

0 - None (no treatment). This code is recorded if a crown and a root are both sound, or if it is decided that a tooth should not receive any treatment.
1 - Caries-arresting care or sealant care
2 - One surface filling
3 - Two or more surface fillings
4 - Crown or bridge abutment
5 - Bridge element, i.e. that portion of a bridge that is replacing the missing tooth
6 - Pulp care
7 - Extraction/indicated for extraction
8/9 - Need for other care. The examiner should specify the types of care for which codes 8 and 9 are used.

Bibliography

1. WHO Oral Health Surveys 3rd edition, 1987.

15C.2 Dentition Status and Treatment Need (WHO 1997)

The criteria for diagnosis and coding were:

0 - Sound crown. A crown is recorded as sound if it showed no evidence of treated or

untreated clinical caries. The stages of caries that precede cavitation, as well as other conditions similar to the early stages of caries, are excluded because they cannot be reliably diagnosed. Thus, a crown with the following defects, in the absence of other positive criteria, should be coded as sound:

- White or chalky spots
- Discolored or rough spots that are not soft to touch with a metal CPI probe
- Stained pits or fissures in the enamel that do not have visual signs of undermined enamel, or softening of the floor or walls detectable with a CPI probe
- Dark, shiny, hard, pitted areas of enamel in a tooth showing signs of moderate to severe fluorosis
- Lesions that, on the basis of their distribution or history, or visual/tactile examination, appear to be due to abrasion.

Sound root: A root is recorded as sound when it was exposed and shows no evidence of treated or untreated clinical caries. (Unexposed roots are coded 8.)

1. Decayed crown: Caries was recorded as present when a lesion in a pit or fissure, or on a smooth tooth surface, has an unmistakable cavity, undermined enamel, or a detectably softened floor or wall. A tooth with a temporary filling, or one which was sealed but also decayed, was also included in this category. In cases where the crown was destroyed by caries and only the root was left, the caries was judged to have originated on the crown and therefore was scored as crown caries only. The CPI probe should be used to confirm visual evidence of caries on the occlusal, buccal and lingual surfaces. Where any doubt existed, caries was not recorded as present.

Decayed root: Caries was recorded as present when a lesion feels soft or leathery to probing with the CPI probe. If the root caries was discrete from the crown and will require a separate treatment, it was recorded as root caries. For single carious lesions affecting both the crown and the root, the likely site of origin of the lesion was recorded as decayed. When it was not possible to judge the site of origin, both the crown and the root was recorded as decayed.

2. Filled crown, with decay: A crown is considered filled, with decay, when it had one or more permanent restorations and one or more areas that were decayed.

Filled root, with decay: A root is considered filled, with decay, when it had one or more permanent restorations and one or more areas that were decayed.

3. Filled crown, with no decay: A crown was considered filled, without decay, when one or more permanent restorations were present and there was no caries anywhere on the crown. A tooth that had been crowned because of previous decay was recorded in this category.

Filled root, with no decay: A root was considered filled, without decay, when one or more permanent restorations were present and there was no caries anywhere on the root.

4. Missing tooth, as a result of caries: This code was used for permanent or primary teeth that were extracted because of caries and was recorded under coronal status.

The root status of a tooth that has been scored as missing because of caries should be coded "7" or "9".

5. Permanent tooth missing, for any other reason: This code was used for permanent teeth judged to be absent congenitally, or extracted for orthodontic reasons or because of periodontal disease, trauma, etc. The root status of a tooth scored 5 should be coded "7" or "9".

6. Fissure sealant: This code was used for teeth in which a fissure sealant was placed on the occlusal surface; or for teeth in which the occlusal fissure has been enlarged with a rounded or "flame shaped" bur, and a composite material placed.

7. Bridge abutment, special crown or veneer: This code was used under coronal status to indicate that a tooth forms part of a fixed bridge, i.e. is a bridge abutment. This code can also be used for crowns placed for reasons other than caries and for veneers or laminates covering the labial surface of a tooth on which there was no evidence of caries or a restoration.

Missing teeth replaced by bridge pontics were coded 4 or 5 under coronal status, while root status is scored 9.

Implant: This code is used under root status to indicate that an implant has been placed as an abutment.

8. Unerupted crown: This classification is restricted to permanent teeth and was used only for a tooth space with an unerupted permanent tooth but without a primary tooth. Unexposed root. This code indicates that the root surface was not exposed, i.e. there was no gingival recession beyond the CEJ.

T- Trauma (facture): A crown was scored as fractured when some of its surface is missing as a result of trauma and there was no evidence of caries.

9. Not recorded: This code was used for any erupted permanent tooth that could not be examined for any reason (e.g. because of orthodontic bands, severe hypoplasia, etc.).

This code was used under root status to indicate either that the tooth has been extracted or that calculus was present to such an extent that a root examination is not possible.

Treatment Needs of Individual Teeth

The codes and criteria for treatment needs were:

0 - None (no treatment). This code is recorded if a crown and a root are both sound, or if it is decided that a tooth should not receive any treatment.
P - Preventive, caries-arresting care
F - Fissure sealant
1 - One surface filling
2 - Two or more surface fillings
3 - Crown for any reason
4 - Veneer or laminate (may be recommended for aesthetic purposes)
5 - Pulp care and restoration
6 - Extraction
7/8 - Need for other care. The examiner should specify the types of care for which codes 7 and 8 are used. The use of these two codes should be kept to a minimum.
9 - Not recorded

Bibliography

1. WHO Oral Health Surveys 4th edition 1997.

15C.3 Prosthetic Status (WHO 1997)

The WHO Oral health assessment form which was prescribed for oral health surveys (WHO 1987, 1997) have provisions to assess prosthetic status and need.

The presence of prostheses should be recorded for each jaw based on the following codes:

0 - No prosthesis
1 - Bridge
2 - More than one bridge
3 - Partial denture
4 - Both bridge(s) and partial denture(s)
5 - Full removable denture
9 - Not recorded

Prosthetic Need (WHO 1997)

A recording should be made for each jaw on the perceived need for prostheses according to the following codes:

0 - No prosthesis needed
1 - Need for one-unit prosthesis (one tooth replacement)
2 - Need for multi-unit prosthesis (more than one tooth replacement)
3 - Need for a combination of one- and/or multi-unit prostheses
4 - Need for full prosthesis (replacement of all teeth)
9 - Not recorded

15C.4 Treatment Need Index

Considering the numerous limitations of the DMF index for its inability to assess treatment need, Mann et al developed a treatment need index. The Index emphasizes actual treatment needs, regardless of what caused the need for treatment (caries, trauma, periodontal disease). Treated teeth not requiring further treatment are not recorded. The use of bite-wing radiographs is preferable as it gives a more accurate estimation of treatment needs, but the index can be used without radiographs. Teeth are categorized according to both the severity of damage and the resulting complexity of treatment required. The assessment of the treatment need of each tooth is based on clinical examination (and radiographs if available) and on the type of treatment required. The tooth is then assigned to one of seven categories described in Table 15.6.

0. **Sound:** No treatment needed.

1. **Fluoride:** A sound dentition, or one requiring no restorative intervention in a subject who would benefit from topical fluoride application (high caries risk, medically at risk, etc.). In this category, the subject and not the tooth is scored.

2. **Sealant:** A tooth with deep fissures or incipient caries for which fissure sealing is indicated.

3. **Initial:** Tooth demanding 'initial' one-surface restoration: A point cavity in which the probe catches on a soft cavity floor; or when a radiograph reveals caries that has not progressed beyond the enamel. This category includes sealant restorations/preventive resin restorations. If use of a probe in this way is considered unacceptable, diagnosis must be based on visual examination only.

4. **Moderate:** Tooth requiring 'moderate' restoration: wider than point cavity (1 mm) but covering less than one-half of the surface involved; or when a radiograph reveals caries that has progressed into the dentine but does not involve the pulp; or when a two-surface restoration is indicated (including cases in which a radiograph shows approximal surface caries confined to enamel).

5. **Advanced:** Tooth requiring 'advanced' restoration: cavitation covering more than half of the involved tooth surface; or when a radiograph discloses that caries has progressed into the dentine but does not involve the pulp and a three-surface restoration or preformed crown is indicated.

6a. **Radical tooth requiring 'radical' dental treatment:** A prosthetic restoration (crown, gold inlay, onlay, bridge or other prosthetic replacement) and not a filling; or when a tooth obviously has clinical or radiographic pulp involvement, or furcation involvement, or has a sinus tract, and endodontic therapy (pulpotomy or pulpectomy) is indicated; or when extraction and prosthetic replacement are planned.

6b. **Extract:** This subdivision of Category 6 can be included when the examiner wants to stipulate teeth indicated clinically or radiographically for extraction without the intent of subsequent prosthetic replacement. Restorations demanding replacement are scored according to the extent of the existing restoration. For example, a 2-surface amalgam restoration with an overhanging margin detected by radiography is scored as '4'. A preformed crown demanding replacement is scored as '5', and a gold onlay demanding replacement is scored as '6'. An endodontic treatment demanding renewal is scored as '6'. Primary teeth are scored in the same way, but are recorded separately as time allocations for pediatric dentistry procedures are different from those of adults. For each individual, the number and the percentage of teeth in each category is recorded.

Table 15.6

Category	Clinical	Radiographic (if available)	Treatment needed
0 Sound	Sound or existing restoration of satisfactory quality	Sound or existing restoration of satisfactory quality	None
1 Fluoride	Subject who would benefit from topical fluoride Sound dentition in	Sound or existing restoration of satisfactory quality	Topical fluoride application
2 Sealant	Deep fissures or incipient fissure canes	Sound-no caries detected on any surfaces	Fissure sealants
3 Initial	Point cavity	Caries limited to enamel	One-surface restoration/ preventive resin restoration
4 Moderate	Area of lesion covers less than half of surface	Occlusal caries penetrating dentine or early proximal caries	One or two-surface restoration
5 Advanced	Area of lesion covers more than half of surface	Caries within dentine but no pulpal involvement detected	Three (or more) surface restoration or preformed crown
6a Radical	Lesion involves pulp or crown totally damaged	Caries process involves pulp	Endodontic or prosthetic or extraction with replacement
6b Extract	As above	As above	No prosthetic replacement intended

Bibliography

1. Mann J, Sgan-Cohen HD, Asher RS, Amir E, Cohen S, Sarnat H. A treatment need index: a pilot study. Int J Paediatr Dent 1993;3:129–34.

15C.5 Index of Treatment Need

This index of treatment need was developed by Hetherington and White for use in school screening procedures to simplify the recording information, facilitate data analysis, reduce inter-examiner variability and reduce inappropriate referrals by excluding teeth which could not be treated. During screening, children are allocated to one of five categories as illustrated in Table 15.7.

Table 15.7: Index of treatment need

Code	Description	Inclusion criteria	Exceptions	Follow-up
0	Disease free	–	–	No follow-up
1	Presence of one or more risk factors	Poor oral hygiene and/or gingivitis; early caries; arrested caries and/or retained roots; caries teeth due to exfoliate		No follow-up
2	Active disease	Cavities in primary teeth	Nursery/reception/year 1: cavities in primary incisors (record as code 1); years 2, 3, 4: cavities in primary canines (record as code 1) years 5 and 6: cavities in primary first molars (record as code 1)	Requires intervention

(Contd).

Table 15.7: Index of treatment need (*Contd.*)

Code	Description	Inclusion criteria	Exceptions	Follow-up
3	Advanced disease	Carious permanent teeth; signs of infection; pulpal involvement and/or multiple cavities in primary teeth		Requires intervention
4	Other oral problems	Oral medical problems; developmental/orthodontic anomalies; trauma; dental erosion		Problem recorded

Bibliography

1. Hetherington I and White DA. The diagnostic accuracy and reproducibility of school dental screening using an index of treatment need. Community Dent Health 2004;21:170–174.

15C.6 Community Caries Index of Treatment Needs

This index is analogous to the Community Periodontal index of treatment needs and was designed for estimating caries treatment needs. The rationale underlying the CCITN should encompass more than restorative need: Emphasis should be on prevention. Active carious lesions in enamel should be arrested. Table 15.8 shows the diagnosis and treatment needs at different levels.

Bibliography

1. Axelsson P. Diagnosis and Risk Prevention of Dental Caries, Volume 2. Quintessence Publishing Co, Inc. 2000. pages 272–4.

Table 15.8: CCITN

Score	Diagnosis	Treatment needs
0	Intact enamel	P
1	Primary active enamel caries	P
2:1	Primary dentin caries without cavitation into dentin	P
2:2	Recurrent (secondary) caries without cavitation	P
3:1	Primary dentin caries with cavitation	P+R?
3:2	Recurrent (secondary) caries with cavitation	P+R
4:1	Primary (active) root caries without cavitation	P
4:2	Recurrent (active) root caries without cavitation	P
5:1	Primary root caries with cavitation	P+R?
5:2	Recurrent root caries with cavitation	P+R?

Modified from Axelsson (1988); P: prevention; R: restoration

16
Miscellaneous Indices

16.1 Gingival Pain Index

It was developed by Garg Subhash, Kapoor KK, Mehrotra KK and Dixit Jaya in 1986. This index depends upon the threshold of patient with respect to pain of gingival origin. The scoring criteria are given in Table 16.1.

Scoring Criteria

Table 16.1: Gingival pain index

Score	Criteria
0	No pain
1	Mild pain; within bearable limit
2	Severe pain, unbearable

Bibliography

1. Garg S, Kapoor KK, Mehrotra KK, Dixit J. Periodontal treatment systems — A clinical assessment and gingival tissue index, gingival pain index and tooth hypersensitivity index. J Indian Dent Asso 1986;58:513–26.

16.2 Retention Index

The purpose of creating a Retention Index System (Björby and Löe, 1967) was to introduce a system for the assessment of the main retentive factors and which expressed the quality of the tooth surface (degree of roughness) adjacent to the gingival tissues. Technically, the retention index is built on principles similar to those underlying the Gingival Index and the Plaque Index. The criteria are based on calculus, plaque and retentive factors (Table 16.2).

Table 16.2: Retention index

Score	Criteria
0	No caries, no calculus, no imperfect margin of dental restoration in a gingival location.
1	Supragingival cavity, calculus or imperfect margin of dental restoration.
2	Subgingival cavity, calculus or imperfect margin of dental restoration.
3	Large cavity, abundance of calculus or grossly insufficient marginal fit of dental restoration in a supra- and/or subgingival location.

Bibliography

1. Löe, H. The gingival index, the plaque index and the retention index systems. J Periodontol 1967;38:610.

16.3 Tooth Hypersenstivity Index

It was developed by Garg Subhash, Kapoor KK, Mehrotra KK and Dixit Jaya in 1986. It takes into account the tolerance threshold of patient with respect to thermal (hot and cold) sensations related to teeth. One score is assigned per segment of dental arches as per the criteria are given in Table 16.3.

Table 16.3: Tooth hypersensitivity index

Score	Criteria
0	No thermal sensations
1	Slight thermal sensations; within bearable limit
2	Sever thermal sensation; unbearable.

Bibliography

1. Garg S, Kapoor KK, Mehrotra KK, Dixit J. Periodontal treatment systems—A clinical assessment and gingival tissue index, gingival pain index and tooth hypersensitivity index. J Indian Dent Asso 1986;58:513-526.

16.4 Irritant Index (II)

Irritant index is a scoring method for plaque and calculus by Timothy O'Leary in 1967 as a component in periodontal screening examination in conjunction with gingival periodontal index.

Method: The scoring is done on all teeth present in which mouth is divided into sextants. Buccal and lingual surfaces are used to record for the presence and extent of plaque or calculus (Table 16.4).

Table 16.4: Irritant Index

Score	Criteria
0	No plaque or calculus (supra or subgingival) on any tooth in the segment
1	A slight amount of plaque or supragingival calculus not extending more than 2 mm from the gingival margin found on any tooth in the segment.
2	Plaque or supragingival calculus covers up to half of the exposed clinical crown on any tooth in the segment
3	Plaque or supragingival calculus covers more than one half of the clinical crown or if or subgingival calculus deposits or overhanging or deficient restorations are detectable by probing

Calculation

Calculation of II: Total of the highest scores in each sextant/number of dentulous sextants

Drawbacks: This index tends to overscore the incisal half of the crown, at the expense of the gingival margin.

Bibliography

1. O'Leary TJ. The periodontal screening examination. J Periodontol 1967;38: 617–24.

16.5 Oral Health Rating Index

Oral rating index (ORI) was developed as a simple scoring system of gingival health care and oral hygiene level for adults (Kawamura 1988). The ORI is based upon examination of four areas: the facial surfaces of the anterior teeth and the lingual surfaces of the right posterior teeth in the mandible and maxilla. Each patient's gingival health care level is recorded as a composite index, which categorizes gingival status and the presence and extent of local irritants (dental plaque and dental calculus) on an ordinal scale from – 2 (very poor) through to + 2 (excellent) (Table 16.5). When in doubt, the examiner assigns the lesser score.

The assessment of the ORI score is weighted by mainly gingival condition, followed by calculus accumulation and plaque accumulation. The ORI uses a set of standard color photographs of each level of the scale, to maintain consistent standards. It is undertaken without hand instruments and using a natural light. It takes around ten seconds to carry out the examination for each patient.

The ORI is not a strict quantitative index for the determination of oral health status, or clinical assessment. Although screening by ORI does not make a specific diagnosis of a periodontal condition, it appears helpful for identifying suspected gingival inflammation and level of oral hygiene need, without any

Table 16.5: Oral health rating index

Score	Criteria
Excellent (+2)	Normal gingivae and no detectable plaque or calculus
Good (+1)	Slight localized inflammatory changes, fairly good oral hygiene
Questionable (0)	Difficult to assign a positive or negative score
Poor (–1)	Overt gingivitis and poor oral hygiene
Very poor (–2)	Severe gingivitis and very poor oral hygiene

extensive instrumentation or additional aide. It does provide a good indicator of a person's commitment to self-care. As such, it appears to be a useful public health tool to classify a person's effective oral health behavior, rather than relying on their stated beliefs, perceptions or practices.

Bibliography

1. Kawamura M, Fukuda S, Inoue C, Sasahara H, Iwamoto Y. The validity and reproducibility of an oral rating index as a measurement of gingival health care and oral hygiene level in adults. J Clin Periodontol 2000; 27: 411–6.

16.6 Mandibular Mobility Index

Helkimo used a mandibular mobility index to evaluate function and dysfunction in the masticatory system.

Four parameters are taken into consideration. Each parameter is scored as per the criteria described in Table 16.6.
1. Maximal opening of the mouth in mm
2. Maximal lateral movement to the right in mm
3. Maximal lateral movement to the left in mm
4. Maximal protrusion in mm.

Bibliography

1. Helkimo M. Studies on function and dysfunction of the masticatory system. II. Index for anamnestic and clinical dysfunction and occlusal state. Swedish Dental Journal 1974;67:101–21.

Table 16.6: Mandibular mobility index

Parameter	Finding	Points
Maximal opening of the mouth in mm	≥ 40 mm	0
	30–39 mm	1
	< 30 mm	5
Maximal lateral movement to the right in mm	≥ 7 mm	0
	4–6 mm	1
	≤ 3 mm	5
Maximal lateral movement to the left in mm	≥ 7 mm	0
	4–6 mm	1
	≤ 3 mm	5
Maximal protrusion in mm	≥ 7 mm	0
	4–6 mm	1
	≤ 3 mm	5

Total score = Sum (points for all 4 parameters)
Interpretation: The higher the score the greater the dysfunction in mandibular mobility (Table 16.7).

Table 16.7 Interpretation of total scores of mandibular mobility index

Total score	Mobility index	Mandibular mobility
0	0	Normal
1 to 4	1	Slightly impaired
5 to 20	5	Severely impaired

16.7 Healing Index

Landry, Turnbull and Howley described an index to describe the extent of healing after periodontal surgery. The criteria are described in Table 16.8.

Table 16.8: Healing index

Healing index	Interpretation	Criteria
1	Very poor	Has 2 or more of the following: Tissue color: ≥ 50% of gingiva red Response to palpation: bleeding Granulation tissue: present Incision margin: not epithelialized, with loss of epithelium beyond incision margin Suppuration present
2	Poor	Tissue color: ≥ 50% of gingiva red Response to palpation: bleeding Granulation tissue: present Incision margin: not epithelialized, with connective tissue exposed

Contd.

Table 16.8: Healing index (*Contd.*)

Healing index	Interpretation	Criteria
3	Good	Tissue color: ≥ 25% and < 50% of gingiva red
		Response to palpation: no bleeding
		Granulation tissue: none
		Incision margin: no connective tissue exposed
4	Very good	Tissue color: < 25% of gingiva red
		Response to palpation: no bleeding
		Granulation tissue: none
		Incision margin: no connective tissue exposed
5	Excellent	Tissue color: all tissues pink
		Response to palpation: no bleeding
		Granulation tissue: none
		Incision margin: no connective tissue exposed

Bibliography

1. Landry RG, Turnbull RS, Howley T. Effectiveness of benzydamyne HCl in the treatment of periodontal post-surgical patients. Research in Clinic Forums 1988;10:105–18.

2. Masse JF, Landry RG, et al. Effectiveness of soft laser treatment in periodontal surgery. Int Dent J 1993;43:121–7.

16.8 Organoleptic Scoring of Halitosis

Table 16.9: Organoleptic scoring

Observer scoring of malodor	Points
No appreciable odor	0
Barely noticeable odor	1
Slight but clearly noticeable odor	2
Moderate odor	3
Strong odor	4
Extremely foul odor	5

17

Indices for Children and Adolescents

INTRODUCTION

Epidemiological data form the basis for planning and evaluation of dental care programs throughout the world. When epidemiological data have been collected the amount of disease found has to be quantified by using dental indices. This holds true even for oral diseases in children. Oral diseases like caries, bleeding gums, periodontitis, alveolar bone loss, dental fluorosis, malocclusion, etc. are often thought as the disease of adulthood and are neglected in children and adolescents. But these diseases are prevalent even in children and young adults.

Indices like simplified oral hygiene index are used in the past for assessment of oral hygiene, but a definitive recording of gingivitis and periodontal health is not carried out routinely. Most of these indices have been developed in order to assess the oral diseases among adults while conducting experimental studies. Primary dentition has differences with respect to many factors like tooth anatomy, position, surface area, size, eruption, exfoliation, etc. when compared to permanent dentition, it is suggested to record the indices separately for primary and permanent dentition wherever applicable. Hence, it is essential to review the indices for potential applicability in children and adolescents.

Indices for Evaluating Gingivitis and bleeding

- PMA Index and its modifications
- Gingival index (GI)
- Sulcus bleeding index (SBI)
- Gingival bleeding index (GBI)
- Gingival bleeding index (GBI – Ainamo and Bay, 1975)
- Papillary bleeding index (PBI)
- Papillary bleeding score (PBS)
- Modified papillary bleeding index (MPBI)
- Bleeding time index (BTI)
- Eastman interdental bleeding index (EIBI)
- Quantitative gingival bleeding index (QGBI)
- Modified gingival index (MGI)
- Bleeding on interdental brushing index (BOIBI)

Indices to Evaluate Periodontal Health

- Periodontal index
- Periodontal disease index
- Gingival periodontal index
- Periodontal disease rate index
- Navy periodontal disease index
- Pocket depth and loss of attachment
- **CPITN/CPI:** This index is WHO preferred method for assessing periodontal diseases in children and adults. For young people up to 19 years, only six index teeth are

considered. The second molars are excluded because of high frequency of false (non-inflammatory associated with tooth eruptions) pockets. In children less than 15 years, pockets are not recorded although probing for bleeding and calculus are carried out. For screening and monitoring in dental practice all teeth in a sextant are examined for adults over age 19 years. Only one score which is the highest is recorded.

Caries Indices

- **DMF**

  It is the most widely used index for reporting dental caries in children and adults. The variations which can be used among children and young adults are as follows:

  ✓ *Primary dentition:* def, dft, dfs, dmfs

  ✓ *Mixed dentition:* dft/DFT, dmft/DMFT, dmfs/DMFS (with respect to scoring caries in mixed dentition, the scores for primary and permanent teeth are reported separately. The index for permanent dentition is usually determined first followed by primary dentition)

  ✓ *Permanent dentition:* DMFT/DMFS

- Stone's index
- Caries severity index (CSI)
- Caries analysis system (CAS)
- Extrapolated carious surface increment index (ECSI)
- RID (Relative increment of decay)
- PUFA/pufa
- ICDAS
- CAST.

Indices for Dental Fluorosis and Enamel opacities

Specific Fluoride Indices

1. Dean's index and its modifications
2. Community fluorosis index (1942)
3. Moller's modification for Dean's index
4. Thylstrup and Fejerskov index and its modification

5. Simplified Thylstrup and Fejerskov index
6. Tooth surface index of fluorosis
7. Fluorosis risk index
8. Chronological fluorosis assessment index
9. Simplified fluoride mottling index
10. Visual Analog scale.

Descriptive Indices for Enamel Opacities

1. Developmental defects of enamel index and its modification
2. Young's classification to classify enamel opacities
3. Al-Alousi and Jackson classification of enamel defects
4. Murray and Shaw criteria for diagnosing enamel opacities
5. Mottling index
6. Enamel defects index.

Indices to Assess Malocclusion

1. Index of tooth position (permanent dentition)
2. Handicapping labio-lingual deviation index and its modifications (permanent dentition)
3. Handicapping malocclusion assessment record (permanent dentition)
4. FDI system — A method for measuring Occlusal traits — COCSTOC (permanent dentition)
5. Occlusal Index (for primary, mixed and permanent teeth)
6. Dental esthetic index (12 years and above in children with no primary teeth)
7. Malocclusion severity index (9 years and above in permanent dentition)
8. WHO method for epidemiological assessment of malocclusion
9. Index of orthodontic treatment outcome/peer assessment rating index (permanent dentition)
10. Swedish medical board index (permanent dentition)
11. Index of orthodontic treatment need (permanent dentition)
12. Modified index of orthodontic treatment need (permanent dentition)

13. Index of complexity, outcome and need (permanent dentition)
14. Norwegian index of orthodontic treatment need (permanent dentition)

Indices to Assess Plaque, Oral Hygiene and Calculus

1. Oral hygiene index and its modification
2. Patient hygiene performance index and its modification
3. Plaque component in Ramfjord index
4. Schick and Ash modification of Ramfjord index
5. Quigley Hein plaque index
6. Plaque index by Silness and Loe
7. Plaque control record
8. Calculus surface index
9. Calculus surface severity index
10. Probe method of calculus assessment
11. Glass's criteria for assessment of calculus
12. Marginal line calculus index.

Indices used to Assess Tooth Wear and Erosion

• Simplified TWI
• Smooth wear assessment

• The Keels-Coffield clinical severity scale of dental erosion
• Erosion criteria from the modified scoring system of Linkosalo and Markkanen
• Aine Index for erosion
• Kunzel Criteria for dental erosion
• Index of erosion for children (Sullivan)

Miscellaneous Indices

• Retention index
• Mobility index by Ramfjord
• Mobility index by Laster.

Bibliography

1. Wei SHS, Lang KP. Periodontal epidemiological indices for children and adolescents: I. Gingival and Periodontal Health Assessments. Pediatric Dentistry 1981;3(4):353–60.

2. Wei SHS, Lang NP. Periodontal epidemiological indices for children and adolescents: II. Evaluation of oral hygiene; III.Clinical Applications. Pediatric Dentistry 1982;4(1):64–73.

3. Poulsen S. Epidemiology and indices of gingival and periodontal disease. Pediatric Dentistry 1981;3:Special issue 82–8.

18

Conclusion

Collecting data and trying to memorize the criteria of an index is a daunting task for most of the researchers. This book would serve as a reliable and easy to use resource for the researchers. The validity and reliability of many of the discussed indices have been established previously. And for many of the newer indices, those factors have to be established. Training and calibration of the examiner alone can improve reliability and validity of an index which can be obtained by repeated sessions of discussions using the criteria with different sets of participants/subjects/patients at different intervals. In most situations even Standardization of the equipment, lighting, etc. should be done to minimize errors.

As a matter of fact, when a new index is chosen or an established index used for a slightly different study design a pilot study should always be conducted to ensure that there are no practical problems associated with the selected index. Based on the analysis of the results and experiences in the pilot study, the main study should be conducted. Examinations for the indices should be done in well illuminated rooms with good lighting and comfortable seating arrangements. Examination of subjects should be limited to a maximum of 25–50 wherever possible to avoid examiner fatigue. A recording clerk increases the efficiency in recording the indices scores.

Every researcher has a specific question for which data is being collected. Indices as such help quantify and qualify such raw data into meaningful, interpretable data which can provide information far from what actually just the numbers mean. The choice of an index for a particular study might be influenced by factors like study design, duration, sample size, resources(man-power and money), reliability, validity and availability of certain instruments, precision and severity of disease, etc. Also each index has its own advantage and disadvantage, indications and contra-indications. Few indices have specific tooth to be scored as a criteria. When an index is chosen considering all the above factors and implemented in the study properly it would fulfill the goals of both the researcher and at a distant level for science itself.

Index